# ANNALS OF THE NEW YORK ACADEMY OF SCIENCES

Volume 765

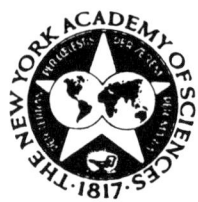

EDITORIAL STAFF

*Executive Editor*
BILL BOLAND

*Managing Editor*
JUSTINE CULLINAN

*Associate Editor*
COOK KIMBALL

The New York Academy of Sciences
2 East 63rd Street
New York, New York 10021

THE NEW YORK ACADEMY OF SCIENCES
(Founded in 1817)
BOARD OF GOVERNORS, July 1994–September 1995

JOSHUA LEDERBERG, *Chairman of the Board*
HENRY M. GREENBERG, *President*
MARTIN L. LEIBOWITZ, *President-Elect*

*Honorary Life Governor*
WILLIAM T. GOLDEN

HENRY A. LICHSTEIN, *Treasurer*

*Governors-at-Large*

| | | |
|---|---|---|
| ELEANOR BAUM | BARRY R. BLOOM | D. ALLAN BROMLEY |
| EDWARD COHEN | SUSANNA CUNNINGHAM-RUNDLES | BILL GREEN |
| SANDRA PANEM | RICHARD A. RIFKIND | DOMINICK SALVATORE |
| DAVID E. SHAW | WILLIAM C. STEERE, Jr. | SHMUEL WINOGRAD |

CYRIL M. HARRIS, *Past Chairman* HELENE L. KAPLAN, *General Counsel* [ex officio]
RODNEY W. NICHOLS, *Chief Executive Officer* [ex officio]

# NEUROPROTECTIVE AGENTS
## CLINICAL AND EXPERIMENTAL ASPECTS

ANNALS OF THE NEW YORK ACADEMY OF SCIENCES
Volume 765

# NEUROPROTECTIVE AGENTS
## CLINICAL AND EXPERIMENTAL ASPECTS

*Edited by Bruce Trembly and William Slikker, Jr.*

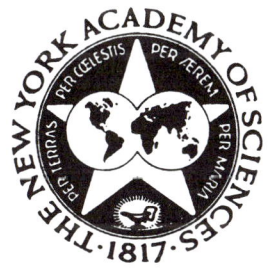

The New York Academy of Sciences
New York, New York
1995

Copyright © 1995 by the New York Academy of Sciences. All rights reserved. Under the provisions of the United States Copyright Act of 1976, individual readers of the Annals are permitted to make fair use of the material in them for teaching or research. Permission is granted to quote from the Annals provided that the customary acknowledgment is made of the source. Material in the Annals may be republished only by permission of the Academy. Address inquiries to the Executive Editor at the New York Academy of Sciences.

Copying fees: For each copy of an article made beyond the free copying permitted under Section 107 or 108 of the 1976 Copyright Act, a fee should be paid through the Copyright Clearance Center, Inc., 222 Rosewood Drive, Danvers, MA 01923. For articles of more than 3 pages, the copying fee is $1.75.

∞ The paper used in this publication meets the minimum requirements of American National Standard for Information Sciences—Permanence of Paper for Printed Library Materials, ANSI Z39.48-1984.

Cover: Fluoro-jade, a fluorochrome recently developed by Dr. Larry Schmued of the Division of Neurotoxicology at the National Center for Toxicological Research (FDA), stains degenerating rat hippocampal neurons yellow-green, while healthy neurons are counterstained red with ethidium bromide.

**Library of Congress Cataloging-in-Publication Data**

Neuroprotective agents : clinical and experimental aspects / edited by Bruce Trembly and William Slikker, Jr.
    p.    cm.—(Annals of the New York Academy of Sciences : v. 765)
    This volume contains the papers from a conference held in Lake George, New York on July 31–August 3, 1994.
    Includes bibliographical references and index.
    ISBN 0-89766-945-2 (cloth : alk. paper).—ISBN 0-89766-946-0 (pbk. : alk. paper)
    1. Neurotoxicology—Congresses.  2. Nervous system—Diseases—Chemoprevention—Congresses.  3. Nervous system—Degeneration—Chemoprevention—Congresses.  I. Trembly, Bruce.  II. Slikker, William.  III. Series.
Q11.N5   vol.765
[RC347.5]
500 s—dc20
[616.8′0475]
                                                                95-21866
                                                                   CIP

MC/PCP
*Printed in the United States of America*
**ISBN 0-89766-945-2 (cloth)**
**ISBN 0-89766-946-0 (paper)**
**ISSN 0077-8923**

ANNALS OF THE NEW YORK ACADEMY OF SCIENCES

Volume 765
September 15, 1995

# NEUROPROTECTIVE AGENTS
## CLINICAL AND EXPERIMENTAL ASPECTS[a]

*Editors and Conference Chairs*
BRUCE TREMBLY AND WILLIAM SLIKKER, JR.

## CONTENTS

Preface. *By* the Editors ............................................. xi

### Part I. Clinical Syndromes Which May Be Suitable for Neuroprotective Agents

Clinical Potential for the Use of Neuroprotective Agents: a Brief Overview. *By* BRUCE TREMBLY ................................. 1

Prophylactic Pharmacologic Neuroprotection against Focal Cerebral Ischemia. *By* SARAN JONAS ...................................... 21

Discussion ........................................................... 26

### Part II. Animal Models and Assessment Approaches

A Fetal Rat Model of Acute Perinatal Ischemia-Hypoxia. *By* ZBIGNIEW BINIENDA ........................................................ 28

Evaluation of the Novel Neuroprotective Agent BW619C89 in the Middle Cerebral Artery Occlusion Model of Focal Ischemia in the Spontaneously Hypertensive Rat and Normotensive Fischer 344 Rat. *By* JEANETTE H. SWAN AND MICHAEL J. LEACH ............... 39

Quantitative Histological Evaluation of Neuroprotective Compounds. *By* ANDREW C. SCALLET ................................................ 47

Discussion ........................................................... 59

### Part III. Mechanisms of Neuronal Degeneration and Modulators of Neuroprotection

Brain Injury and Inflammation: a Putative Role of TNFα. *By* BABAK ARVIN, LEWIS F. NEVILLE, FRANK C. BARONE, AND GIORA Z. FEUERSTEIN ........................................................ 62

---

[a] This volume contains the papers from a conference entitled *Second International Conference on Neuroprotective Agents: Clinical and Experimental Aspects,* which was held by the National Center for Toxicological Research/FDA, Jefferson, Arkansas and the Department of Veterans Affairs Medical Center, Togus, Maine at Lake George, New York on July 31–August 3, 1994.

Comparison of Glutamine-Enhanced Glutamate Release from Slices and Primary Cultures of Rat Brain. *By* JOHN F. BOWYER, GEORGE W. LIPE, JOHN C. MATTHEWS, ANDREW C. SCALLET, AND DAVID L. DAVIES ................................................. 72

Effect of Hypocapnia on Extracellular Glutamate and Glycine Concentrations during the Periischemic Period in Rabbit Hippocampus. *By* KYU TAEK CHOI, JUNG KIL CHUNG, CHUN SIK KWAK, AND HAE KYU KIM ................................. 86

Discussion ........................................................ 98

### Part IV. Antioxidants and Free Radical Scavengers

Neuroprotective Effects of Free Radical Scavengers and Energy Repletion in Animal Models of Neurodegenerative Disease. *By* JÖRG B. SCHULZ AND M. FLINT BEAL ........................ 100

Neuroprotective Effects of Radical Scavengers in an Intact Dorsal Root Ganglion Hypoxia Model. *By* P. R. BÄR ................. 111

Discussion ........................................................ 116

### Part V. Calcium Channel Antagonists: Theoretical and Clinical Aspects

Short-Term Regulation of Neuronal Calcium Channels by Depolarization. *By* JAI LIU, ALETA RUTLEDGE, AND DAVID J. TRIGGLE ........ 119

Potential Interactions between Nimodipine and Adrenal Hormones. *By* ROBERT L. ISAACSON AND JULIE A. VARNER ............... 134

The Effects of Nimodipine on the EEG of Substance Abusers. *By* RONALD I. HERNING, XIAOYAN GUO, AND W. ROBERT LANGE .... 143

Nimodipine Improves Information Processing in Substance Abusers. *By* RONALD I. HERNING, XIAOYAN GUO, AND W. ROBERT LANGE .... 152

Discussion ........................................................ 160

### Part VI. Other Agents as Neuroprotectants

Adenosine: a Prototherapeutic Concept in Neurodegeneration. *By* DAG K. J. E VON LUBITZ, MARGARET F. CARTER, MARK BEENHAKKER, RICK C-S. LIN, AND KENNETH A. JACOBSON ............... 163

Dexamethasone and the Prevention of Neonatal Hypoxic-Ischemic Brain Damage. *By* URSULA I. TUOR ............................... 179

Discussion ........................................................ 196

### Part VII. Risk Assessment and Regulatory Concerns with Respect to Neuroprotective Agents

Risk Assessment Strategies for Neuroprotective Agents. *By* WILLIAM SLIKKER, JR. AND DAVID W. GAYLOR ........................ 198

Discussion ........................................................ 209

### Part VIII. NMDA Antagonists: Theoretical Considerations

Neuroprotective Use-Dependent Blockers of $Na^+$ and $Ca^{2+}$ Channels Controlling Presynaptic Release of Glutamate. *By* STANLEY M. GOLDIN, KATRAGADDA SUBBARAO, RAHUL SHARMA, ANDREW G. KNAPP, JAMES B. FISCHER, DEBORAH DALY, GRAHAM J. DURANT,

N. LAXMA REDDY, LAIN-YEN HU, SHARAD MAGAR, MICHAEL E. PERLMAN, JUN CHEN, STEVEN H. GRAHAM, W. F. HOLT, DAVID BERLOVE, AND LEE D. MARGOLIN. . . . . . . . . . . . . . . . . . . . . 210

Receptor Subtypes Linked to Metabotropic Glutamate Receptor Agonist-Mediated Limbic Seizures in Mice. *By* JOSEPH P. TIZZANO, KELLY I. GRIFFEY, AND DARRYLE D. SCHOEPP . . . . . . . . . . . . . . . . . . . . 230

Neuroprotective Properties of the Uncompetitive NMDA Receptor Antagonist Remacemide Hydrochloride. *By* GENE C. PALMER, EDWARD F. CREGAN, ALFONSO R. BORRELLI, AND FRANCES WILLETT . . . . . . . . . . . . . . . . . . . . . . . . . . . . . . . . . . . . . . . 236

Discussion . . . . . . . . . . . . . . . . . . . . . . . . . . . . . . . . . . . . . . . . 248

## Part IX. NMDA Antagonists: Clinical Aspects

Safety, Tolerability and Pharmacokinetics of the *N*-Methyl-D-Aspartate Antagonist Ro-01-6794/706 in Patients with Acute Ischemic Stroke. *By* THE DEXTRORPHAN STUDY GROUP AND HOFFMANN-LA ROCHE . . 249

The Rationale for Glutamate Antagonists in the Treatment of Traumatic Brain Injury. *By* J. S. MYSEROS AND R. BULLOCK . . . . . . . . . . . 262

Stratgies for Neuroprotection with Glutamate Antagonists: Extrapolating from Evidence Taken from the First Stroke and Head Injury Studies. *By* R. BULLOCK . . . . . . . . . . . . . . . . . . . . . . . . . . . . . . . . . . 272

Clinical Pharmacology of CNS 1102 in Volunteers. *By* KEITH W. MUIR, DONALD G. GROSSET, AND KENNEDY R. LEES . . . . . . . . . . . . 279

Evidence for Prolonged Release of Excitatory Amino Acids in Severe Human Head Trauma: Relationship to Clinical Events. *By* R. BULLOCK, A. ZAUNER, J. S. MYSEROS, A. MARMAROU, J. J. WOODWARD, AND H. F. YOUNG . . . . . . . . . . . . . . . . . . . . . . . 290

Discussion . . . . . . . . . . . . . . . . . . . . . . . . . . . . . . . . . . . . . . . . 298

## Poster Papers

The Neuroprotective Effect of Calcitonin Gene-Related Peptide following Subarachnoid Hemorrhage. *By* B. ANTHONY BELL, FOR THE EUROPEAN CGRP IN SUBARACHNOID HAEMORRHAGE STUDY GROUP 299

A Small Animal Model of Focal Cerebral Ischemia for Studying Neuroprotective Agents. *By* JEREMY P. HOLLAND AND B. ANTHONY BELL . . . . . . . . . . . . . . . . . . . . . . . . . . . . . . . . . . . . . . . . . . 301

Quantitative Histological Evaluation of Neurotoxic Hippocampal Damage. *By* ANDREW C. SCALLET . . . . . . . . . . . . . . . . . . . . . 303

Perinatal Brain Injury: Pathophysiology and Therapeutic Intervention. *By* CHRIS WILLIAMS, CARINA MALLARD, WILLIAM TAN, BARBARA JOHNSTON, ALISTAIR GUNN, KYLA MARKS, AND PETER GLUCKMAN 304

The Role of the Growth Factors IGF-1 and TGF$\beta_1$ after Hypoxic-Ischemic Brain Injury. *By* CHRIS WILLIAMS, JIAN GUAN, ODETTE MILLER, ERICA BEILHARZ, HEATHER MCNEILL, ERNEST SIRIMANNE, AND PETER GLUCKMAN . . . . . . . . . . . . . . . . . . . . . . . . . . . . 306

Oxidative Brain Damage in Aged Mice: Protection by Caloric Reduction. *By* HARBANS LAL, MICHAEL J. FORSTER, AND RAJ S. SOHAL . . . . . 308

The Role of Hyperthermia in Amphetamine's Interactions with NMDA Receptors, Nitric Oxide, and Age to Produce Neurotoxicity. *By* JOHN F. BOWYER ............................. 309

Lack of Mitigation of Methamphetamine-Induced Neurotoxicity by Ganglioside $GM_1$ or Vitamin E. *By* SYED F. ALI ............. 311

Structural-Functional Correlates of Neuroprotection in the Aging Rabbit by a Calcium Channel Blocker: Nimodipine Reverses Neocortical Dendritic Atrophy and Improves Memory Retention. *By* RONALD F. MERVIS, N. KUNTZ, D. BURTON, R. DVORAK, R. TANDON, L. HOOVER, M. S. WOOD, AND P. R. SOLOMON ............. 312

Neoprotective Activity of HU-211, a Novel Nonpsychotropic Synthetic Cannabinoid. *By* A. BIEGON ......................... 314

A Randomized, Double-Blind, Placebo-Controlled Pilot Trial of Intravenous Magnesium Sulfate in Acute Stroke. *By* KEITH W. MUIR AND KENNEDY R. LEES ........................... 315

Efficacy and Tolerability of Lifarizine in Acute Ischemic Stroke: a Pilot Study. *By* I. B. SQUIRE, K. R. LEES, W. PRYSE-PHILLIPS, A. KERTESZ, AND J. BAMFORD, FOR THE LIFARIZINE STUDY GROUP ... 317

Considerations in the Design of Preclinical Safety Evaluation Programs for Novel Therapeutics Used in Neurologic Diseases. *By* J. A. CAVAGNARO AND S. LIU ........................... 319

Sensitization and Desensitization of the NMDA Receptor Complex: Implications for Therapy. *By* LINDA H. FOSSOM AND PHIL SKOLNICK ................................... 320

Initial Experience with Remacemide Hydrochloride in Patients with Acute Ischemic Stroke. *By* KEITH W. MUIR AND KENNEDY R. LEES  322

The Tolerability, Pharmacokinetics and Pharmacodynamics of Increasing Intravenous Doses of 619C89, a Novel Compound for the Acute Treatment of Stroke, in Healthy Volunteers. *By* A. J. MERCER, R. J. LAMB, Z. HUSSEIN, S. HOBBIGER, AND J. POSNER .......... 324

*N*-Methyl-D-Aspartate Receptor Participation in Parkinson's Disease, a Neurodegenerative Disorder. *By* ANITA VERMA AND S. K. KULKARNI .................................. 327

A Randomized, Double-Blind, Placebo-Controlled Ascending Dose Tolerance Study of 619C89 in Acute Stroke. *By* KEITH W. MUIR, KENNEDY R. LEES, STEVEN J. C. HAMILTON, CHARLES F. GEORGE, STEPHEN F. HOBBIGER, AND MARTIN W. LUNNON .......... 328

Disposition and Pharmacokinetics of Remacemide Hydrochloride in Male Sprague-Dawley Rats. *By* STEPHEN CURRY, DENNIS J. MCCARTHY, KEN R. CASE, MARK S. EISMAN, MATTHEW R. MARLER, AND NIK A. MAHMOOD ................................. 330

The Cerebral Hemodynamic and Metabolic Effects of the Noncompetitive NMDA Antagonist CNS 1102 in Humans with Severe Head Injury. *By* A. WAGSTAFF, G. M. TEASDALE, G. CLIFTON, AND L. STEWART ...................... 332

Effects of Nimodipine and Verapamil on Cerebral Blood Flow and Cerebrovascular Reactivity in Conscious Rabbits. *By* GUSTAV B. WEINSTEIN ................................. 334

Clinical Pharmacology of CNS 1102 in Man. *By* KEITH W. MUIR, DONALD G. GROSSET, AND KENNEDY R. LEES . . . . . . . . . . . . . 336

Low Environmental Temperatures or Pharmacologic Agents That Produce Hypothermia Decrease Methamphetamine Neurotoxicity in Mice. *By* S. F. ALI, G. D. NEWPORT, R. R. HOLSON, W. SLIKKER, JR., AND J. F. BOWYER . . . . . . . . . . . . . . . . . . . . . . . . . 338

Biologically Based Dose-Response Model for Neurotoxicity Risk Assessment. *By* WILLIAM SLIKKER, JR. AND DAVID W. GAYLOR . . . 339

Role of Reactive Oxygen Species (ROS) in Neuronal Degeneration: Modulation by Protooncogene Expression. *By* M. ANTHONY VERITY, D. E. BREDESEN, AND T. SARAFIAN . . . . . . . . . . . . . . . . . . 340

Phospholipase $A_2$ Regulation in Neural Function and Injury. *By* M. ANTHONY VERITY . . . . . . . . . . . . . . . . . . . . . . . . . . . 341

Subject Index . . . . . . . . . . . . . . . . . . . . . . . . . . . . . . . 343

Index of Contributors . . . . . . . . . . . . . . . . . . . . . . . . . . 347

**Financial assistance was received from:**
- THE NATIONAL CENTER FOR TOXICOLOGICAL RESEARCH/FDA, JEFFERSON, ARKANSAS
- DEPARTMENT OF VETERANS AFFAIRS MEDICAL CENTER, TOGUS, MAINE

The New York Academy of Sciences believes it has a responsibility to provide an open forum for discussion of scientific questions. The positions taken by the participants in the reported conferences are their own and not necessarily those of the Academy. The Academy has no intent to influence legislation by providing such forums.

# Preface

This volume contains the papers and posters from the Second International Meeting on Neuroprotective Agents, which was held at Lake George, New York on July 31–August 3, 1994. The first such conference was in Rockland, Maine in September, 1991, and the third, in keeping with the international flavor of these meetings, will be held at Lake Como, Italy September 8–12, 1996.

These conferences provide a broad, informal and unique forum for researchers in basic sciences as well as in clinical disciplines. Attendees and speakers from all over the world have the opportunity to exchange ideas with others from widely divergent backgrounds. Clinicians learn of new trends in neurochemistry, and neuropharmacologists learn of new clinical applications for their work.

The purpose of this conference was to bring together clinical and basic science researchers in a multidisciplinary and multinational forum to exchange ideas and data related to this expanding field of interest, examine recent clinical and experimental data pertaining to neuroprotective agents, clarify safety and effectiveness issues of these agents, suggest future research and clinical applications and survey the possible regulatory aspects with respect to these agents.

We are grateful to the New York Academy of Sciences for the opportunity to share these proceedings with others.

*Bruce Trembly*
*William Slikker, Jr.*

# Clinical Potential for the Use of Neuroprotective Agents

## A Brief Overview

BRUCE TREMBLY

*Section of Neurosurgery*
*VA Medical Center*
*Togus, Maine 04330*

Clinical studies elaborating the use of neuroprotective agents have necessarily followed at arm's length the numerous laboratory and animal investigations of several classes of neuroprotective agents. The potential for improvement in the neurologic outcome of patients with various injuries to the central nervous system (CNS) continues to increase as new agents develop and survive clinical protocols. These injuries have traditionally included ischemic stroke, aneurysmal rupture, and traumatic brain and spinal cord injury. However, in the light of recent investigations, the range of potentially applicable clinical syndromes may gradually encompass even more of clinical practice in neurology and neurosurgery. This brief review serves only to outline some present and speculative future applications of neuroprotective agents.

## BACKGROUND

As noted in some of the papers in this volume, ischemic, traumatic, or hemorrhagic injury to the CNS results in death of neurones in a portion of the lesion. However, there remains a residual adjacent mass of neuronal and glial tissue, the *ischemic penumbra*, that suffers from varying degrees of decreased blood flow, bioenergy/metabolic insufficiency, free oxygen radical permeation, toxic extracellular accumulations of excitatory neurotransmitters, vasogenic and cytotoxic edema, and influx of calcium and other ions through altered cell membrane channels. Ginsberg[1] described the ischemic penumbra as " . . . an evolving zone of bioenergetic upheaval." That the ischemic penumbra remains amenable to therapy for a short time after injury provides considerable impetus to clinical research. The changes just noted may be altered individually by various pharmacologic agents whose functions are generally described as neuroprotective. These agents include calcium channel blockers, free radical scavengers, corticosteroids, antagonists of glutamate at *N*-methyl-D-aspartate (NMDA) and non-NMDA receptors, moderate hypothermia, and various thrombolytic agents.

The inevitable cascade of injurious events begins within minutes of ischemia, and permanent neuronal injury may occur in the center of the ischemic area within 6–8 minutes.[2] However, a variable window of therapeutic opportunity probably continues for several hours after injury, at least with respect to peripheral portions of the ischemic penumbra. Fisher and Bogousslavsky[3] emphasized that as each therapeutic agent affects only one of several mechanisms in the cascade of cellular destruction, " . . . it is likely that multiple therapies will be needed and will prove to be better than a single approach."

Early investigation of pharmacological protection against cerebral ischemia dates from 1964 when Wright and Ames[4] reported that the maximum period of global ischemia that could be reversibly sustained in cats was 5–7.5 minutes. Their model involved occlusion of all arterial supply to the brain in two stages, with subsequent bilateral carotid temporary occlusion. The maximum period of total reversible occlusion could be doubled by the intraarterial carotid injection of sodium pentobarbital (12 mg/kg) just prior to carotid occlusion. Recent evidence, 30 years later, suggests a pharmacologic basis for neuroprotective action of certain barbiturates against neuronal degeneration. Barbiturates, including diazepam, block glutamate (NMDA and non-NMDA) receptors and may reduce cellular damage in ischemia.[5]

## Ischemic Stroke

The major clinical impetus with respect to use of neuroprotective agents has been in acute spontaneous ischemic stroke. A large multicenter clinical trial of nimodipine (a lipophylic calcium channel blocker) was reported in 1992 as showing no effect of nimodipine (30 mg po qid) when instituted up to 48 hours after onset of symptoms. However, a subset of patients treated within 18 hours of onset of symptoms showed " . . . statistically significant positive effects of possible clinical significance."[6] Another recent report found no benefit from nimodipine in a carefully controlled, 350 patient randomized stroke study, and again, treatment may have been started too late.[7] It is now apparent that a 48-hour time delay is much too long and that a 3- to 4-hour maximum time window after onset of symptoms is more realistic with respect to potential for treatment.[1,3]

To this end, another multicenter university and community hospital prospective analysis of patient admissions to hospital reveals that 59% of patients arrived at the emergency room within three hours of onset of symptoms, and two thirds arrived within 4 hours. The extensive use of 911 emergency call, public and physician education, legislative action and prompt attention by a member of the stroke evaluation team may result in an improved cohort of stroke patients well suited to clinical trials of various neuroprotective agents.[8]

In a recent report, Gomez *et al.* established a "Code Stroke" alert system within a large university hospital in an effort to give stroke patients the same rapidly available team approach to evaluation and early treatment afforded to cardiac emergencies. The average time from onset of symptoms to arrival at the hospital was 118 minutes; the average time from arrival to activation of "Code Stroke" was 41 minutes; the average time from the "code" to arrival at bedside by a member of the stroke team was 4.8 minutes; and the average time to institution of treatment was 30 minutes. The mean total time was 3.2 hours, barely within the present concept of the therapeutic time window. Further efforts in this direction, and dissemination of the need for these procedures to all hospitals should result in greatly improved access for patients with ischemic stroke to neuroprotective and other treatment in the future.[9] The rationale for this urgency is elaborated in an exhaustive current review by Camarata et al., in which they emphasize that the cost to society of strokes in our population is "staggering." Imaging techniques for the acute patient, interventional methods and emergency surgical procedures (if any might be indicated) are discussed with emphasis upon urgent medical management.[10]

## Neuroprotective Agents in Ischemia

The role of calcium ions in ischemic cell damage and survival of viable but jeopardized cells during reperfusion after ischemia is elaborated in early reviews by Siesjo and Cheung, et al.[11,12] Calcium channel blockers are briefly discussed under *subarachnoid hemorrhage*, below. Hypothermia is also discussed below *(traumatic brain injury)*, but it should be noted here that in animal studies of global ischemia, "Lowering of the brain temperature by only a few degrees during ischemia confers a marked protective effect."[13] Also in animal studies of global ischemia, brain temperature was found to fall spontaneously during ischemia by several degrees, also suggesting that, " . . . postinsult hypothermia may ameliorate brain damage due to trauma or transient ischemia."[14]

The role of antioxidants and corticosteroids in neural injury is discussed under *spinal cord trauma*. However, even though there has been no demonstrated clinical benefit from postischemic administration of corticosteroids, dexamethasone (0.1 mg/kg) was found to be neuroprotective in neonatal rats, when given 6 hours prior to global hypoxia. Pretreatment by 3 hours was not effective, nor were calcium channel blockers.[15] Continued clinical studies of corticosteroids within the therapeutic window of 3-4 hours after onset of ischemia may eventually demonstrate some benefit from these agents, especially in the light of Hall's hypothesis that high-dose methylprednisolone (MPS) actually inhibits oxygen free radical-induced lipid perioxidation.[16] The significance of this process is that, "There is extensive experimental support for the early occurrence and pathophysiological importance of oxygen radical formation and cell membrane lipid perioxidation in the injured nervous system."[17]

NMDA and other alpha-amino-3-hydroxy 5-methyl-4-isoxazole proprinate (AMPA)[18] receptor antagonists are showing considerable promise as neuroprotective agents in ischemia. Bullock and Fugisawa summarize animal evidence supporting the reduction in ischemic damage by excitatory amino acid (EAA) antagonists. In most of the 26 studies cited, the agent was administered prior to ischemia, but two agents (MK-801 and GYKI 52466) were effective when given up to 2 hours post-event.[20]

Choi hypothesizes that under normal conditions, glutamate is present in extracellular space as part of its role as an excitatory neurotransmitter. Under conditions of ischemia, cellular energy stores are depleted and neurones are depolarized with resultant increased release of glutamate from excitatory terminals. Cellular mechanisms for uptake and deactivation of glutamate are also impaired in the face of ischemic loss of energy. The resulting toxic build up of extracellular glutamate produces further neuronal injury.[21] As noted in several reports in this volume, some NMDA antagonists are in early clinical trials with respect to safety, pharmacokinetics, and efficacy.[22–24] In another report in this volume, Palmer *et al.* note that remacemide, a weak NMDA antagonist, is well tolerated by patients with acute ischemic stroke, and its effectiveness in animal stroke models is thought to be due to the ability of remacemide to limit activity at excitatory amino acid receptors of the NMDA type.[25]

Lyden and Lonzo found that the combination of a glutamate antagonist (MK-801) and a gamma-aminobutyric acid (GABA) agonist (muscimol) was more effective in combination than either agent alone with respect to ipsilateral hemisphere size after microsphere carotid injection-embolization on one side in rats. This combination is also "highly effective" in protecting visual-spatial learning after unilateral embolic lesioning in the same rats (Morris water maze). GABA blocks the voltage-gated intracellular calcium influx associated with glutamate.[26] In an editorial discussing that paper, Traystman argued that since there are multiple mechanisms involved in cerebral injury, " . . . it is likely that we will need to use a 'cocktail' agent that has a number of different pharmacologic qualities, or perhaps effective treatment may be a matter of simultaneous or sequential treatment with several different pharmacologic agents."[27] So, here we have such a combination of NMDA antagonist and a GABA agonist that blocks ingress of calcium ions into the neurone, and this two-headed approach may well be the future of neuroprotective agents in clinical practice.

It appears probable that only in acute *ischemic* stroke will thrombolytic agents be *safely* used to reperfuse penumbral tissue before the peri-infarct penumbra becomes progressively encompassed within the enlarging, irreversibly damaged ischemic core. Early restoration of even marginal perfusion in the penumbral zone may allow better penetration of other neuroprotective agents along with oxygen and glucose. A recent report describing the effect of Ancrod (Arvin, Knoll Pharmaceutical Co.), a purified fraction of Malayan pit viper venom, which dissolves fibrinogen and allows increased local blood flow after infarction, emphasizes the potential value of improved perfusion in ischemic stroke. This multicenter study concluded that in humans, intravenously-administered Ancrod did not increase bleeding, and in a subgroup of patients, whose 6-hour fibrinogen levels were 130 mg/dL or less, the neurologic outcome was marginally significantly better than in placebo-treated patients. As with other agents, it was necessary to administer Ancrod within 6 hours of ischemic stroke.[28] Perhaps an even narrower therapeutic window of 3 to 4 hours after onset will prove of greater value with respect to potential benefit of early reperfusion.

*Prophylactic Neuroprotection in Focal Ischemia*

As opposed to studying and treating patients *after* acute ischemic stroke, an opposite tack is suggested by Jonas in the next paper, in which he discusses the concept and practical aspects of prophylactic neuroprotection against focal cerebral ischemia. He proposes using patients undergoing coronary artery bypass surgery (CABS) as ideal subjects for prophylactic neuroprotective trials. These patients frequently sustain some degree of ischemic/embolic insult during surgery, often measured by changes in neuropsychological testing before and after operation.[29] At least one neuroprotective agent (remacemide) is already undergoing clinical trials in a group of CABS patients.[25]

Similar reasoning may also apply to patients undergoing carotid endarterectomy because of atheromatous plaque formation in the neck. In various studies, as many as one-fourth of these patients demonstrate some evidence of embolic particulate shower during mobilization of the artery, insertion of internal shunts and especially during reestablishment of flow in the internal carotid artery, as measured by intraoperative transcranial Doppler.[30,31] More important, perhaps, is detection of deficient flow in the middle cerebral artery (MCA) as when an internal shunt may, unknown to the surgeon, be kinked or blocked, or when the mean flow in the MCA is below approximately 30 cm/sec, and a shunt may be required.[31] Doppler detection of both defective flow and embolic shower has served to alert surgeons to intraoperative problems, stimulating improved surgical techniques with overall reduction in surgical morbidity. The incidence of computerized tomography (CT)-demonstrated cerebral infarction after carotid endarterectomy ranges from <3 to about 8 percent overall, but ulcerated or tightly stenotic lesions have a postoperative risk of demonstrable cerebral infarction of 30–90%.[32] In patients who demonstrate middle cerebral artery blood flow deficits or evidence of particulate embolism, intraoperative prophylactic administration of a neuroprotective agent may be of value. Bullock (personal communication[33]) has suggested that an agent with rapid brain penetration and action, as well as rapid clearance, such as CNS-1102 (Cambridge Neuroscience), a noncompetitive NMDA antagonist, or CP-101606 (Pfizer), may be worth intraoperative trials in high-risk carotid endarterectomy patients. Jonas also proposes, with fine logic, that a large cohort of carotid endarterectomy patients be prospectively and empirically started on neuroprotective agents prior to surgery, emphasizing that valuable statistical information could be gathered in a relatively short time.[29] Fischer *et al.* elaborate further the topic of prophylactic neuroprotection, extending potential future application to patients with chronic conditions, such as hypertension, atrial fibrillation and transient ischemic attacks (who may not be surgical candidates), and who may possibly benefit from long-term neuroprotective therapy.[34]

### *Subarachnoid Hemorrhage*

Subarachnoid hemorrhage (SAH) associated with ruptured cerebral aneurysm remains a source of significant morbidity and mortality, for such hemorrhage usually produces local and generalized vasospasm, often severe enough to delay surgery and induce irreversible changes in cerebral perfusion. Operative intervention may further prompt immediate and delayed focal ischemia by virtue of arterial manipulation in the region of the aneurysm and parent vessel, and by necessary retraction and exposure. Over many years, various techniques to reduce these effects have evolved, including hypothermia *(vide infra)*, delay of surgery until vasospasm has subsided, and the use of neuroprotective agents.

In the early 1980s investigators began using calcium channel blocking agents, nimodipine and nicardipine, in an effort to reduce vasospasm in subarachnoid hemorrhage, and to promote early operation to remove the threat of further hemorrhage.[35,36] Subsequent larger studies in Great Britain and the United States demonstrated that oral nimodipine reduced the number of cerebral infarcts, the incidence of poor outcome (although increase in good outcome was marginal), and possibly also the incidence of rebleeding.[37] Intravenous nicardipine, on the other hand, significantly reduced the overall incidence of demonstrable vasospasm (angiography/middle cerebral artery flow velocity)[38] as well as symptomatic vasospasm in patients with aneurysmal SAH, but this did not translate into improved overall late outcome.[39]

If, in addition to improved cerebral perfusion by reducing vasospasm, toxic influx of calcium into ischemic neurones can be reduced by use of calcium channel blocking agents, any beneficial cellular effect will probably be only in those cells that have been subjected to relatively short periods of ischemia within the present therapeutic window of 3–4 hours after onset.[17] Hence, the rationale for early administration of calcium channel blocking agents in patients with SAH. Nimodipine (60 mg po q4h around the clock for 21 days) in patients with SAH is often used in current neurosurgical practice, and this is the only Federal Drug Administration (FDA) approved indication for nimodipine at present.

Lipid perioxidation has also been implicated in the process of vasospasm in SAH. Antioxidant agents, including U74006F (Upjohn), ameliorate vasospasm by reducing lipid perioxidation in primates,[40] although little clinical information has emerged.

Palmer *et al.* (this volume)[25] cite two unpublished studies in which autologous blood was injected into the subarachnoid space in animals. The NMDA antagonist, remacemide (Fisons Pharmaceuticals), significantly reduced extravasation of dye in the hemisphere injected with blood and also reduced the amount of resultant vasospasm. This latter effect is attributed to action of remacemide on the NMDA receptors in cerebral microvessels, which may mediate trauma-induced breakdown of the blood-brain barrier. There have been no published clinical trials as yet with respect to NMDA antagonists in subarachnoid hemorrhage.

*Traumatic Brain Injury*

Bullock *et al.* (this volume) describe an elegant microdialysis technique of measuring patterns of excitatory amino acid (EAA) release in human cortex following acute head injury, as well as the time course and relationship between EAA release and increased intracranial pressure, cerebral perfusion pressure, and ionic changes. Glutamate and aspartate rapidly accumulate in severely injured, contused, and ischemic brain in amounts that are destructive to neuronal and glial cells, and persist in patients with secondary and focal ischemia for 4+ days. They conclude that these head-injured patients would be candidates for prolonged EAA antagonist therapy, and suggest several appropriate agents.[41] Mechanisms of damage by excitotoxic neurotransmitters, glutamate and aspartate, are elaborated in reviews by Olney,[42,43] and by Myseros and Bullock in this volume,[44] as well as in other recent trauma literature.[20,45] "The prospect of achieving a major reduction in head injury-induced morbidity and mortality is at last becoming tangible."[44] On the basis of these studies, milder head injuries may be appropriately treated with an EAA antagonist as "coverage" for 12 hours or so, and in severe head injuries with evidence of contusion or significant ischemia, prolonged use of EAA antagonists over a period of 4–6 days, may reduce the sometimes overwhelming neurologic consequences of head injury. The urgency of beginning treatment within the therapeutic window is emphasized; some NMDA antagonists rapidly enter the brain[24] and some are effective in animal models when given up to 2 hours after injury.[20,44] The sedative, analgesic, and anticonvulsant effects of certain of these agents, some of which also increase cerebral blood flow, are also beneficial properties when dealing with severe human head injury.[44]

The symptomatic side effects of glutamate/aspartate antagonists may tend to restrict their use in mildly obtunded or awake patients. In volunteers, these side effects include disagreeable symptoms such as flushing, diaphoresis, pallor, paraesthesiae, nausea and vomiting, as well as behavioral changes such as disorientation, paranoia, anxiety, vivid hallucinations, somnolence, confusion, even catatonia. These effects are not necessarily dose related, and usually subside as the drug is cleared, and vary with the specific agent used. Moderate elevation of blood pressure and increased cerebral blood flow are beneficial effects of certain of these agents,[24] but hypotension has been noted with others.[22] Muir *et al.* in this volume[24] note that the side effects of another NMDA receptor blocker, CNS 1102 (Cerestat, Cambridge Neuroscience) in normal volunteers, were not observed in phase II studies in stroke and traumatic brain injury patients. In addition, a new category of NMDA antagonists, which block glutamate *release* from synaptic vesicles, and which appear to lack the severe side effects of other NMDA antagonists, is being tested in animals.[44] Perhaps a shorter duration of NMDA antagonist treatment of less than 24 hours would reduce side effects, and still remain therapeutic.

Several NMDA antagonists, including ketamine and phencyclidine (PCP), also produce pathomorphologic changes in certain cortical areas, such as cingulate and retrosplenial areas in rats, transient at low doses, but permanent at higher doses. Barbiturates, scopalamine and diazepam block some of the psychomimetic symptoms associated with some NMDA antagonists, and more importantly, block the pathomorphologic changes produced by NMDA antagonists, presumably by exerting gamma-aminobutyric acid (GABA)-mimetic activity that is stronger than the NMDA antagonist activity.[5] Concomitant administration of an NMDA antagonist and a GABA-mimetic agent may offer neuroprotection from injury without drug-induced side effects and neuronal damage.

*Hypothermia*

Brain temperature directly influences the extent of histopathological injury in vulnerable brain regions under conditions of even transient global ischemia in animals, independently of rectal temperature.[13] Furthermore, with respect to global ischemia, the neuroprotective effects of agents such as MK-801 and nicardipine appear to be dependent upon hypothermic brain conditions. Under conditions of transient global ischemia followed by recirculation, preischemic-administered MK-801 itself produces hypothermia as low as 34.5°C with no associated ischemic hippocampal damage. Postischemic external cooling alone under the same conditions also prevented hippocampal damage. MK-801 administered under normothermic conditions failed to protect the hippocampus from damage.[46] On the other hand, as noted above, global ischemia itself will reduce deep brain temperature by 4–5°C, even when the skull is warmed.[14] Furthermore, again in animal studies, the blocking effect of MK-801 on methamphetamine-induced toxicity appears partly due to MK-801's ability to block the hyperthermia associated with methamphetamine.[47] The cytoprotective action of mild hypothermia was found not to be mediated by attenuation of the rise in interstitial concentrations of aspartate and glutamate after brain trauma; indeed, concentration of these excitatory amino acids increased under hypothermic conditions.[48] On the other hand, Busto *et al.* found that hypothermia does attenuate postischemic glutamate release, as well as free radical production.[49] But hypothermia attenuates glutamate-induced hyperexcitability and oxygen free radical-induced lipid peroxidation,[50] both of which are neurotoxic. Even 30-minute (but not 60-minute) delayed induction of mild whole body hypothermia in animals significantly reduced infarct volume, independently of cortical blood flow during the period of ischemia.[51] These observations illustrate the complex interactions between EAA release/toxicity and cerebral functions, such as temperature regulation. MK-801 has been withdrawn from clinical trials, but it may typify the actions of some of the NMDA antagonists. However, new "second generation" glutamate antagonists with fewer side effects are in phase II clinical trials.[44]

In human studies, Sternau *et al.* found that deep brain temperature (lateral ventricle) was 0.2–0.5°C higher than cortical temperature and both were 0.5°C higher than bladder temperature. In severely head-injured patients, brain temperature was 0.5–2.5°C higher than body temperature, and elevations in core brain temperature coincided with increasing intracranial pressure.[52] Interest in brain temperature in human injury dates from as early as 1943, when Fay proposed "generalized refrigeration" (to 91–92°F) as a treatment modality in severe traumatic brain injury.[53] Profound hypothermia to 10–15°C, however, with circulatory arrest has been long discarded in clinical practice.[54] Moderate brain hypothermia (to 30°C), induced prior to fluid percussion brain injury, reduces mortality significantly over 33 and 36°C hypothermia groups, and improves postinjury behavioral scores in rats. In this study, total time at reduced temperature was increased at lower brain temperatures as well, and may have been an additional factor. The authors emphasize the potential clinical benefit of moderate hypothermia in severely head-injured patients.[55]

Dietrich has extensively reviewed much recent data with respect to the protective effects of hypothermia, synergistic with those of other neuroprotective agents, and the adverse effects of core brain hyperthermia. " . . . it is obvious that abnormalities in brain temperature may represent a manageable consequence of human cerebral injury."[56]

An alternative method of inducing hypothermia is proposed by Hall *et al.*, who demonstrated the protective effect of a muscarinic cholinergic partial agonist (U80816E), which reduced brain temperature by as much as 2.2°C in Mongolian gerbils, with significant improvement in survival of hippocampal neurones after

10 minutes of global ischemia. Maintaining brain temperature by external means during the ischemic process completely abolished the neuroprotective action of this compound.[50] This has clinical significance in the future, for as purely pharmacologic hypothermic agents develop and survive clinical feasibility and toxicology studies, they may be added to the armentarium of the clinician dealing with all forms of potential neuronal damage from many precipitating events.

The increasing relevance of hypothermia as a therapeutic modality is illustrated by a recent 2-day conference on this subject in Pittsburgh, Pennsylvania in September 1994.

### *Traumatic Spinal Cord Injury*

In a review of mechanisms of spinal cord injury, Tator and Fehlings discuss at length the concept of secondary cord injury. They argue that the primary mechanical injury rarely causes complete transection, even in the face of total functional loss caudal to the lesion. Posttraumatic cord ischemia and infarction may be potentially altered by restoration of systemic blood pressure, and specifically by improvement in microcirculation in the segments of spinal cord above and below the lesion. By means of elegant colloidal carbon angiography, they demonstrated luxuriant microcirculation within the uninjured central grey matter, and the propensity for hemorrhages to occur in the grey matter with "especially severe" ischemia in adjacent white matter shortly following trauma. They list in detail the vascular and electrolyte changes, loss of cord autoregulation, biochemical alterations, edema, and loss of energy metabolism which comprise the "secondary injury."[57]

However, acute spinal cord injury (SCI) had not been ameliorated by any form of medical therapy until the Second National Acute Spinal Cord Injury Study (NASCIS-II), which was the first clinical trial to demonstrate improvement in neurologic recovery after medical therapy in the acute stage. In this study, methylprednisolone (MPS) given in large doses (30 mg/kg IV at once and 5.4 mg/kg q1hr × 24 hours) to patients with incomplete spinal cord lesions, and started within 8 hours of injury, gave significantly better neurologic recovery than similar patients given placebo. MPS given to similar patients starting more than 8 hours after injury produced significantly worse neurologic recovery than similar patients given placebo.

Complete lesions were not improved by MPS.[58] Because of a difference in outcome of the two *placebo* groups (those entering the study before 8 hours and those entering more than 8 hours after injury), and because many patients in the first MPS treatment group were clustered close to the 8-hour cut off starting time, the results of NASCIS II have been questioned. Ducker carefully examined the data from this study and concluded that the earlier a glucosteroid is given after injury (*even in the ambulance*—author's emphasis), the better the outcome. Ducker also advocates discontinuing high-dose corticosteroid therapy after 8 hours.[59] A shorter duration of therapy (8 versus 24 hours) may reduce the increased incidence of pneumonia, wound infections, longer hospital stay, and undesirable effects upon the immune system associated with high-dose steroids noted in some recent reports.[60]

In 1982, Hall suggested that a single massive dose (30 mg/kg) of methylprednisolone may actually reduce free-radical reactions, reduce lipid peroxidation and enhance the activity of $(Na^+ + K^+)$-ATPase with beneficial effects in early spinal cord contusion.[61] In 1992, Hall *et al.* elaborated upon the effects of antioxidants in brain and spinal cord injury. Alpha tocopherol (vitamin E) attenuates progressive posttraumatic spinal cord ischemia, but requires extensive pretreatment because of slow uptake in the CNS. The optimal initial dose of MPS remains 30 mg/kg iv in animals, and presumably in humans. Higher doses are deleterious because the cell membrane concentration at this dose is " . . . apparently necessary to protect the membrane from posttraumatic insult, whereas higher concentrations produced by even more massive doses can cause membrane instability." New and novel antioxidants, including the nonglucocorticoid steroid analogs of MPS, the 21-aminosteroids, "lazaroids," are more potent and effective inhibitors of lipid peroxidation than previous steroid compounds, and have shown considerable promise in spinal cord injury.[62]

A high-dose steroid regimen administered as soon as possible after acute spinal cord injury apparently offers the present optimum potential recovery to the unfortunate SCI patient, and this regimen will probably be supplemented in the future by the addition of other neuroprotective agents.

Calcium channel antagonists (nimodipine, nicardipine, and nifedipine) have demonstrated variable results in numerous animal studies of spinal cord injury, with reports of increased cord blood flow in uninjured animals,[63] but maintenance of a normal mean systemic blood pressure by the use of adrenalin was necessary.[64] However, no significant improvement in functional results or reduction in lesion size was noted following nicardipine administration at various doses after injury.[65] Thus far, there have been no clinical studies suggesting value in acute administration of calcium channel antagonists in spinal cord injury.

Another aspect of spinal cord injury is related to extensive thoracic-abdominal aortic vascular procedures, and in spontaneous dissection of the thoracic-abdominal aorta, with ischemic damage to the dorsal spinal cord. Either can result in total paraplegia. Marsala *et al.* demonstrated that mechanically lowered regional temperature can preserve function in rat studies, as measured by lesion histology and behavioral function.[66] The mechanics of this particular approach seem to obviate its use in humans, but perhaps a pharmacological hypothermic agent administered shortly after surgery (or even prophylactically, in elective surgical procedures) would be of protective value (see the report of Hall noted above[50]). A more radical approach in the acute human spinal cord-injured patient might involve introducing a cool saline intrathecal infusion via a percutaneous high cervical catheter, with lumbar catheter drainage (providing there was no cerebrospinal fluid block), perhaps resulting in direct cord cooling, along with other pharmacologic neuroprotective agents, should animal research indicate their possible clinical value.

Considering the relatively small neuronal population contained within the spinal cord, even faint improvement in cell and axonal viability may result in significant functional improvement in the injured patient.

## Surgical Retraction Injury

Collins described neurosurgery as "planned trauma."[67] Avoidance of additional, superimposed injury requires the use of a number of techniques, some established, some of recent development. During the surgical approach to deeply situated lesions, brain retraction by means of fixed or hand-held retractors is inevitable and can be injurious. In a recent, extensive review, Andrews and Bringas emphasized that "brain injury secondary to retraction occurs in approximately 10% of major cranial base tumor procedures and 5% of intracranial aneurysms or cranial tumor (other than base) procedures." Pressure injury beneath the retractor is increased as retraction pressure is increased, but with fixed retraction pressure, the brain seems to adjust to the blade, and retraction pressure diminishes to about 50% of initial value. Intermittent retraction with relaxation of the blade every 10–15 minutes allows reperfusion, and keeping retraction pressure below 40 mg Hg is superior to constant and high pressure retraction.[68] Neuroprotection can be assisted by a wide range of techniques, some within standard surgical practice. These include positioning of the patient so as to facilitate venous drainage, extensive bone removal at the cranial base so as to reduce brain retraction, cerebrospinal fluid drainage, anesthetic agents such as isoflurane and propofol, and hypothermia. In addition, mannitol (an osmotic diuretic) has been used alone for years to assist in exposure by reducing intracranial fluid volume, and although it may mildly reduce mean arterial pressure, it appears also to reduce blood viscosity during the first hour after administration and to slightly improve cerebral blood flow. Mannitol administered by constant infusion appears to better preserve electrical activity, and may be better than when given in a series of bolus infusions.[69]

Hyperventilation has long been used by neurosurgeons to reduce cerebral edema, especially in the face of acute, severe intraoperative swelling, with visible reduction in mass within minutes of initiation of hyperventilation. These disasterous events seem to be less frequent with the routine preoperative use of corticosteroids and sometimes mannitol during induction of anesthesia. However, hyperventilation reduces cerebral blood flow and produces alkalosis, which may be neurotoxic under conditions of hypoxia. Under these circumstances, the combination of mannitol and nimodipine appears to be neuroprotective, in that cerebral blood flow and evoked potentials are preserved during retraction.[70,71] Nimodipine is not clinically available in intravenous form, but preoperative oral administration of nimodipine (in doses comparable to those used in acute SAH) may be of value, combined with mannitol as a slow intravenous drip during surgery. Some surgeons are using nimodipine perioperatively in more difficult brain cases, but there has been no controlled clinical trial to evaluate its possible value. The hypotheses that brain edema (including that encountered in surgery) can be reduced by inhibiting blood-to-brain sodium transport—and possibly also chloride ions, which accumulate in ischemic brain in parallel with edema formation—may be partly supported by the known effects of dexamethasone and progesterone in the treatment of brain edema, in addition to any possible free radical scavenger function of corticosteroids.[72]

## Epilepsy

Seizures are associated with excessive neuronal discharge, and resultant excessive release of excitatory neurotransmitters. Limbic structures, especially the hippocampus, are especially seizure-prone, and contain high concentrations of NMDA receptors. Activation of metabotropic glutamate receptors by extrinsic glutamate agonists leads to limbic seizures.[73] When endogenous extracellular concentrations of glutamate and aspartate are elevated, limbic discharges are increased, and may propagate to similar areas on the opposite side, as well as throughout the neocortex. In status epilepticus, near-continuous seizure activity produces markedly elevated EAA concentrations, and probably secondary transient and permanent excitotoxic damage. It appears likely that the exhaustion phenomenon of "Todd's paralysis" after a prolonged seizure, and the mechanisms of "kindling" of seizures are related to glutamate/aspartate toxic effects. There has been recent interest in using NMDA antagonists as anticonvulsants. Remacemide is a weak NMDA antagonist, which limits activity at excitatory amino acid receptors, has relatively mild side effects, and is undergoing clinical evaluation in patients with intractable epilepsy.[25] Bullock briefly discusses the rationale for clinical use of NMDA antagonists in epilepsy.[23] The considerable recent literature implicating GABA and GABA-ergic compounds in reducing excessive neuronal discharges in clinical control of epilepsy is exciting, but beyond the scope of this review.

## Neurodegenerative Diseases

"In the aging brain, loss of calcium homeostasis is believed to be a key factor underlying neuronal damage associated with dendritic atrophy and, ultimately, cell death."[74] As dendrites atrophy, intercellular synaptic connections are progressively lost, and brain circuitry becomes increasingly disrupted. Kowalska and Disterhoft hypothesize that as calcium accumulates in injured (anoxia, ischemia, hypoglycemia, status epilepticus, trauma, neurotoxicity, etc.) or aging neurones, deficits in learning and memory become manifest.[75] Increased intracellular calcium appears to participate in memory deficits associated with senility and Alzheimer's disease (AD). Dendritic branching loss seems to characterize the histologic appearance of these states, and may represent an anatomic basis for cognitive dysfunction in aging brain.[74,76]

Olney discusses the relationship of excitatory amino acid toxicity to the histopathologic changes in AD, hypothesizing that degeneration of various types of neurones in this disease can be explained by an excitotoxic process, and that the characteristic plaques and dendritic tangles might be a secondary response to the primary EAA-induced neurodegenerative process. Furthermore, he considers the scenario of "normal" loss of neurones beginning in middle age as being related to age-linked alteration of balance between excitotoxic agonist and antagonist forces playing upon NMDA and non-NMDA receptors. These receptors appear to be situated on various types of neurones, including cholinergic, adrenergic, and somatostatinergic, and all can be damaged by EAA toxicity. These receptors may become less efficient in removing extracellular glutamate and other EAAs in aging brain, possibly subjecting these neurones to increased excitotoxic damage and eventual death.[43]

These two postulated mechanisms of neuronal degeneration probably represent only a part of the whole picture, but thus far, only calcium channel blockers have received clinical attention in age-related degenerative diseases.

Nimodipine is a remarkably well tolerated calcium channel blocker, discussed under *subarachnoid hemorrhage* (above), and is presumed to be effective by blocking L-type calcium channels on the neural membrane, and bringing the intracellular calcium back toward normal levels. This apparently allows neurones to function in a more normal manner, as demonstrated in aging rabbits. Nimodipine does not exert its effect on normal "healthy" cells, whose calcium homeostasis is undisturbed. Nimodipine's action appears also to be on the basis of improved microcirculation, and Kowalska and Disterhoft demonstrated that increased cerebral blood flow was seen in the same nimodipine dose range that was effective in enhancing behavioral learning rate.[75] Herning *et al.* (this volume) cite evidence that nimodipine alters the electroencephalogram (EEG) of geriatric patients toward a more normal pattern.[76]

Parnetti *et al.* gave relatively low doses of nimodipine (30 mg orally three times daily) for 3 or 6 months in a multicenter trial involving 755 patients. They demonstrated dose-related improvement in orientation, language, attention/calculation, information, memory, calculation, registration and recall. This was not a controlled study, but measurement of improvement was by four specific psychobehavioral scales and psychometric tests. Reduction in blood pressure in hypertensive patients by nimodipine appeared to be synergistic with the effects of standard hypotensive drugs.[77]

In an earlier study, Tollefson reported a randomized, double-blind, placebo-controlled, multicenter study involving 227 patients with Alzheimer's disease who were treated with low-dose nimodipine. Patients were evaluated with an elaborate battery of measures before and after 12 weeks of treatment, 8 of which improved significantly from baseline testing. Several placebo group scores also increased over the 12 weeks. "These findings appear to support the possibility that 30 mg of nimodipine three times daily prevented further deterioration across several cognitive and social parameters. This apparent benefit, however, was not manifest at the 60-mg dosage."[78]

Mervis *et al.* (poster paper, this volume) have demonstrated reversal of age-related atrophy of cortical dendritic branching (Golgi staining) by nimodipine in high doses, with significantly better retention of a standard conditioned eye blink response as compared with controls. More importantly, they concluded, " . . . chronic high dose nimodipine treatment completely reversed age-related atrophic changes: both total dendritic length and distribution of dendritic material of the aging rabbits were the same as in young controls." This treatment also reversed age-related atrophy of the soma.[74] Perhaps the Fountain of Youth has a nimodipine spout!

Although cholinesterase inhibitors are being evaluated in clinical trials in patients with Alzheimer's disease, their function is not strictly neuroprotective.

These agents simply increase the available amount of brain acetylcholine, with improvement in several test measures.

Keeping in mind potential prophylactic application of neuroprotective agents in certain clinical populations, a cohort of patients with sleep apnea dementia might be appropriate for a low-dose, long-term, placebo-controlled nimodipine prospective study.

### Parkinson's Disease and Huntington's Disease

Palmer *et al.* (this volume) cite evidence that "excessive stimulation by excitatory amino acid transmitters at critical neuronal connections within the brain has been linked to both Parkinson's and Huntington's disorders." They suggest that excitatory glutamate projections from the subthalamus to the globus pallidus and substantia nigra become "overactive," contributing to the clinical expression of these diseases and suggesting that glutamate receptor antagonists might reduce the consequences of this overactivity. NMDA receptor antagonists potentiate the action of levodopa (L-dopa), and in conjunction with the latter, may permit better clinical management.[25] In rhesus monkeys rendered moderately parkinsonian, remacemide plus levodopa/carbidopa produced a substantially better clinical score than did levodopa/carbidopa alone. The major part of the anti-parkinson action of remacemide appears to be at the postsynaptic (from subthalamic nucleus) level in both the internal segment of the globus pallidus and substantia nigra pars reticulata.[79] Greenberg suggests that if underlying metabolic defects in specific neuronal populations (basal ganglia), possibly produced by glutamate-induced neuronal degeneration, NMDA antagonists such as remacemide may not only reduce the clinical symptoms in Parkinson's disease, but may also slow actual progression of the disease by reducing cell destruction by glutamate excitotoxicity.[80]

Olney *et al.* report that L-dopa is itself a weak excitotoxin, and that its derivative, 6-OH-dopa is a powerful excitotoxin. They postulate that an aberrant mechanism which allows buildup of L-dopa, or its excitotoxic derivative, in the nigrostriatal dopaminergic terminals may allow leakage of the dopa-derived excitotoxin, into extracellular space. In conjunction with endogenous glutamate, accumulation of L-dopa may produce degeneration of striatal neurons in the pattern seen in Huntington's disease.[80] This is, of course, a sketchy and possibly incorrect interpretation (on the part of this author) of very complex data. However, from Olney's concept, a neuroprotective agent may eventually evolve to alter the formidable curse of a dreadful inherited disease before the full syndrome becomes manifest.[81]

### Substance Abuse

In two papers in this volume, Herning *et al.* describe the potential use of nimodipine in chronic substance abusers. Cocaine abusers have increased deficits in cerebral blood flow and increased beta activity in the electroencephalogram (EEG), consistent with those seen in the aging brain. They demonstrate that nimodipine increases alpha EEG activity and mildly reduces beta activity after single and multiple oral doses, these changes being in the direction of normal. Nimodipine also reduces craving in drug-deprived abusers, and may play a role in treatment of chronic cocaine abuse.[76] Subjects were also tested using auditory and visual programmed stimulation, which is picked up on the EEG as an event-related potential (ERP), specifically its P3 component. Alterations in the P3 component are seen in fatigue or boredom in normal subjects, and are thought to measure ability to evaluate task-relevant stimuli and to update recent memory. Chronic cocaine use tends to improve this measure, and abstinence to diminish it. Herning *et al.* found improvement in information processing, as measured by the P3 component, in cocaine abusers after a single dose of nimodipine (30 mg po), but, inexplicably, not with a 60-mg dose. They conclude that nimodipine may assist in drug-abuse treatment by alleviating the cognitive deficits seen during abstinence.[82]

## Reflex Sympathetic Dystrophy

Recent evidence demonstrates release of glutamate at bipolar sensory nerve endings at the periphery, as well as centrally in the dorsal horn, after injury along the course of a nerve, and upon even the faintest sensory stimulation. Glutamate injected into the paws of normal rats sharply reduced the latency of withdrawal from a standard heat source, as compared with controls.[83] Perhaps this may in part account for the otherwise poorly explained phenomenon of reflex sympathetic dystrophy (RSD). Patients with this dismal problem usually have sustained a partial injury to a peripheral nerve, and gradually develop severe, intractable hyperalgesia and pain, swelling and blanching and autonomic changes in the distal affected extremity. Pain is sympathetically maintained in the early stages, but later is independent of sympathetic stimulation. This often evolves into a permanent disability, sometimes requiring amputation, although helped in early stages by sympathetic block or sympathectomy. Schwartzman decodes the enigma of RSD in part by noting in his extensive review that in an uninjured nerve, sympathetic stimulation has a suppressor effect on C fiber activity. "If the C fibers have been sensitized from a tissue injury and are firing spontaneously, they are driven by sympathetic stimulation and the application of noradrenaline."[84] Could it be that glutamate released at the peripheral terminals of the sensory nerve is the sensitizing factor, augmented by sympathetic stimulation?

## ADDENDUM

Several reports describing an emerging *calpain hypothesis* have appeared in very recent literature, and bear notation here. Calpain, a normal intracellular cytosolic protease, is activated by excess intracellular calcium, and may serve as a site of action for neuroprotective agents. Ischemic injury damages calcium homeostasis, and excessive calcium entering the cell (by NMDA/AMPA receptors, voltage-gated ionic channels, or even activated intracellular calcium pools) initiates intracellular proteolysis by calpain. Calpain thus appears to be a "final common pathway," for when activated, it destroys intracellular and membrane proteins.

Bartus demonstrated that two different calpain inhibitors (AK-275 and AK-295) dramatically reduced infarct size in a rate model of focal ischemia.[85,86] Hong et al. suggest further that proteolytic inhibition (by calpain antagonists) may be useful in treating a variety of neurodegenerative diseases in which glutamate-receptor toxicity is a common factor.[87]

## SUMMARY

"Stroke treatment seems to be entering a golden age . . . ."[3] Fisher's observation not only applies to ischemic stroke, but to all the conditions described above, and in the future, possibly (and quite speculatively), to other neurologic diseases, such as multiple sclerosis, amyotrophic lateral sclerosis, even radiation therapy and Bell's palsy. Physicians must sharpen their criteria for decisions regarding therapy and must " . . . be prepared to accept what is actually known from scientific data . . . rather than to rely on instinct, clinical impression, or the need to do something rather than nothing."[2]

## REFERENCES

1. GINSBERG, M. D. & W. A. PULSINELLI. 1994. The ischemic penumbra, injury thresholds, and the therapeutic window for acute stroke (editorial). Ann. Neurol. **36:** 553–554.
2. SCHEINBERG. 1994. Stroke: the way things really are. Stroke **25:** 1290–1294.
3. FISHER, M. & J. BOGOUSSLAVSKY. 1993. Evolving toward effective therapy for acute ischemic stroke. JAMA **270:** 360–364.
4. WRIGHT, R. H. & A. AMES, III. 1964. Measurement of maximal permissable cerebral ischemia and a study of its pharmacological prolongation. J. Neurosurg. **7:** 567–574.
5. OLNEY, J. W., L. LABRUYERE, G. WANG, D. F. WOZNIAK, M. T. PRICE & M. A. SESMA. 1991. NMDA antagonist neurotoxicity: Mechanism and prevention. Science **254:** 1515–1518.
6. THE AMERICAN NIMODIPINE STUDY GROUP. 1992. Clinical trial of nimodipine in acute ischemic stroke. Stroke **23:** 3–8.
7. KASTE, M., R. FOGELHOLM, T. ERILA, H. PALOMAKI, K. MURROS, A. RISSANEN & S. SARNA. 1994. A randomized, double-blind, placebo-controlled trial of nimodipine in acute ischemic hemispheric stroke. Stroke **25:** 1348–1353.
8. BARSAN, W. G., T. G. BROTT, J. P. BRODERICK, E. C. HALEY, D. E. LEVY & J. R. MARLER. 1993. Time of hospital presentation in patients with acute stroke. Arch. Int. Med. **153:** 2558–2561.
9. GOMEZ, C. R., M. D. MALKOFF, C. M. SAUER, R. TULYAPRONCHOTE, C. M. BURCH & G. A. BANET. 1994. Code stroke. An attempt to shorten inhospital therapeutic delays. Stroke **25:** 1920–1923.
10. CAMARATA, P. J., R. C. HEROS & R. E. LATCHAW. 1994. "Brain Attack": the rationale for treating stroke as a medical emergency. Neurosurgery **34:** 144–158.
11. SIESJO, B. K. 1988. Historical overview. Calcium, ischemia and death of brain cells. Ann. N.Y. Acad. Sci. **522:** 638–661.
12. CHEUNG, J. Y., J. V. BONVENTRE, C. D. MALIS & A. LEAF. 1986. Calcium and ischemic injury. N. Engl. J. Med. **314:** 1670–1676.
13. BUSTO, R., W. D. DIETRICH, M. Y-T. GLOBUS, I. VALDES, P. SCHEINBERG, & M. D. GINSBERG. 1987. Small differences in intraischemic brain temperature critically determine the extent of ischemic neuronal injury. J. Cereb. Blood Flow Metab. **7:** 729–738.

14. MINAMISAWA, H., P. MELLERGARD, M-L. SMITH, F. BENGTSSON, S. THEANDER, F. BORIS-MOLLER & B. K. SIESJO. 1990. Preservation of brain temperature during ischemia in rats. Stroke **21:** 758–764.
15. CHUMAS, P., M. R. DEL BIGIO, J. M. DRAKE & U. I. TUOR. 1993. A comparison of the protective effects of dexamethasone to other potential prophylactic agents in a neonatal rat model of cerebral hypoxia-ischemia. J. Neurosurg. **79:** 414–420.
16. HALL, E. D. 1992. The neuroprotective pharmacology of methylprednisolone. J. Neurosurg. **76:** 13–22.
17. HALL, E. D. 1993. Lipid antioxidants in acute central nervous system injury. Ann. Emerg. Med. **22:** 1022–1027.
18. BULLOCK, R., D. I. GRAHAM, S. SWANSON & J. MCCULLOCH. 1994. Neuroprotective effect of the AMPA receptor antagonist LY-293558 in focal cerbral ischemia in the cat. J. Cereb. Flow Metab. **14:** 466–471.
19. BUCHAN, A. M., H. LESIUK, K. A. BARNES, H. LI, Z-G. HUANG, K. E. SMITH & D. XUE. 1993. Ampa antagonists: do they hold more promise for clinical stroke trials than NMDA antagonists? Stroke **24**(Suppl. 1):I-148–I-152.
20. BULLOCK, R. & H. FUJISAWA. 1992. The role of glutamate antagonists for the treatment of CNS injury. J. Neurotrauma **9**(Suppl. 2):S443–S462.
21. CHOI, D. W. 1989. Toward a new pharmacology of ischemic neuronal death. *In* Selective Vulnerability of the Brain: New Insights into the Pathophysiology of Stroke. R. C. Collins, Moderator. Ann. Intern. Med. **110:** 992–1000.
22. THE DEXTRORPHAN STUDY GROUP & HOFFMAN-LA ROCHE. 1995. Safety, tolerability and pharmacokinetics of the *N*-methyl-D-aspartate antagonist, RO-01-6794/706 in patients with acute ischemic stroke. Ann. N. Y. Acad. Sci. This volume.
23. BULLOCK, R., A. KOTAKE & H. FALECK. 1995. Strategies for neuroprotection with glutamate antagonists: extrapolating from evidence taken from the first stroke and head injury studies. Ann. N. Y. Acad. Sci. This volume.
24. MUIR, K. W., D. G. GROSSET & K. R. LEES. 1995. Clinical pharmacology of CNS 1102 in volunteers. Ann. N. Y. Acad. Sci. This volume.
25. PALMER, G. C., E. F. CREGAN, A. R. BORRELLI & F. WILLET. 1995. Neuroprotective properties of the uncompetitive NMDA receptor antagonist remacemide hydrochloride. Ann. N. Y. Acad. Sci. This volume.
26. LYDEN, P. D. & L. LONZO. 1994. Combination therapy protects ischemic brain in rats. Stroke **25:** 189–196.
27. TRAYSTMAN, R. J. 1994. Editorial comment. Stroke **25:** 196.
28. THE ANCROD STROKE STUDY INVESTIGATORS. 1994. Ancrod for the treatment of acute ischemic brain infarction. Stroke **25:** 1755–1759.
29. JONAS, S. 1995. Prophylactic pharmacologic neuroprotection against focal cerebral ischemia. Ann. N. Y. Acad. Sci. This volume.
30. SPENCER, M. P., G. I. THOMAS, S. C. NICHOLLS & L. R. SAUVAGE. 1990. Detection of middle cerebral artery emboli during carotid endarterectomy using transcranial Doppler ultrasonography. Stroke **21:** 415–423.
31. NAYLOR, A. R., J. A. W. WILDSMITH, J. MCCLURE, A. MCL. JENKINS & C. V. RUCKLEY. 1991. Transcranial Doppler monitoring during carotid endarterectomy. Br. J. Surg. **78:** 1264–1268.
32. HABOZIT, B. 1990. The silent brain infarct before and after carotid surgery. Ann. Vasc. Surg. **4:** 485–489.
33. BULLOCK, R. 1994. Personal communication, letter dated November 9, 1994.
34. FISHER, M., S. JONAS & R. L. SACCO. 1994. Prophylactic neuroprotection for cerebral ischemia. Stroke **25:** 1075–1080.
35. ALLEN, G. S. *et al.* 1983. Cerebral arterial spasm: a controlled trial of nimodipine in patients with subarachnoid hemorrhage. N. Engl. J. Med. **308:** 616–624.
36. HANDA, J., M. MATSUDA, Y. NAKASU, S. NAKASU, M. KIDOOKA & K. WATANABE. 1984. Early operation of aneurysmal subarachnoid hemorrhage. Use of nicardipine, a calcium channel blocker. Arch. Jpn. Chir. **53:** 619–630.
37. PICARD, J. D., G. D. MURRAY, R. ILLINGWORTH, M. D. M. SHAW, G. M. TEASDALE, P. M. FOY, P. R. D. HUMPHREY, D. A. LANG, R. NELSON, P. RICHARDS, J. SINAR, S. BAILEY & A. SKENE. 1989. Effect of oral nimodipine on cerebral infarction and

outcome after subarachnoid haemorrhage: British aneurysm nimodipine trial. Br. Med. J. **298:** 636–642.
38. HALEY, E. C., JR., N. F. KASSELL, J. C. TORNER & the participants. 1993. A randomized trial of nicardipine in subarachnoid hemorrhage: angiographic and transcranial Doppler ultrasound results. A report of the Cooperative Aneurysm Study. J. Neurosurg. **78:** 548–553.
39. HALEY, E. C., JR., N. F. KASSELL, J. C. TORNER & the participants. 1993. A randomized controlled trial of high-dose intravenous nicardipine in aneurysmal subarachnoidal hemorrhage. A report of the Cooperative Aneurysm Study. J. Neurosurg. **78:** 537–547.
40. KANAMARU, K., B. K. A. WEIR, I. SIMPSON, T. WITBECK & M. GRACE. 1991. Effect of 21-aminosteroid U-74006F on lipid perioxidation in subarachnoid clot. J. Neurosurg. **74:** 454–459.
41. BULLOCK, R., A. ZAUNER, J. S. MYSEROS, A. MARMAROU, J. J. WOODWARD & H. F. YOUNG. 1995. Evidence for prolonged release of excitatory amino ACIDS IN severe human head trauma: relationship to clinical events. Ann. N. Y. Acad. Sci. This volume.
42. OLNEY, J. W. 1982. The toxic effects of glutamate and related compounds in the retina and the brain. Retina **2:** 341–358.
43. OLNEY, J. W. 1990. Excitotoxin-mediated neuron death in youth and old age. Prog. Brain Res. **86:** 37–51.
44. MYSEROS, J. S. & R. BULLOCK. 1995. The rationale for glutamate antagonists in the treatment of traumatic brain injury. Ann. N. Y. Acad. Sci. This volume.
45. BULLOCK, R. 1993. Opportunities for neuroprotective drugs in clinical management of head injury. J. Emerg. Med. **11:** 23–30.
46. BUCHAN, A. & W. A. PULSINELLI. 1990. Hypothermia but not the $N$-methyl-D-aspartate antagonist, MK-801, attenuates neuronal damage in gerbils subjected to transient global ischemia. J. Neurosci. **10:** 311–316.
47. BOWYER, J. F. 1995. The role of hyperthermia in amphetamine's interaction with NMDA receptors, nitric oxide and age to produce neurotoxicity (Abstr.). Ann. N. Y. Acad. Sci. This volume.
48. PALMER, A. M., D. W. MARION, M. I. BOTSCHELLER & E. E. REDD. 1993. Therapeutic hypothermia is cytoprotective without attenuating the traumatic brain injury-induced elevations in interstitial concentrations of aspartate and glutamate. J. Neurotrauma **10:** 363–372.
49. BUSTO, R., M. Y-T. GLOBUS, W. D. DIETRICH, E. MARTINEZ. I. VALDES & M. D. GINSBERG. 1989. Effect of mild hypothermia in ischemia-induced release of neurotransmitters and free fatty acids in rat brain. Stroke **20:** 904–910.
50. HALL, E. D., P. K. ANDRUS & K. E. PAZARA. 1993. Protective efficacy of a hypothermic pharmacological agent in gerbil forebrain ischemia. Stroke **24:** 711–715.
51. KARIBE, H., J. CHEN, G. J. ZAROW, S. H. GRAHAM & P. R. WEINSTEIN. 1994. Delayed induction of mild hypothermia to reduce infarct volume after temporary middle cerebral artery occlusion in rats. J. Neurosurg. **80:** 112–119.
52. STERNAU, L., C. THOMPSON, W. D. DIETRICH, R. BUSTO, M. Y-T. GLOBUS & M. D. GINSBERG. 1991. Intracranial temperature observations in the human brain. J. Cereb. Blood Flow Metab. **11**(Suppl. 2): S123.
53. FAY, T. 1943. Observations on generalized refrigeration in cases of severe cerebral trauma. Assoc. Res. Nerv. Ment. Dis. Proc. **24:** 611–619.
54. DRAKE, C. G., H. W. K. BARR, J. C. COLES & N. F. GERGELY. 1964. The use of extracorporeal circulation and profound hypothermia in the treatment of ruptured intracranial aneurysm. J. Neurosurg. **21:** 575–581.
55. CLIFTON, G. L., J. Y. JIANG, B. G. LYETH, L. W. JENKINS, R. J. HAMM & R. L. HAYES. 1991. Marked protection by moderate hypothermia after experimental traumatic brain injury. J. Cereb. Blood Flow Metab. **11:** 114–121.
56. DIETRICH, W. D. 1992. The importance of brain temperature in cerebral injury. J. Neurotrauma **9**(Suppl. 2): S475–S485.

57. TATOR, C. H. & M. G. FEHLINGS. 1991. Review of the secondary injury theory of acute spinal cord trauma with emphasis on vascular mechanisms. J. Neurosurg. **75:** 15–26.
58. BRACKEN, M. B. *et al.* 1992. Methylprednisolone or naloxone treatment after acute spinal cord injury: 1-year follow-up data. Results of the Second National Acute Spinal Cord Injury Study. J. Neurosurg. **76:** 23–31.
59. DUCKER, T. B. & S. M. ZEIDMAN. 1994. Spinal cord injury. Role of steroid therapy. Spine **19:** 2281–2287.
60. GALANDIUK, S., G. RAQUE, S. APPEL & H. C. POLK, JR. 1993. The two-edged sword of large-dose steroids for spinal cord trauma. Ann. Surg. **218:** 419–427.
61. HALL, E. D. & J. M. BRAUGHLER. 1982. Effects of intravenous methylprednisolone on spinal cord lipid perioxidation and ($Na^+$ + $K^+$)-ATPase activity. J. Neurosurg. **57:** 247–253.
62. HALL, E. D., M. BRAUGHER & J. M. MCCALL. 1992. Antioxidant effects in brain and spinal cord injury. J. Neurotrauma. **9**(Suppl. 1): S165–S172.
63. GUHA, A., C. H. TATOR & I. PIPER. 1985. Increase in rat spinal cord blood flow with the calcium channel blocker, nimodipine. J. Neurosurg. **63:** 250–259.
64. GUHA, A., C. H. TATOR & I. PIPER. 1987. Effect of a calcium channel blocker on posttraumatic spinal cord blood flow. J. Neurosurg. **66:** 423–430.
65. BLACK, P., R. S. MARKOWITZ, S. D. FINKELSTEIN, K. MCMONAGLE-STRUCKO & J. A. GILLESPIE. 1988. Experimental spinal cord injury: Effect of a calcium channel antagonist (nicardipine). Neurosurgery **22:** 61–66.
66. MARSALA, M., I. VANICKY & T. L. YAKSH. 1994. Effect of graded hypothermia (27° to 34°C) on behavioral function, histopathology, and spinal blood flow after spinal ischemia in rat. Stroke **25:** 2038–2046.
67. COLLINS, W. F. 1993. Discussion in Galandiuk *et al.*[60]
68. ANDREWS, R. J. & J. R. BRINGAS. 1993. A review of brain retraction and recommendations for minimizing intraoperative brain injury. Neurosurgery **33:** 1052–1064.
69. ANDREWS, R. J., J. R. BRINGAS & R. P. MUTO. 1993. Effects of mannitol on cerebral blood flow, blood pressure, blood viscosity, hematocrit, sodium and potassium. Surg. Neurol. **39:** 218–222.
70. ANDREWS, R. J. & R. P. MUTO. 1992. Retraction brain ischemia: mannitol plus nimodipine preserves both cerebral blood flow and evoked potentials during normoventilation and hyperventilation. Neurol Res. **14:** 19–25.
71. ANDREWS, R. J. & R. P. MUTO. 1992. Retraction brain ischemia: cerebral blood flow, evoked potentials, hypotension and hyperventilation in a new animal model. Neurol. Res. **14:** 12–18.
72. BETZ, A. L. & H. C. COESTER. 1990. Effect of steroids on edema and sodium uptake of the brain during focal ischemia in rats. Stroke **21:** 1119–1204.
73. TIZZANO, J. P., K. I. GRIFFEY & D. D. SCHOEPP. 1995. Receptor subtypes linked to metabotropic receptor agonist mediated limbic seizures in mice. Ann. N. Y. Acad. Sci. This volume.
74. MERVIS, R. F., N. KUNTZ, D. BURTON, R. DVORAK, R. TANDON, L. HOOVER, M. S. WOOD & P. R. SOLOMAN. 1995. Structural-functional correlates of neuroprotection in the aging rabbit by a calcium channel blocker: nimodipine reverses neocortical dendritic atrophy and improves memory retention (Abstr.) Ann. N. Y. Acad. Sci. This volume.
75. KOWALSKA, M. & J. F. DISTERHOFT. 1994. Relation of nimodipine dose and serum concentratioon to learning enhancement in aging rabbits. Exp. Neurol. **127:** 159–166.
76. HERNING, R. I., X. GUO & W. R. LANGE. 1995. The effects of nimodipine on the EEG of substance abusers. Ann. N. Y. Acad. Sci. This volume.
77. PARNETTI, L., U. SENIN, M. CAROSI, H. BAASCH AND THE NIMODIPINE STUDY GROUP. 1993. Mental deterioration in old age: results of two multicenter, clinical trials with nimodipine. Clin. Ther. **15:** 394–406.
78. TOLLEFSON, G. D. 1990. Short-term effects of the calcium channel blocker nimodipine (Bae-e-9736) in the management of primary degenerative dementia. Biol. Psychiatry **27:** 1133–1142.
79. GREENAMYRE, J. T., R. V. ELLER, Z. ZHANG, A. OVADIA, R. KURLAN & D. M. GASH.

1994. Antiparkinsonian effects of remacemide hydrochloride, a glutamate antagonist, in rodent and primate models of Parkinson's disease. Ann. Neurol. **35:** 655–661.
80. GREENBERG, D. A. 1994. Glutamate and Parkinson's disease. Ann. Neurol. **35:** 639.
81. OLNEY, J. W., C. F. ZORUMSKI, G. R. STEWART, M. T. PRICE, G. WANG & J. LABRUYERE. 1990. Excitotoxicity of -dopa and 6-OH-dopa: implications for Parkinson's and Huntington's diseases. Exp. Neurol. **108:** 269–272.
82. HERNING, R. I., X. GUO & W. R. LANGE. 1995. Nimodipine improves information processing in substance abusers. Ann. N. Y. Acad. Sci. This volume.
83. JACKSON, D. L., J. D. RICHARDSON & K. M. HARGREAVES. 1994. Peripheral administration of excitatory amino acids modulates nociceptive behavior in rats. Soc. Neurosci. (Abstr.) **20**(part 2): 1390.
84. SCHWARTZMAN, R. J. 1993. Reflex sympathetic dystrophy. Curr. Opin. Neurol. Neurosurg. **6:** 531–536.
85. BARTUS, R. T., K. L. BAKER, A. D. HEISER, S. D. SAWYER, R. L. DEAN, P. J. ELLIOTT & J. A. STRAUB. 1994. Post-ischemic administration of AK275, a calpain inhibitor, provides substantial protection against focal ischemic brain damage. J. Cereb. Blood Flow Metab. **14:** 537–544.
86. BARTUS, R. T., N. J. HAYWARD, P. J. ELLIOTT, S. D. SAWYER, K. L. BAKER, R. L. DEAN, A. AKIYAMA, J. A. STRAUB, S. L. HARBISON, Z. LI & J. POWERS. 1994. Calpain inhibitor AK295 protects neurones from focal brain ischemia. Effects of postocclusion intra-arterial administration. Stroke **25:** 2265–2270.
87. HONG, S-C., Y. GOTO, G. LANZINO, S. SOLEAU, N. F. KASSELL & K. S. LEE. 1994. Neuroprotection with a calpain inhibitor in a model of focal cerebral ischemia. Stroke **25:** 663–669.

# Prophylactic Pharmacologic Neuroprotection against Focal Cerebral Ischemia

SARAN JONAS[a]

*Department of Neurology*
*New York University School of Medicine*
*New York, New York 10016*

### The Concept of Prophylactic Pharmacologic Neuroprotection

The theory of pharmacologic neuroprotection posits the existence of agents that will minimize the effects of ischemia on the brain. Through the present, the focus of clinical and much animal work in neuroprotection has been the stroke model, in which treatment is given after an artery supplying the brain has been occluded. I will emphasize the very obvious theoretical ceiling to benefit from this approach and will discuss the theoretical advantage of prophylactic pharmacologic neuroprotection, that is, giving neuroprotective agents to people before they have a stroke.

When an artery supplying the brain has been occluded, the core of the ischemic volume may develop irreversible damage from the sequence of biochemical events that we call the ischemic cascade, whereas the outer zone of ischemic tissue closer to the collateral circulation, called the ischemic penumbra, has a better chance of recovery. The aim of neuroprotective maneuvers is to influence the ischemic cascade so as to maximize the proportion of ischemic volume that will survive and recover.

Unfortunately, as Scheinberg[1] has pointed out, irreversible damage can begin within 6–8 minutes after the onset of ischemia. The window for obtaining a perfect result, therefore, can be dauntingly small. In addition, the window for even partial benefit with regard to glutamate- and calcium-induced damage may be limited to 1–3 hours.[2] Thus, the core of an ischemic region may become unsalvageable before any postischemic treatment can be given, because many patients do not reach the hospital for many hours. (According to Ferro *et al.*,[3] 58% of stroke patients in Lisbon from 1991–1992 reached the university hospital 6 or more hours after the event.)

Obviously, minimizing the time before the neuroprotective agent reaches an optimal level in ischemic brain tissues is crucial. The best time interval clearly would be zero. Because there is always a delay between stroke onset and initiation of poststroke treatment, the only way to obtain a zero interval is to have the agent in the brain before the stroke occurs. This is prophylactic neuroprotection. An analogy to the treatment of epilepsy is useful; we can attempt emergency room

---

[a] Mailing address: Department of Neurology, Bellevue Hospital Center, Room 7-West-11, 462 First Avenue, New York NY 10016.

TABLE 1. Annual Stroke Rate in Various Populations[a]

| Population | Annual Stroke Rate |
|---|---|
| Warsaw community 1991–92;[6] age in years | |
| 45–54 | 0.1 |
| 55–64 | 0.3 |
| 65–74 | 0.6 |
| 75–79 | 0.9 |
| 80+ | 1.8 |
| TIA or minor stroke patients | |
| On ticlopidine[7] | 3.4 |
| Intact after carotid endarterectomy, on APT[8] | 3.4 |
| With nonvalvular AF, on anticoagulant[9] | 3.9 |
| On aspirin[7] | 4.2 |

[a] AF = atrial fibrillation; APT = antiplatelet therapy; TIA = transient ischemic attack. Calculations of stroke rates during follow-up for TIA or minor stroke patients: on ticlopidine: 172 strokes in 1529 patients during a mean follow-up of 1197 days: (172/1529/1197)(365) = 3.4% per year; on aspirin: (212/1540/1187)(365) = 4.2%; in patients intact after carotid endarterectomy: 16 strokes in 328 patients during a mean follow-up of 17 months: (16/328/17)(12) = 3.4% per year; for nonvalvular AF patients: 20 strokes in 507 patient-years of follow-up: (20/507) = 3.9% per year.

management of status epilepticus in a person who is not on prophylactic anticonvulsant treatment, but seizure patients live better lives if they already have adequate anticonvulsant concentrations on the surfaces of their neurons when epileptogenic events occur in their brains.

### *Practical Aspects of the Development of a Prophylactic Pharmacologic Neuroprotection Regimen*

Identification of an agent with potential for prophylactic neuroprotection is a matter for the animal laboratory; the model would allow treatment for a suitable interval before induction of cerebral arterial occlusion. Techniques exist for inducing suitable occlusions and infarcts in animals and for studying both infarct size and motor function.

To test the prophylactic value of such an agent in humans at risk for stroke presents logistic problems. Because of the low event rate per unit time, even in "high risk" groups (TABLE 1), many people would have to be treated and followed up for long periods so that enough strokes could be observed to permit meaningful analysis of outcomes. Dr. Ralph Sacco's calculations for our paper on prophylactic neuroprotection[4] show the number of patients required to generate the occurrence of stroke in 127 patients in order to give the randomized trial of agent versus placebo an 80% chance to demonstrate (at the 0.05 level of statistical significance, two-sided test) a 50% difference in outcome. From a population with a 4.2% annual stroke rate a cohort of 3024 patients would be needed to generate 127 strokes in a year. This would be a reasonable size for a definitive clinical trial, but not for screening trials. Clearly, less cumbersome and costly screening trials in humans would be desirable for selecting from animal studies drugs for efficacy, safety, and tolerability, for dose etc.

In this regard there is a group of patients not particularly high in stroke occurrence who nevertheless have a very high rate, per unit of time, of recognized acute cerebral ischemia: patients undergoing cardiopulmonary bypass (CPB) for cardiac surgery (CS). There is strong evidence that CS-CPB (cardiac surgery under cardiopulmonary bypass) produces showers of microemboli to the brain. The number of microemboli entering the cerebral circulation (as determined by ultrasound monitoring) correlates with the degree of impairment in mental function demonstrated by postoperative versus preoperative neuropsychological test (NPT) scores.[5] This impairment is believed to reflect multiple tiny regions of focal ischemia in the brain. It disappears after some months, and can be considered a mild transient dementia, bearing the same relationship to multi-infarct dementia that TIA (transient ischemic attack) bears to stroke. Its rate of occurrence for one week of observation (the immediate post-op week: it can be identified by NPT at 7 days after the procedure) is generally given as 75%. Even if one takes a very conservative estimate of 50%, one is dealing with an occurrence rate at least 600 times that of the weekly stroke rate in a population with a 4.2% annual stroke risk.

In theory, a neuroprotective agent should reduce the degree of decline in NPT scores for a given severity of embolization. An 80% chance to demonstrate (at $p < 0.05$) a 50% difference in treatment versus control NPT scores at one week would require less than 2 weeks of study per patient (baseline NPT and pretreatment, plus repeat NPT testing a week after CS-CPB) in 254 CPB patients. We have demonstrated the logistical feasibility of such a protocol in two small randomized trials (phenytoin, $G_{M1}$) totaling 42 patients easily recruited at NYU. (We saw no difference between treatment and control outcomes in these protocol development trials.)

It is our concept that demonstration that an agent is neuroprotective against cognitive decline after CS-CPB would (in addition to providing a useful benefit for CS-CPB patients in the future) justify a clinical trial against actual strokes in humans. We think that the cohort in which such a trial could most efficiently be accomplished would be composed of patients undergoing carotid endarterectomy (CE). These people are easily accessed for recruitment in a medical center, and have an incidence of actual stroke of about 5% during surgery and in the first postoperative month. The protocol would be similar to that of the CS-CPB protocol, except that a stroke severity scale would replace the NPT battery. A cohort size of 2540 would provide an 80% chance of showing a 50% difference at the 0.05 level. An answer could be gained in four weeks of follow-up per patient: less than a tenth as much clinical follow-up time as would be needed in a study of spontaneous stroke patients.

With a demonstration of efficacy in ameliorating the consequences of immediate postsurgical strokes in the CE cohort, one would be justified in going on to a long-term spontaneous stroke study protocol using outcome measures similar to those used in the CE protocol. From Table 1 it can be seen that an efficient approach would be the long-term follow-up of the population recruited for the 1-month CE trial. At an annual stroke rate of 3.4%, 3735 patients could provide a demonstration of efficacy during a mean observation time of one year.

Because strokes occurring in long-term follow-up after CE do not differ from spontaneous strokes in the nonvascular surgery population, it may be that no further clinical trials will be needed to justify the use of a demonstrably successful agent for prophylactic neuroprotection in the other classes of patients (as shown in TABLE 1) who previously suffered TIA or minor stroke. One might then consider a trial of the drug—if it appears to be suitably low in cost, side effects, and complications—in people who do not have a specific neurologic or medical risk profile for stroke. People over a certain age (see TABLE 1 for age-related risks) would be an obvious choice. Such trials would have to be very large, of course: 12,700 people followed for two years, if the expected stroke rate is 0.5% per year.

## FOR THE FUTURE

If several agents can be shown to be neuroprotective when used alone one could, as Grotta has suggested for poststroke treatment, consider trials in which agents operating on different levels of the ischemic cascade are combined. Also, a similar study to evaluate the effect of prophylactic neuroprotection on the efficacy and safety of poststroke thrombolytic treatment would be of potential value.

## SUMMARY

The crucial importance of the earliest possible treatment of ischemic stroke has been stressed. This leads to the concept of prophylactic neuroprotection: long-term administration of neuroprotective agents to people at risk for stroke, so that the effects of focal ischemia are countered from the moment of onset of vascular occlusion.

We at NYU (and researchers at several other centers) have been testing possible neuroprotective agents in the cardiopulmonary bypass setting. We believe that by such means we can rapidly and economically screen agents and dose schedules for efficacy. We believe that an agent demonstrably reducing mental impairment after cardiopulmonary bypass suggests that testing such an agent in a prospective manner in people at risk for stroke would be productive, and we propose a sequence for such trials: people during and in the first month after carotid endarterectomy, then postcarotid endarterectomy patients during long-term follow-up, and finally populations at risk for spontaneous stroke in the nonvascular surgery setting.

## REFERENCES

1. SCHEINBERG, P. 1994. Stroke: the way things really are. Stroke **25:** 1290–1294.
2. GROTTA, J. 1994. The current status of neuronal protective therapy: why have all neuronal protective drugs worked in animals but none so far in stroke patients? Cerebrovasc. Dis. **4:** 115–120.
3. FERRO, J. M., T. P. MELO, V. OLIVEIRA, M. CRESPO, P. CANHAO & A. N. PINTO. 1994. An analysis of the admission delay of acute strokes. Cerebrovasc. Dis. **4:** 72–75.
4. FISHER, M., S. JONAS & R. L. SACCO. 1994. Prophylactic neuroprotection for cerebral ischemia. Stroke **25:** 1075–1080.

5. PUGSLEY, W. B., L. KLINGER, C. PASCHALIS, T. TREASURE, M. HARRISON & S. NEWMAN. 1994. The impact of microemboli during cardiopulmonary bypass on neuropsychological functioning. Stroke **25:** 1393–1399.
6. CZLONKOWSKA, A., D. RYGLEWICZ, T. WEISSBEIN, M. BARANSKA-GIERUSZCZAK & D. HIER. 1994. A prospective community-based study of stroke in Warsaw, Poland. Stroke **25:** 547–551.
7. HASS, W. K., J. D. EASTON, H. P. ADAMS, W. PRYSE-PHILLIPS, B. A. MOLONY, S. ANDERSON & B. KAMM FOR THE TICLOPIDINE ASPIRIN STROKE STUDY GROUP. 1989. A randomized trial comparing ticlopidine hydrochloride with aspirin for the prevention of stroke in high-risk patients. N. Engl. J. Med. **321:** 501–507.
8. NORTH AMERICAN SYMPTOMATIC CAROTID ENDARTERECTOMY TRIAL COLLABORATORS. 1991. Beneficial effect of carotid ondarterectomy in symptomatic patients with high-grade carotid stenosis. N. Engl. J. Med. **325:** 445–453.
9. EAFT (EUROPEAN ARTERIAL FIBRILLATION TRIAL) STUDY GROUP. 1993. Secondary prevention in non-rheumatic atrial fibrillation after transient ischemic attack or minor stroke. Lancet **342:** 1255–1262.

# Discussion

S. GOLDIN (*Cambridge Neuroscience*): What is your perspective on the time-window for therapy in head trauma following the event?

R. BULLOCK (*Medical College of Virginia*): Clearly, therapy should begin as soon as possible after injury, and should continue as long as glutamate is elevated in the extracellular fluid (ECF). For trials, a compromise between the practical and the ideal must be achieved. Most current head trauma trials with glutamate antagonists aim at a 6–8-hour enrollment window and 4 or more days of therapy.

W. KOZACHUK (*Wallace Laboratories, Princeton, NJ*): By using the terms transient ischemic attack (TIA)/reversible ischemic neurologic deficit (RIND), which imply a reversible neuronal damage, are you not minimizing the fact that neuronal cell death occurs and promoting the popular conception that such events are clinically benign? Prospective neuroimaging studies have shown abnormal brain metabolism for weeks after a TIA?

S. JONAS (*New York University*): I agree with you fully. I mentioned the terms to introduce them to the nonclinicians, not to imply mechanism or lack of structural change. TIA/RIND-minor stroke as defined have been the selection criteria for almost all secondary prevention studies. Stroke neurologists now agree that there is no differential prediction value for clinical prognosis or structural lesion among the three categories. They have historical rather than scientific value in stroke research.

D. K. J. E. VON LUBITZ (*National Institute of Diabetes and Digestive and Kidney Diseases, NIH, Bethesda, MD*): In terms of intraoperative and postoperative control of cerebral blood flow, attention ought to be drawn to the studies of Sollevi *et al.* at the Karolinska Institutet in Stockholm, who showed impressive improvement following adenosine infusion. The advantages offered by adenosine acting at $A_{2A}$ receptors (vasodilation) may be considered very seriously in view of the fact that, as "ADENOCARD™," adenosine has been recently approved by the FDA for cardiological use.

L. S. LESKO (*Hoffmann-La Roche, Nutley, NJ*): With calcitonin gene-related peptide (CGRP), did you define hypotension and did you specify what levels of hypotension were troublesome for the investigators?

B. A. BELL (*University of London*): The hypotensive effect of CGRP in patients who have suffered a subarachnoid hemorrhage is a mean fall of approximately 15% in systolic and diastolic pressures. This reflects the decrease in vascular resistance produced by the peptide, and there is no evidence that cerebral blood flow falls. The investigators tended to regard even small changes in blood pressure as a cause for concern, and tended to ignore the fact that these changes in blood pressure were not associated with neurological deteriorations.

A. J. MERCER (*Wellcome Research Laboratories, Beckenham, UK*): Was the scale used to measure outcome in the CGRP study sensitive enough to show a difference between treatments given the high percentage of good recovery in both treated and placebo groups?

BELL: The outcome scale used is relatively coarse with five points between normality and death (the Glasgow outcome scale). Minor improvements in the treatment or placebo groups in the trial could not be detected by this scale.

VON LUBITZ: Many problems with screening drugs active in stroke/ischemia arise from our inability to assess neurologic damage in animal models. Apart from the Morris water maze, there are hardly any methods that are sensitive enough to detect subtle cognitive effects known to accompany milder ischemic/traumatic events. Therefore, many therapies that have no impact on massive damage and which have been abandoned for that very reason may be quite useful in less intense events.

BULLOCK: I agree. The rat brain, with its limitations for behavioral studies, cannot always predict effects in higher gyroencephalic species.

KOSACHUK: Recent studies using autoradiographic techniques have suggested a decrease in $N$-methyl-D-aspartate (NMDA) receptors in the spinal cord of amyotrophic lateral sclerosis (ALS) patients. Is there any evidence that NMDA receptors contribute to spinal cord damage?

BULLOCK: Yes. Faden *et al.* about 7–8 years ago demonstrated glutamate effects after spinal cord injury, which were ameliorated by an NMDA antagonist. Dense ischemia of the contused segment of the cord has been shown by Tator's group, and suggests a role for glutamatergic blockade.

# A Fetal Rat Model of Acute Perinatal Ischemia-Hypoxia

ZBIGNIEW BINIENDA

*Division of Neurotoxicology*
*National Center for Toxicological Research*
*Food and Drug Administration*
*Jefferson, Arkansas 72079-9502*

## INTRODUCTION

Perinatal cerebral hypoxia has been implicated in neonatal morbidity and mortality as well as in brain dysfunctions and neurological handicaps in adulthood.[1-3] Although the fetus is thought to be relatively protected from hypoxia,[4] this protection may be suppressed and damage may occur under the ischemic-hypoxic conditions accompanying placental insufficiency due to maternal stress, drug abuse, placental abruption, or umbilical cord compression. In addition, a growing body of evidence suggests that rather than hypoxia alone, it is the combination of ischemia-hypoxia that is harmful to brain tissues during the perinatal period.[5] Against this background, a need evidently exits for an animal model of ischemia-hypoxia that would adequately simulate conditions that sometimes occur during human pregnancy. Such a model would permit not only a study of the neurotoxic effects of hypoxia, but also an evaluation of the safety and efficacy of potential neuroprotective agents.

As there is currently no ideal model that addresses all sides of the multifactorial mechanism of human perinatal hypoxic brain damage over time, a variety of animal models using various endpoints have been developed to study this problem.[6] The particular model presented here permits evaluation of the energy deficient induced by ischemia-hypoxia in the fetal rat near term. Accordingly, the effect of an ischemic-hypoxic insult on several biomarkers of hypoxia was studied. These included biochemical markers (enzymes of energy metabolism, stress proteins, and free fatty acids) and also some behavioral markers (negative geotaxis, olfactory discrimination, and open field activity) as possible consequences of such an insult.

## MATERIALS AND METHODS

### Animals

Sprague-Dawley date-mated rats obtained from the NCTR breeding colony of Charles River CD strain (Kingston, New York) were used in these studies. Individual nulliparous dams were housed with singly-caged experienced male breeders. The day of vaginal plug detection was designated gestational day (GD) 0. Pregnant dams were housed individually and kept under controlled environmental conditions (temperature 22°C, relative humidity 50%, and 12-hour light:dark cycle with lights out at 1800 hours). They were given free access to a standard diet and water.

### Experimental Procedure

Pregnant dams (GD 20) were anesthetized with halothane, and laparotomy was performed. Ischemic-hypoxic conditions were induced by ligating either uterine vessel of one pregnant horn at the ovarian and cervical ends for 10–45 minutes. The adjacent horn was not ligated and those fetuses served as sham-operated within-dam controls. Pups from both horns were then delivered by cesarean section at the end of the ischemic-hypoxic insult. Another group of pregnant dams (GD 21) was exposed to carbon dioxide for 45 seconds and sacrificed by cervical dislocation. A modified technique described by Bjelke et al.[7] was applied in this group to induce fetal ischemia-hypoxia by submerging the entire horn dissected from a dam in saline solution for 15 minutes. Pups from the adjacent control horn were delivered immediately after laparatomy was performed. All live pups scheduled for biochemical analyses were frozen in liquid nitrogen, they were transferred onto aluminum dishes placed on dry ice, and their brains and livers were dissected and stored at $-80°C$ for subsequent enzyme and free fatty acid analyses.

### Liver and Brain Enzyme Analyses

Glycolytic enzymes (lactate dehydrogenase and fructose diphosphate aldolase), Krebs cycle enzymes (malate dehydrogenase and isocitrate dehydrogenase), enzymes of amino acid metabolism (glutamate dehydrogenase), and lipid metabolism (fatty acid synthetase) were determined in whole liver and brain tissue homogenates by spectrophotometry using a Microcentrifugal Analyzer (Instrumentation Laboratory, Lexington, Massachusetts) with absorbance measured at 340 nm, reflecting the production or loss of either NADPH or NADH.[8]

### Brain Free Fatty Acids Analyses

Fetal brain total free fatty acids (FFA) concentration was measured in extracts of whole brain homogenates by column chromatography. Two or three whole brains were pooled for one sample to obtain the minimum 200 mg of tissue required for extraction. Free fatty acids were subsequently derivatized to esters and quantified by gas chromatography.[9]

### Neurohistological Assessment

Newborn pups scheduled for neurohistological assessment were allowed 80 minutes of reperfusion (maintained in an incubator at 37°C), followed by pentobarbital sodium anesthesia and perfusion (5 ml/min for 12 minutes with 4% formaldehyde in 0.1 M potassium phosphate buffer). Fifty-micron sagittal sections of whole brain were cut on a microslicer (DTK-3000W, Ted Pella, Inc., Redding, California). The immunostaining procedure used to localize c-fos and HSP-72 protein was a modification of the peroxidase-antiperoxidase method.[10,11]

### Behavioral Assessment

Pups from both the control and saline submerged horn scheduled for behavioral assessment were placed with surrogate dams on postnatal day (PND) 0. They were tested at various PNDs for the following early behaviors: negative geotaxis (PND 6–7), olfactory discrimination (PND 9–11), and open field activity (PND 19–22).

### Brain Dissection and Regional Brain Weight Analysis

On PND 30, two pups from each litter (one control and one hypoxic) were sacrificed and their brains harvested. Each brain was dissected into the following regions: olfactory bulbs, caudate nucleus, frontal cortex, diencephalon, hippocampus, cerebellum, brain stem, and remnant. The weight of each brain region was determined gravimetrically to the nearest 0.1 mg.

### Statistical Analyses

Data were analyzed by one-way ANOVA or Student $t$ test using a significance level of $p < 0.05$. Behavioral data were subjected to within-litter analysis of variance, with treatment (control or hypoxic) and sex as between factors. For olfactory discrimination and open field tests, sessions were a repeated measure in the analysis of variance.

## RESULTS AND DISCUSSION

To date, several animal models using different species and different techniques of insult have been used to study the various factors that play a role in perinatal hypoxic brain damage.[6] The experimental model proposed here takes advantage of the type of rat uterus (uterus duplex) that allows induction of ischemia-hypoxia in fetuses of one uterine horn, while fetuses of the adjacent horn serve as within-animal control. In its current stage of development, this model allows the researcher to focus on the biomarkers of energy deficit caused by hypoxic conditions. The model may be useful not only for studying the primary consequences of perinatal ischemia-hypoxia on the developing brain, but also for testing the effectiveness of possible neuroprotective agents.

The mechanism of cerebral hypoxic injury is complex and still poorly under-

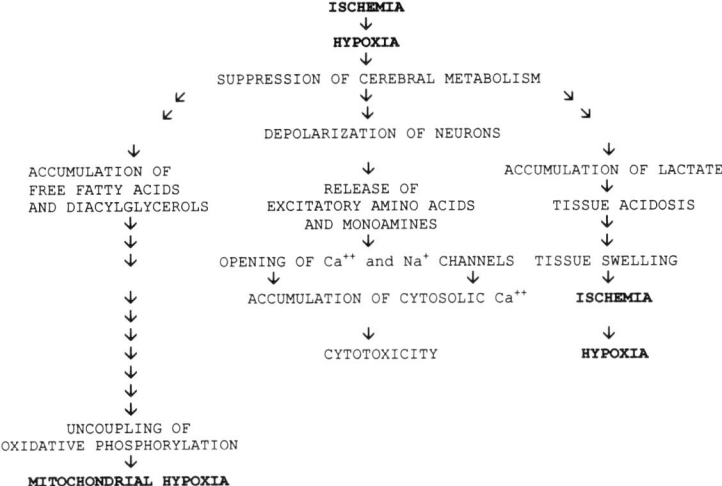

**FIGURE 1.** Simplified mechanism of ischemic-hypoxic brain damage. Note secondary hypoxic conditions perpetuated by initial ischemia-hypoxia.

stood. Data generated in this study will be discussed in terms of the working model of cerebral hypoxic injury presented in FIGURE 1.

The effect of vascular ligation on fetal survival is shown in TABLE 1. Whereas no mortality was observed in control fetuses, vascular ligation was associated with fetal death. Furthermore, the incidence of fetal death increased with the duration of ligation.

Data from a preliminary study indicated that the surgical preparation itself stimulated selected enzyme activity in control fetuses.[12] Specifically, liver fatty acid synthetase was increased significantly 30 minutes following surgery in within-dam control fetuses compared to independent control fetuses. On the other hand, in the present study, fatty acid synthetase activity 15 minutes following ligation was lower in hypoxic fetuses than in within-dam control fetuses (FIG. 2). This inhibitory effect of 15 minutes of ischemia-hypoxia was particularly significant for fetuses submerged in saline solution (TABLE 2). Brain fatty acid synthetase activity showed trends similar to those observed in the liver, that is, increased activity in

TABLE 1. Incidence of Fetal Mortality after Ischemic-Hypoxic Insult due to Ligation of Uterine Vessels on Day 20 of Gestation

| Dams (n) | Duration of Insult (Min) | Number of Fetuses | | Percent Mortality | |
|---|---|---|---|---|---|
| | | Hypoxic | Control | Hypoxic | Control |
| 5 | 10 | 15 | 25 | 0 | 0 |
| 9 | 15 | 64 | 60 | 3 | 0 |
| 5 | 20 | 39 | 36 | 21 | 0 |
| 4 | 30 | 34 | 26 | 12 | 0 |
| 3 | 45 | 24 | 15 | 83 | 0 |

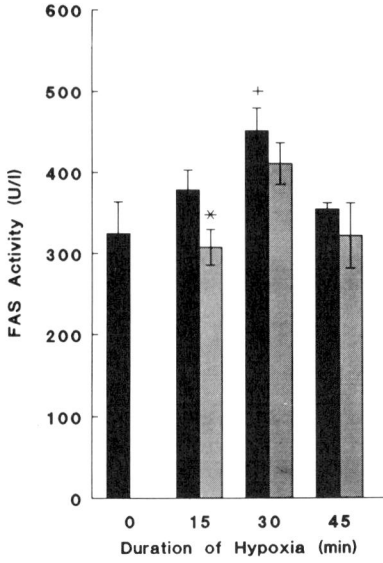

**FIGURE 2.** Fatty acid synthase activity in fetal control (■) and hypoxic (▨) rat liver following ischemic-hypoxic insult induced by ligation of uterine blood vessels. Mean ± SEM; $^*p$ <0.05 compared with within-dam control, $^+p$ <0.05 compared with independent control.

TABLE 2. Effect of 15 Minutes of Ischemia-Hypoxia on Fetal Liver Metabolic Enzyme Activity[a]

| Enzyme | HAL (Cont) (n = 25) | | HAL (Hyp) (n = 34) | | % | $CO_2$ (Cont) (n = 22) | | $CO_2$ (Hyp) (n = 21) | | % |
|---|---|---|---|---|---|---|---|---|---|---|
| LDH | 2,401 | (208) | 2,204 | (180) | −8 | 3,183 | (255) | 1,888 | (222) | −40* |
| FDP | 1,252 | (682) | 951 | (324) | −24 | 828 | (104) | 525 | (68) | −37* |
| MDH | 3,882 | (166) | 3,666 | (204) | −6 | 3,821 | (175) | 3,224 | (186) | −16 |
| ICD | 795 | (221) | 788 | (180) | −1 | 804 | (62) | 531 | (71) | −34* |
| GDH | 533 | (95) | 495 | (89) | −7 | 540 | (70) | 408 | (65) | −25 |
| FAS | 318 | (52) | 242 | (41) | −24 | 301 | (22) | 195 | (18) | −35* |

[a] % = reduction of enzyme activity in hypoxic pups as percent of control; HAL (Cont) = control group (halothane anesthesia, sham-operated); HAL (Hyp) = hypoxic group (halothane anesthesia and vascular ligation); $CO_2$ (Cont) = control group (45 seconds of exposure to carbon dioxide); $CO_2$ (Hyp) = hypoxic group (45 seconds of exposure to carbon dioxide solution followed by submersion of ligated uterine horn into warm saline solution for 15 minutes. Data presented as mean (SEM); *$p$ <0.05. Abbreviations: LDH = lactate dehydrogenase; FDP = fructose diphosphate aldolase; MDH = malate dehydrogenase; ICD = isocitrate dehydrogenase; GDH = glutamate dehydrogenase; FAS = fatty acid synthetase.

within-dam control fetuses after 15 minutes of ischemia-hypoxia, and activity in hypoxic fetuses was significantly lower than that in within-dam controls within 15 minutes following uterine ligation (FIG. 3).

In neonatal rats, the activity of some enzymes of brain energy metabolism (*e.g.*, cytochrome oxidase in the hippocampus) decreased after acute ischemia-hypoxia induced by umbilical cord compression.[13] Similarly, cytochrome oxidase or malate dehydrogenase activity in hippocampus, corpus striatum, and cerebellum is reportedly decreased following intermittent hypoxia in adult rats, reflecting

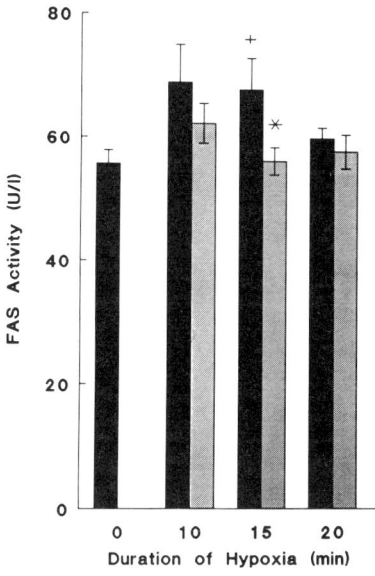

**FIGURE 3.** Fatty acid synthase activity in fetal control (■) and hypoxic (▨) rat brain following ischemic-hypoxic insult induced by ligation of uterine blood vessels. Mean ± SEM; * $p < 0.05$ compared with within-dam control, + $p < 0.05$ compared with independent control.

some adaptation to hypoxic conditions.[14] In the present study, enzyme activity related to energy metabolism in the liver showed a decreasing trend after ischemia-hypoxia induced by vascular ligation. This suppression of enzyme activity became significant when the stimulatory effect of surgical stress was removed by submerging in saline solution. Compared to that of the liver, the response of brain enzymes to ischemia-hypoxia was marginal, although a similar trend of decreasing enzyme activity (fatty acid synthetase) was observed.

Free fatty acids are useful markers of degradation of neuronal membranes and they have a direct toxic effect in the pathogenesis of ischemic-hypoxic brain damage.[15] Studies have shown arachidonic acid liberation and prostaglandin production in fetal brain during the reoxygenation that follows brain ischemia-hypoxia induced by clamping uterine blood vessels.[16,17] In the present study, total brain free fatty acids increased significantly in fetuses exposed to 15 minutes of ischemia-hypoxia induced by submerging in saline solution (FIG. 4). Although the rise in concentration of brain arachidonic acid calculated as a percentage of total free fatty acids did not reach statistical significance, it was previously reported that arachidonate concentrations increase during reoxygenation following 20 minutes of ischemia.[16] In the present study, free fatty acids were measured directly after a 15-minute insult without reperfusion and reoxygenation.

Ischemic-hypoxic conditions stimulate the synthesis of stress proteins in both infant and adult rats.[18,19] In the present study, the activities of c-fos and HSP-72 were induced in near-term fetal rats after either vascular ligation or submerging in saline solution.[20,21] Immunoreactivity of c-fos was particularly evident in the nuclei of the hippocampus (subfield CA1) and neocortex (FIG. 5). Furthermore, HSP-72 immunoreactivity was detected in the cytoplasm of adjacent hippocampal areas (subfield CA3; FIG. 6).

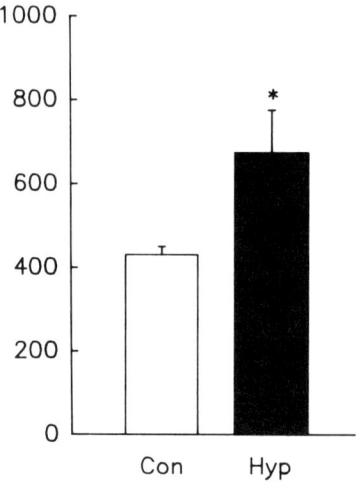

FIGURE 4. Concentration of total free fatty acids in control (□) and hypoxic (■) rat brain following 15 minutes of ischemic-hypoxic insult induced by submerging of the uterine horn in saline solution for 15 minutes. Mean ± SEM; * $p < 0.05$.

A reduction in adult rat brain volume has been observed by other investigators as a long-term effect of ischemia-hypoxia induced by umbilical cord compression.[13] In the present study, ischemia-hypoxia induced by submerging the uterine horn in saline solution for 15 minutes was associated with a significant reduction in weight of the caudate nucleus ($p < 0.02$) and brain stem regions ($p < 0.01$) at PND 30. A significant reduction in caudate nucleus and brain stem weight was observed in male as well as female hypoxic pups. Also, cerebellar weight was marginally affected by hypoxia ($p < 0.07$).

Weight reduction in brain regions of hypoxic rats was not strongly manifested in the behaviors assessed in this study.[22] Within-litter analyses indicated no significant differences between control and hypoxic pups in measures of negative geotaxis or olfactory discrimination. However, the activity in the open field on PND 19, as measured by the number of sectors entered, was significantly lower in male hypoxic pups ($p < 0.03$) than in controls (FIG. 7). Perinatal hypoxia reportedly results in hyperactivity in male rats in an open field,[13] but this effect disappears by PND 20.[23]

## CONCLUSIONS

1. With regard to biochemical markers, ischemic/hypoxic insult as applied in the currently proposed model was accompanied by the following responses:
   a. a reduction in the activity of enzymes of energy metabolism in the brain (marginally) and liver (significantly);
   b. a significant increase in the concentration of total free fatty acids in the brain;
   c. induced synthesis of stress proteins c-fos and HSP-72 in the hippocampus and neocortex;

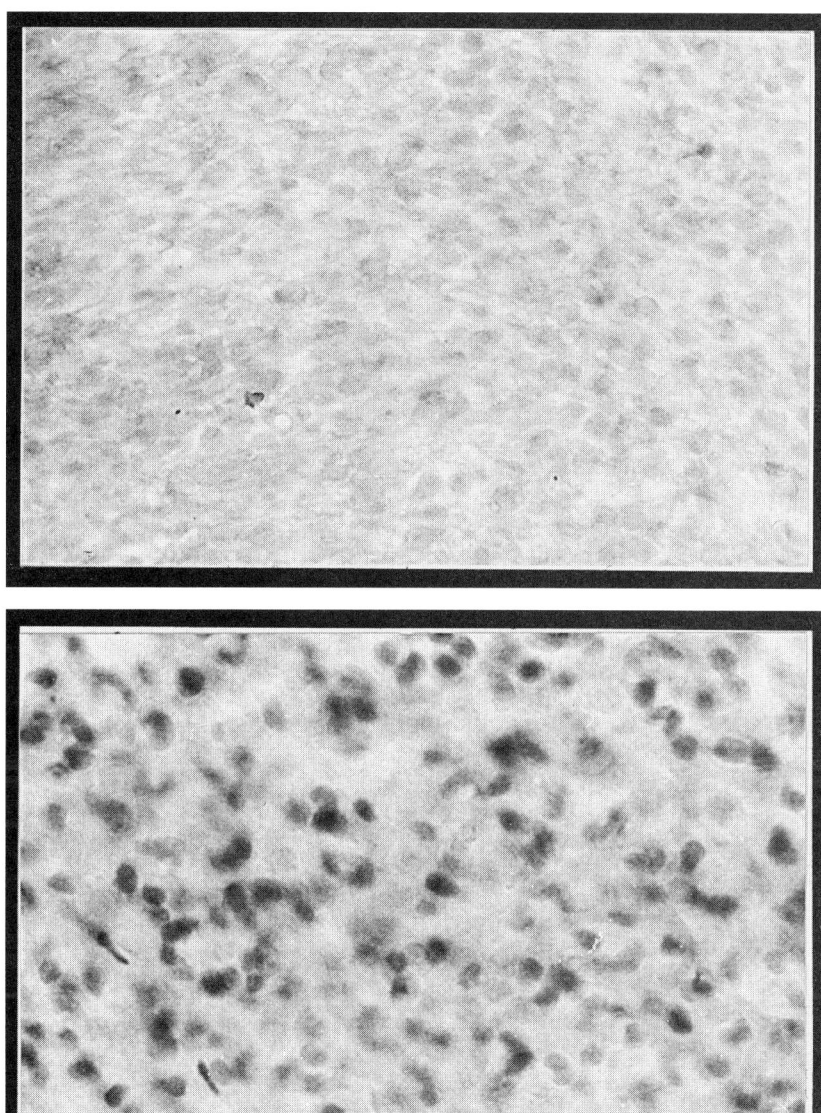

**FIGURE 5.** Sagittal section of transitional region between hippocampal subiculum and cortex of fetal control *(top)* and hypoxic *(bottom)* rat brain at GD 21. Note cell nuclei immunostained for c-fos in the hypoxic brain. Magnification 585X. (From Binienda & Scallet.[21] Reprinted by permission from the *International Journal of Developmental Neuroscience*.)

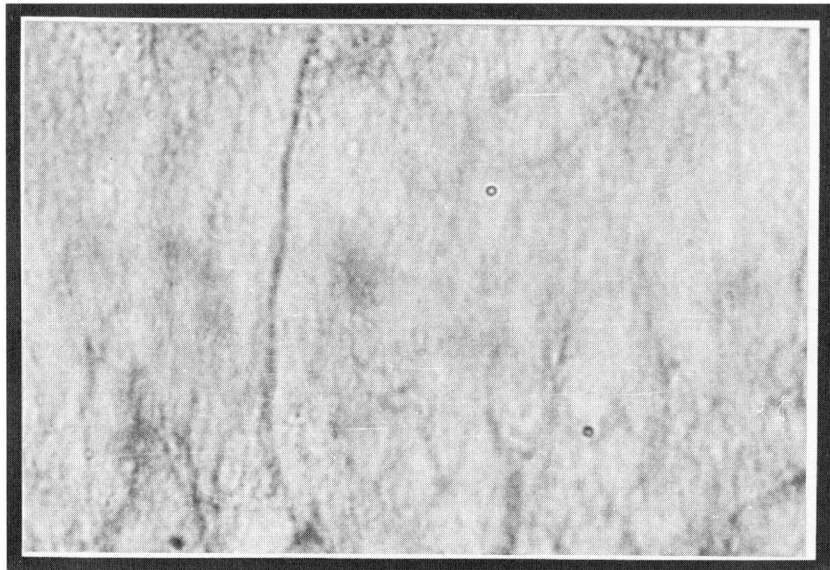
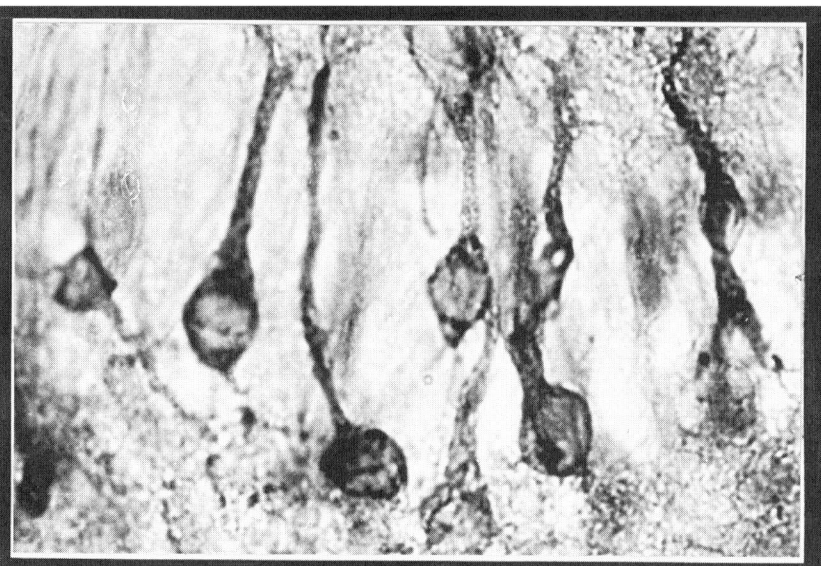

**FIGURE 6.** Sagittal section of the CA3 subfield of fetal control *(top)* and hypoxic *(bottom)* rat brain at GD 21. Note cytoplasm of hippocampal pyramidal cells immunostained for HSP-72 in the hypoxic brain. Magnification 585X. (From Binienda and Scallet.[21] Reprinted by permission from the *International Journal of Developmental Neuroscience*.)

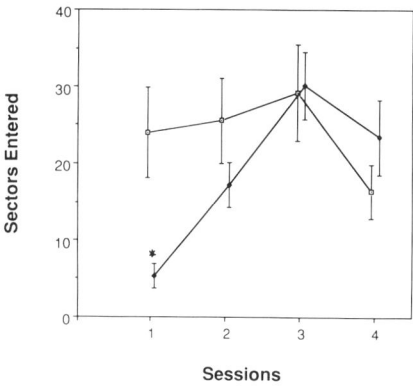

**FIGURE 7.** Activity in an open field of control (□) and hypoxic (■) male rats at PND 19–22. Mean ± SEM; * $p < 0.05$.

   d. a significant reduction in the weight of the caudate nucleus and brain stem regions at PND 30.
2. With regard to behavioral markers, ischemic-hypoxic insult as applied in the currently proposed model was accompanied by the following responses:
   a. a significant reduction in open field activity on PND 19 in male hypoxic pups;
   b. no significant change in negative geotaxis or olfactory discrimination. It is presently unclear what type of behavioral alterations might be accompanied by weight reduction of the brain regions detected in this study.
3. Submerging the uterine horn in saline solution circumvented surgical stress, which by itself stimulates the enzymes of energy metabolism, offsetting the inhibitory effect of ischemia-hypoxia.

## ACKNOWLEDGMENTS

The author thanks Drs. R. Robert Holson, Sherry A. Ferguson, Ritchie J. Feuers, Chung S. Kim, Thomas Flynn, Andrew C. Scallet, and William Slikker, Jr. for their collaboration on various aspects of this study.

## REFERENCES

1. VOLPE, J. J. 1987. Hypoxic-ischemic encephalopathy: neuropathology and pathogenesis. *In* Neurology of the Newborn. M. Markowitz, Ed. 209–235. W. B. Saunders Co. Philadelphia.
2. VANNUCCI, R. C. 1990. Current and potentially new management strategies for perinatal hypoxic-ischemic encephalopathy. Pediatrics **85:** 961–968.
3. PASTERNAK, J. F. 1993. Hypoxic-ischemic brain damage in the term infant. Ped. Clin. North Am. **40:** 1061–1072.
4. LAGERCRANTZ, H. & T. A. SLOTKIN. 1986. The "stress" of being born. Sci. Am. **254:** 100–107.

5. VANNUCCI, R. C. 1992. Cerebral carbohydrate and energy metabolism in perinatal hypoxic-ischemic brain damage. Brain Pathol. **2:** 229–234.
6. RAJU, T. N. K. 1992. Some animal models for the study of perinatal asphyxia. Biol. Neonate **62:** 202–214.
7. BJELKE, B., K. ANDERSSON, S. O. ÖGREN, & P. BOLME. 1991. Asphyctic lesion: proliferation of tyrosine hydroxylase-immunoreactive nerve cell bodies in the rat substantia nigra and functional changes in dopamine neurotransmission. Brain Res. **543:** 1–9.
8. FEUERS, R. J., R. R. DELONGCHAMP, D. A. CASCIANO, J. G. BURKHART & H. W. MOHRENWEISER. 1980. Assay for mouse tissue enzymes: levels of activity and statistical variation for 29 enzymes of liver or brain. Anal. Biochem. **101:** 123–130.
9. DINNAUER, M. 1991. Omega-3 highly unsaturated fatty acid methyl esters on DB-23 and DB-WAX. The J&W Separation Times **5:** 10–12.
10. STERNBERGER, L. A. 1982. Immunocytochemistry, 2nd Edit. Wiley. New York.
11. SCALLET, A. C., G. W. LIPE, S. F. ALI, R. R. HOLSON, C. H. FRITH & W. SLIKKER, JR. 1988. Neuropathological evaluation by combined immunohistochemistry and degeneration-specific methods: application to methylenedioxymethamphetamine. Neuro Toxicology **9:** 529–538.
12. BINIENDA, Z., R. R. HOLSON, C. S. KIM, T. FLYNN, W. SLIKKER, JR. & R. J. FEUERS. 1992. Fatty acid synthetase (FAS) in fetal rat brain and liver during placental ischemia. Abstr. Soc. Neurosci. 1(Abstr. 68.21): 155.
13. SHEN, Y., R. L. ISAACSON & W. P. SMOTHERMAN. 1991. The behavioral and anatomical effects of prenatal umbilical cord clamping in the rat and their alteration by the prior maternal administration of nimodipine. Rest. Neurol. Neurosci. **3:** 11–22.
14. SMIALEK, M. & A. HAMBERGER. 1970. The effect of hypoxia and ischemia on cytochrome oxidase activity and protein synthesis in brain mitochondria. Brain Res. **17:** 369–371.
15. NEMOTO, E. M., R. W. EVANS & P. M. KOCHANEK. 1992. Free fatty acid liberation in the pathogenesis and therapy of ischemic brain damage. *In* Neurochemical Correlates of Cerebral Ischemia. N. G. Bazan, P. Braquet & M. D. Ginsberg, Eds. Chapt. 10: 183–218. Plenum Press. New York.
16. KUNIEVSKY, B., N. G. BAZAN & E. YAVIN. 1992. Generation of arachidonic acid and diacylglycerol second messengers from polyphosphoinositides in ischemic fetal brain. J. Neurochem. **59:** 1812–1819.
17. MAGAL, E., E. GOLDIN, S. HAREL & E. YAVIN. 1988. Acute uteroplacental ischemic embryo: lactic acid accumulation and prostaglandin production in the fetal rat brain. J. Neurochem. **51:** 75–80.
18. GUNN, A. J., M. DRAGUNOW, R. L. M. FAULL & P. D. GLUCKMAN. 1990. Effects of hypoxia-ischemia and seizures on neuronal and glial-like c-fos protein levels in the infant rat. Brain Res. **531:** 105–116.
19. DWYER, B. E. & R. N. NISHIMURA. 1992. Heat shock proteins in hypoxic-ischemic brain injury: a perspective. Brain Pathol. **2:** 245–251.
20. BINIENDA, Z., R. L. ROUNTREE, N. L. TAYLOR, W. SLIKKER, JR. & A. C. SCALLET. 1994. The effects of reduced perfusion and reperfusion on c-fos protein immunohistochemistry in gestational day 21 rat brains. Ann. N.Y. Acad. Sci. **723:** 457–461.
21. BINIENDA, Z. & A. C. SCALLET. 1994. The effects of reduced perfusion and reperfusion on c-fos and HSP-72 protein immunohistochemistry in gestational day 21 rat brains. Int. J. Dev. Neurosci. **12:** 605–610.
22. BINIENDA, Z., S. A. FERGUSON, F. D. RACEY, N. R. TAYLOR, W. SLIKKER, JR. & R. R. HOLSON. 1993. The effect of prenatal hypoxic insult on regional brain weight and behavior in rats. Abstr. Soc. Neurosci. 2(Abstr. 679.13): 1659.
23. NYAKAS, C., E. MARKEL, T. SCHUURMAN & P. G. M. LUITEN. 1991. Impaired learning and abnormal open-field behaviors of rats after early postnatal anoxia and the beneficial effect of the calcium antagonist nimodipine. Eur. J. Neurosci. **3:** 168–174.

# Evaluation of the Novel Neuroprotective Agent BW619C89 in the Middle Cerebral Artery Occlusion Model of Focal Ischemia in the Spontaneously Hypertensive Rat and Normotensive Fischer 344 Rat

JEANETTE H. SWAN AND MICHAEL J. LEACH

*Systems Pharmacology*
*Division of Biology*
*Wellcome Research Laboratories*
*Beckenham, Kent BR3 3BS, United Kingdom*

## INTRODUCTION

BW619C89 [4-amino-2-(4-methyl- 1 - piperazinyl)-5 -(2,3, 5-trichlorophenyl) pyrimidine] is a novel neuroprotective agent with efficacy in models of global and focal ischemia.[1-3] Like the related compounds lamotrigine and BW1003C87, BW619C89 appears to act at voltage sensitive sodium channels, inhibiting ischemia-induced rise in glutamate in both cortex and caudate following middle cerebral artery occlusion,[3] and reducing both ischemia-induced glutamate release and neuronal cell loss in the hippocampal CA1 region and striatum in the 4-VO (combined bilateral common carotid and vertebral artery occlusion) model of global cerebral ischemia.[2]

Lamotrigine (LTG; 3,5-diamino-6-[2,3-dichlorophenyl]-1,2,4-triazine) is a new antiepileptic drug, being a use-dependent blocker of voltage-gated $Na^+$ channels and inhibiting veratrine but not $K^+$-stimulated glutamate release.[4-6] BW1003C87 (5-[2,3,5-trichlorophenyl]-2,4-diamino pyrimidine) is a more potent inhibitor of veratrine-stimulated glutamate release, protecting against global and focal ischemic brain damage.[7-9] However, due to its antifolate properties, BW1003C87 is an unsuitable candidate for stroke therapy. BW619C89, a structural analogue of BW1003C87, is devoid of such antifolate activities and has been shown to be an effective cerebroprotective agent particularly in the middle cerebral artery occlusion (MCAO) model of focal ischemia.[1-3] Previous studies with BW619C89 have used the permanent MCAO model in the normotensive Fischer 344 or Sprague-Dawley rat.[1,3] The spontaneously hypertensive rat is arguably a more appropriate strain of rat, as it produces a consistently larger infarct than the normotensive rat,[10,15] and especially since arterial hypertension is a known risk factor in human stroke. BW619C89 has now been evaluated in the permanent MCAO model in the spontaneously hypertensive rat (SHR) to compare with the normotensive Fischer 344 rat.

## METHODS

The method used for MCAO was essentially as described previously.[1,23] Briefly, adult male Fischer 344, or spontaneously hypertensive Sprague-Dawley (SHR) rats weighing 270–360 g were anesthetized with 2% halothane in a mixture of 30% oxygen and 70% nitrous oxide. The left femoral artery and vein were cannulated to enable continuous blood pressure monitoring, blood gas sampling and intravenous administration of drugs. Animals were then intubated and ventilated on 0.5–1% halothane. Body temperature was maintained at 37 ± 0.5°C using a Harvard homeothermic blanket system. Blood gases were monitored throughout the surgery and maintained at $PaCO_2$ 35–45 mm Hg, $PaO_2$ > 100 mm Hg, and pH 7.4 ± 0.05.

The neuroprotective efficacy of BW619C89 was investigated in three separate experiments: (1) Dose response study (Fischer 344): BW619C89 mesylate (5, 10, 20, and 40 mg kg$^{-1}$) or distilled water diluent, was administered 5 min postocclusion (0 h). (2) Delayed administration study (Fischer 344): BW619C89 mesylate (10 mg kg$^{-1}$) was administered at 0 h, 1 h, 2 h or 4 h postocclusion, and distilled water diluent at 0 h postocclusion. (3) Neuroprotection in the spontaneously hypertensive rat: BW619C89 mesylate (20 mg kg$^{-1}$) was administered 5 min postocclusion (0 h).

In all experiments BW619C89 was administered as the mesylate salt with dose corrected to base compound and infused intravenously over 10 min. The infusion rate was kept constant at 0.05 ml min$^{-1}$. Each rat therefore received a constant volume of 0.5 ml with concentration varying to accommodate rat weight variation. During the 10-min infusion period, all rats were lightly anesthetized with 0.5% halothane. The control (distilled water) and all 0 h groups were still artificially ventilated, whereas the delayed infusion groups (1 h, 2 h, 4 h) were spontaneously breathing. Five min. postinfusion the cannulae were removed, anesthesia discontinued, all wounds sutured, artificial ventilation withdrawn, and the animal allowed to recover whilst breathing oxygen-enriched air. When mobility returned, the animal was returned to a cage with access to food and water.

At 48 h, the rats were assessed in a blinded manner for neurological deficit using a grading scale of 0–3, to assess the effects of occlusion.[11] Animals were then reanesthetized with pentobarbitone (60 mg kg$^{-1}$ ip) and perfusion stained with 3% 2,3,5-triphenyltetrazolium chloride (TTC) for image analysis and determination of infarct volume as previously described.[1]

## RESULTS

### Physiological Variables

*Dose Response and Delayed Administration of BW619C89*

An immediate or delayed 10-min intravenous infusion of BW619C89 to MCAO rats produced small transient reductions in mean arterial blood pressure (MABP) and a longer lasting reduction in heart rate (HR). These effects were only statistically significant at the immediate postocclusion dose of 40 mg kg$^{-1}$. At this dose MABP decreased by 17 ± 4 mm Hg (15 ± 4% reduction, n = 8, $p$ <0.05) and HR reduced by 41 ± 3 bpm (13 ± 4% reduction, n = 8, $p$ <0.05).

*Spontaneously Hypertensive Rats*

SHR animals with MABP below 170 mm Hg were excluded from the experiments. The MABP for all animals used (n = 16 in total) was 175 ± 2 mm Hg. A 10-min infusion of BW619C89 (20 mg kg$^{-1}$ iv) to MCAO rats produced small transient reductions in MABP and a longer lasting, but nonsignificant reduction in HR. Infusion of BW619C89 did not produce significant changes in pH, $pCO_2$ or $PO_2$ in either SHR or Fischer 344 rats.

## *Effect of BW619C89*

*Normotensive Fischer 344 Rats*

All doses of BW619C89 (5–40 mg kg$^{-1}$ iv) significantly ($p$ <0.001) reduced total infarct volume (FIG. 1). Control animals (n = 13) had a mean total volume of 129 ± 6 mm$^3$. BW619C89 at 5, 10, 20 and 40 mg/kg iv (n = 8) dose-dependently reduced this volume to 71 ± 13 mm$^3$ (45%, $p$ <0.001), 53 ± 8 mm$^3$ (59%, $p$ <0.001), 48 ± 10 mm$^3$ (63%, $p$ <0.001) and 37 ± 7 mm$^3$ (71%, $p$ <0.001), respectively. Neurological scores were also significantly reduced in a dose-related manner (FIG. 1).

Cortical infarct volumes were significantly reduced at all doses. Control animals had a mean cortical infarct volume of 86 ± 4 mm$^3$. BW619C89 at 5, 10, 20, and 40 mgkg iv reduced this volume to 44 ± 7 mm$^3$ (49%, $p$ <0.01), 30 ± 5 mm$^3$ (65%, $p$ <0.001) 31 ± 7 mm$^3$ (64%, $p$ <0.001) and 27 ± 5 mm$^3$ (69%, $p$ <0.001), respectively. Delayed administration of BW619C89 (10 mg kg$^{-1}$ iv) produced a significant reduction in total infarct volume at 0, 1, and 2 h postocclusion (FIG. 2). Control animals (n = 8) had a mean total infarct volume of 139 ± 7 mm$^3$. BW619C89 at 0, 1 and 2 h (n = 8) reduced this volume to 57 ± 9 mm$^3$ (59%, $p$ <0.001), 61 ± 8 mm$^3$ (56%, $p$ <0.001), 90 ± 13 mm$^3$ (35%, $p$ <0.01), respectively. BW619C89 at 4 h (n = 5) did not significantly reduce total infarct volume.

*Spontaneously Hypertensive Rats*

Control total infarct volume following MCAO in the SHR (173 ± 10 mm$^3$) was significantly ($p$ <0.001) greater than that produced in the normotensive rat (129 ± 6 mm$^3$). BW619C89 (20 mg kg$^{-1}$ iv) reduced total infarct volume by 32% from 173 ± 10 mm$^3$ (n = 8) to 118 ± 9 mm$^3$ (n = 8, $p$ <0.001) compared with 63% in the normotensive Fischer rat. Neurological deficit was also significantly reduced (control = 1.9 ± 0.1; BW619C89 = 1.3 ± 0.2: $p$ <0.01). The effect of BW619C89 (20 mg kg$^{-1}$) on sectional infarct areas following MCAO in the SHR compared with the Fischer 344 rat is shown in FIGURE 3.

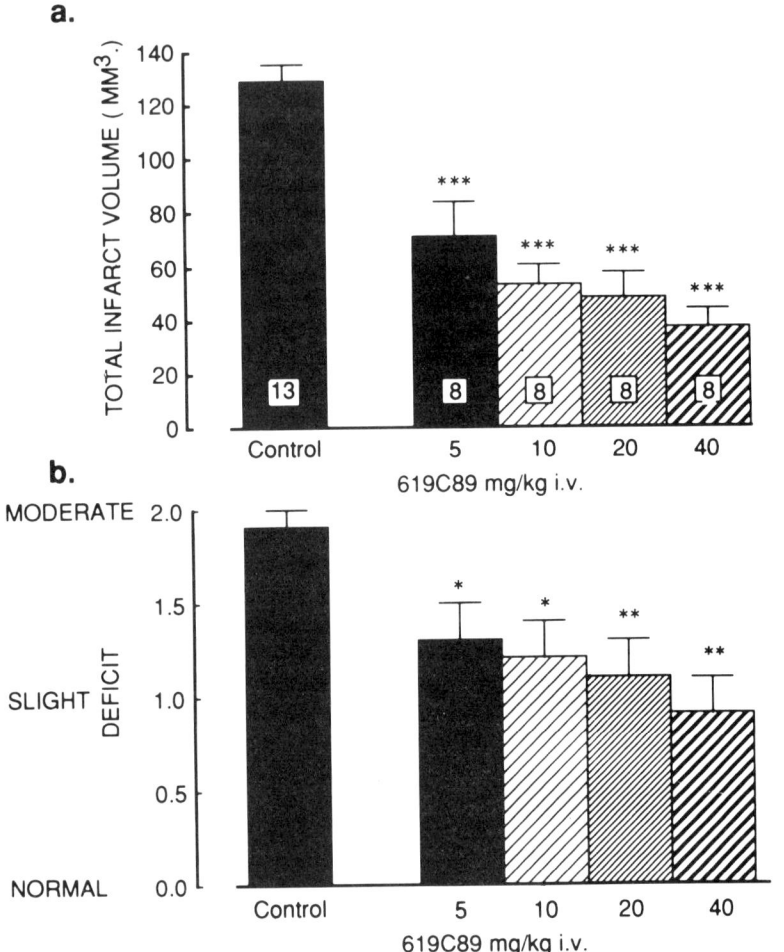

**FIGURE 1.** Effect of BW619C89 (5–40 mg kg$^{-1}$) on (**a**) total infarct volume and (**b**) neurological scores following MCAO in the Fischer 344 rat. Data are mean ± SEM with number of animals as indicated. *$p$ <0.05; **$p$ <0.01; ***$p$ <0.001, compared to control.

## DISCUSSION

This present study further demonstrates the neuroprotective action of BW619C89 in both the normotensive and hypertensive rat. We previously showed in the normotensive rat that a short (1–2-min) bolus injection of BW619C89 (5–40 mg kg$^{-1}$) produces a bell-shaped dose-response curve for reduction of total infarct volume. However, by lengthening the infusion period to 10 min a superior neuroprotection is achieved (59% reduction in total infarct volume at 10 mg kg$^{-1}$ follow-

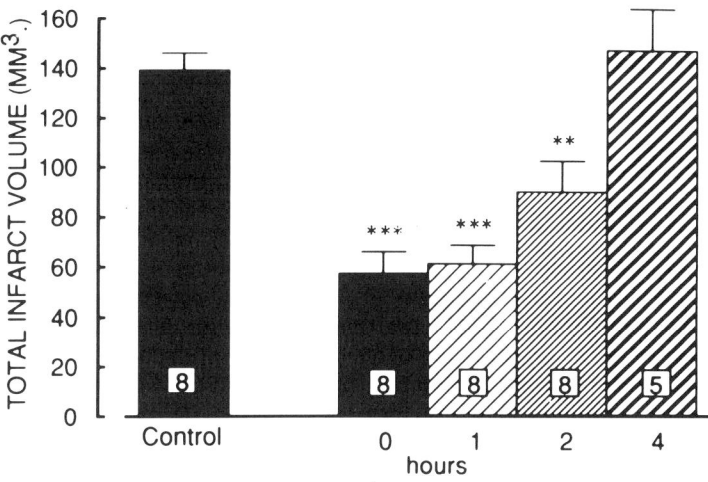

FIGURE 2. Effect of delayed administration of BW619C89 (10 mg kg$^{-1}$) on total infarct volume following MCAO in the Fischer 344 rat. Data are mean ± SEM with number of animals as indicated. **$p$ <0.01; ***$p$ <0.001, compared to control.

ing 10 min iv infusion administration, compared with 57% reduction at 20 mg kg$^{-1}$ following short bolus injection), with significant salvage of brain tissue at all doses tested, there being no evidence of a bell-shaped dose response for reduction of total infarct volume. This difference in efficacy may relate to differing CNS penetration rates, rate of metabolism, and hypotension induced at high doses over a short infusion period which could compromise drug bioavailability or exacerbate brain damage. Previous studies have shown BW619C89 to be effective when given up to 1 h postinsult.[2,3] In the present experiments we extended the window of therapeutic opportunity to 2 h in the normotensive rat. This is consistent with the known pathology in this rat model of focal ischemia where increased metabolism occurs early and evolves to decreased metabolism and infarction within 30 min in "core" tissue and 120 min in penumbral tissue.[12] The efficacy of BW619C89 following delayed administration is similar to that seen with NMDA antagonists which are neuroprotective in the rat MCAO when administered within 1–2 h postocclusion.[13]

Permanent MCAO in the SHR produced a 1.3-fold increase in total infarct volume when compared with the normotensive animal. This may be due to the difference in the morphology and physiology of the cerebral vasculature. The SHR exhibits impaired collateral circulation from pial anastomoses[14] and cortical surface arteries,[20] which both have lumen diameters that are 30–40% smaller than in normotensive animals. Therefore, a greater reduction in cerebral circulation in the ischemic territory is very probable. In addition the lower limit of cerebral autoregulation is substantially elevated in this strain (62 mm Hg in normotensive rats to 95 mm Hg in the SHR).[19] These cerebrovascular differences may also

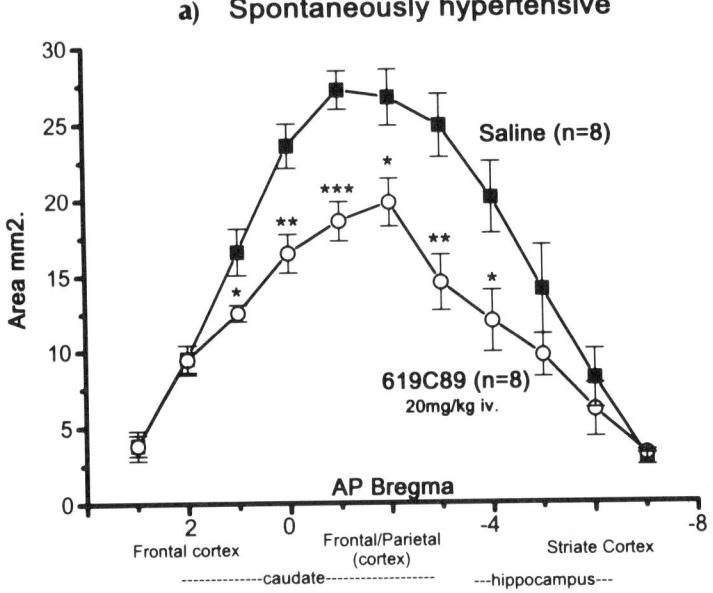
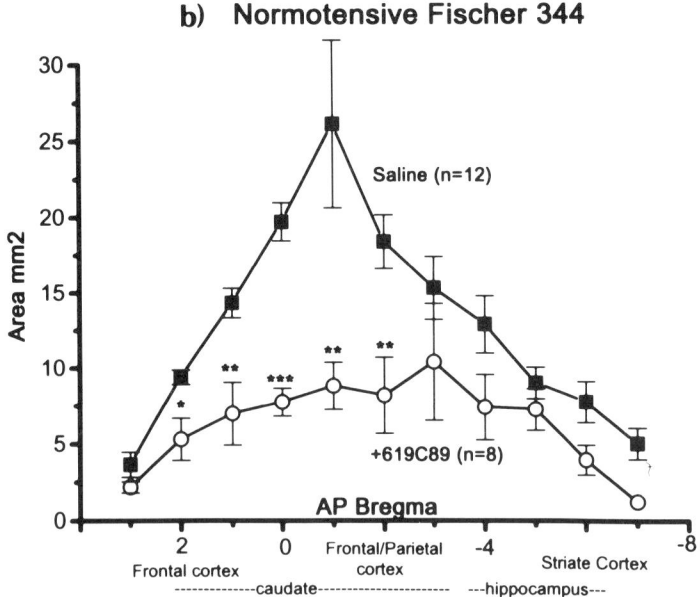

**FIGURE 3.** Effect of BW619C89 (20 mg kg$^{-1}$) on individual sectional infarct areas following MCAO in (a) the SHR and (b) Fischer 344 rat. Data are mean ± SEM with number of animals as indicated. *$p$ <0.05; **$p$ <0.01; ***$p$ <0.001.

contribute to the reduced efficacy of neuroprotective agents in this rat strain. Agents such as MK 801, kyneurenate and nitric oxide synthase inhibitors, which are neuroprotective in the normotensive rat, have proved inconsistent or ineffective in the SHR.[16–18,22] In contrast, the present data show that following permanent MCAO, BW619C89 effectively reduces total infarct volume and neurological deficit in the SHR. The protection, although significant is not as dramatic as in the normotensive strain, with efficacy being reduced by half. Because the SHR has a higher susceptibility to a larger infarct, it is more difficult to elicit neuroprotection. Also blood flow in the vicinity of the occluded vessel is lower in hypertensive animals than in normotensive rats,[21] thus compromising the amount of drug available to dying neurones.

## CONCLUSIONS

In the normotensive rat BW619C89 (5–40 mg kg$^{-1}$) reduces total infarct volume and neurological deficit in a dose-dependent manner when administered immediately after MCAO or following 1 h or 2 h, but not 4 h post-occlusion. In the SHR permanent MCAO produces a larger total infarct when compared with the normotensive animal. Impaired collateral circulation in the ischemic territory may account for this difference, and may contribute to the reduced efficacy of those neuroprotective agents which afford protection to normotensive animals. BW619C89 (20 mg kg$^{-1}$) effectively reduces total infarct volume and neurological deficit in the SHR as well as the normotensive animal.

## REFERENCES

1. LEACH, M. J., J. H. SWAN, D. EISENTHAL, M. DOPSON & M. NOBBS. 1993. BW619C89, a glutamate release inhibitor, protects against focal cerebral ischaemic damage. Stroke **24:** 1063–1067.
2. SMITH, S. E., D. LEKIEFFRE, P. SOWINSKI & B. MELDRUM. 1993. Cerebroprotective effect of BW619C89 after focal or global cerebral ischaemia in the rat. NeuroReport **4:** 1339–1342.
3. GRAHAM, S. H., J. CHEN, J. LAN, M. J. LEACH & R. SIMON. 1994. Neuroprotective effects of a use-dependent blocker of voltage-dependent sodium channels, BW619C89 in rat middle cerebral artery occlusion. J. Pharmacol. Exp. Ther. **269:** 854–859.
4. LEACH, M. J., C. M. MARDEN & A. A. MILLER. 1986. Pharmacological studies on lamotrigine, a novel potential antiepileptic drug. 2. Neurochemical studies on the mechanism of action. Epilepsia **27:** 490–497.
5. LEES, G. & M. J. LEACH. 1993. Studies on the mechanism of action of the novel anticonvulsant lamotrigine (Lamictal) using primary neuroglial cultures from rat cortex. Brain Res. **612:** 190–199.
6. LANG, D. G., C. M. WANG & B. R. COOPER. 1993. Lamotrigine, phenytoin and carbamazepine interactions on the sodium current present in N4TG1 mouse neuroblastoma cells. J. Pharmacol. Exp. Ther. **266:** 829–835.
7. GRAHAM, S. H., J. CHEN, F. R. SHARP & R. P. SIMON. 1993. Limiting ischaemic injury by inhibition of excitatory amino acid release. J. Cereb. Blood Flow Metab. **13:** 88–97.
8. MELDRUM, B. S., J. H. SWAN, M. J. LEACH, M. H. MILLAN, R. GWINN, K. KADOTA,

S. H. GRAHAM, J. CHEN & R. P. SIMON. 1992. Reduction of glutamate release and protection against ischemic brain damage by BW1003C87. Brain Res. **593:** 1–6.
9. LEKIEFFRE, D. & B. S. MELDRUM. 1993. The pyrimidine-derivative BW1003C87, protects CA1 and striatal neurons following transient severe forebrain ischaemia in rats. A microdialysis and histological study. Neuroscience **56:** 93–99.
10. DUVERGER, D. & E. T. MACKENZIE. 1988. The quantification of cerebral infarction following focal ischaemia in the rat: influence of strain, arterial pressure, blood glucose concentration and age. J. Cereb. Blood Flow Metab. **8:** 449–461.
11. BEDERSON, J. B., L. H. PITTS, M. TSUJI, M. C. NISHIMURA, R. L. DAVIS & H. BARTKOWSKI. 1986. Rat middle cerebral artery occlusion: Evaluation of the model and development of a neurologic examination. Stroke **17:** 472–476.
12. SIMON, R. 1990. Treatment of brain ischaemia: from preclinical pharmacology to clinical practice. *In* Advances in the Biosciences. Excitatory Amino Acids and Brain Ischaemia, Pharmacological and Clinical Aspects. G. Biggio, P. F. Spano, G. Toffano & G. L. Gessa, Eds. Vol. 78: 79–91. Pergamon Press. Oxford, UK.
13. MELDRUM, B. 1990. Protection against ischaemic neuronal damage by drugs acting on excitatory neurotransmission. Cereb. Brain Metab. Rev. **3:** 27–57.
14. COYLE, P. 1987. Spatial relations of dorsal anastomoses and lesion border after middle cerebral artery occlusion. Stroke **18:** 1133–1140.
15. GINSBURG, M. D. & R. BUSTO. 1989. Rodent models of cerebral ischaemia. Stroke **20:** 1627–1642.
16. ROUSSEL, S., E. PINARD & J. SEYLAZ. 1992. Effect of MK-801 on focal brain infarction in normotensive and hypertensive rats. Hypertension **19:** 40–46.
17. PULSINELLI, W., U. DIRNAGL, M. JACEWICZ & A. BUCHAN. 1992. Antagonists of excitatory amino acid neurotransmitters: a comparison of their effects on global versus focal ischaemia. *In* Drug Research Related to Neuroactive Amino Acids. Alfred Benzon Symposium. A. Schousboe, N. Diemer & H. Kofod, Eds. Vol. 32: 225–238. Munksgaard. Copenhagen.
18. BUCHAN, A. M., S. Z. GERTLER, Z.-G. HUANG, H. LI, E. CHAUNDY & D. XUE. 1994. Failure to prevent sensitive CA1 neuronal death and reduce cortical infarction following cerebral ischaemia with inhibition of nitric oxide synthase. Neuroscience **61:** 1–11.
19. FUJISHAMA, M. & T. OMAE. 1976. Lower limit of cerebral autoregulation in normotensive and spontaneously hypertensive rats. Experentia **32:** 1019–1021.
20. JOHANSSON, B. B., L. M. AUER & I. SAYAMA. 1985. Reaction of pial arteries and veins to hypercapnia in hypertensive and normotensive rats. Stroke **16:** 320–323.
21. COYLE, P. & D. D. HEISTAD. 1986. Blood flow through cerebral collateral vessels in hypertensive and normotensive rats. Hypertension 8(Suppl. II): II-67–II-71.
22. ROUSSEL, S., E. PINARD & J. SEYLAZ. 1990. Kynurenate does not reduce infarct size after middle cerebral artery occlusion in spontaneously hypertensive rats. Brain Res. **518:** 353–355.
23. TAMURA, A., D. I. GRAHAM, J. MCCULLOCH & G. M. TEASDALE. 1981. Focal cerebral ischaemia in the rat. I. Description of technique and early neuropathological consequences following middle cerebral artery occlusion. J. Cerb. Blood Flow Metab. **1:** 53–60.

# Quantitative Histological Evaluation of Neuroprotective Compounds

ANDREW C. SCALLET

*Experimental Neuropathology Laboratory*
*Division of Neurotoxicology*
*National Center for Toxicological Research*
*Jefferson, Arkansas 72079*

## INTRODUCTION

Measurement is an essential part of the experimental procedure in histological studies of neuroprotective drugs. Although measuring images is difficult, since the advent of stereological methods some years ago (*e.g.,* "Weibel's Bible"[1]) tremendous progress has been made. At present, numerous commercial image analysis systems are available to support the conduct of quantitative neurohistological evaluation of the efficacy of neuroprotective agents. My aim here is to briefly review the experimental design and stereological principles underlying morphometric studies, to describe some neurohistological tissue preparation approaches of particular utility to screening the efficacy of neuroprotective compounds, and to exemplify their quantitation and statistical analysis.

## EXPERIMENTAL DESIGN AND STATISTICAL ANALYSIS OF MORPHOMETRIC STUDIES

### *Numbers of Animals and Number of Samples/Animal*

The number of animals (n) required per experimental group to detect an effect, as in any study, depends on the minimum difference one would like to detect (precision) as well as the underlying variability (as represented by the standard deviation "sigma") of the measured quantity. More precisely, the difference between group means (an estimate of the magnitude of the effect), when divided by the standard error of such differences (computed as sigma/square root of n), provides a Student *t* statistic which determines the probability that the means were that far apart by chance alone. The smaller the standard error, the larger the *t* statistic and the less likely the effect is due to chance alone. The magnitude of the effect is *a priori* unknown, but it *is* known that the standard error (in the denominator) decreases as the square root of the sample size, n, increases. For this reason, as the sample size increases, the value of the *t* statistic for a given magnitude of effect increases, but only as the square root of the sample size. For this reason, increasing n from 5 to 20 per group is required to merely double *t*. This law of diminishing returns with increased sample size is mitigated partially by the increase in degrees of freedom (reducing the *t* value required for a given level of significance) with sample size. The n for treatment comparisons is always based on the number of animals, which should be a minimum of 5–10 per group, but it is also necessary to decide the number of anatomical areas and samples per area. As a practical matter, the cost of morphometric sampling and analysis must be divided in some ratio between all the samples chosen from the same anatomical site or fewer samples divided among a broader range of anatomical sites sampled. For this reason, an n of 5 samples per region is suggested as a minimum for an initial experiment for most applications, where the precise region of greatest anatomical sensitivity to neurotoxicity may be unknown. Then, within-lab replication of any important (but statistically marginal) effects should be undertaken. Also, the desired sample size (and anatomical location) of subsequent experiments may then be better predicted on the basis of power computations, once the variability has been estimated from the initial experiment.

### *Experimental Design and Statistics*

Although anatomical measurements usually require a more complex design than a simple *t* test, the basic principles of experimental design and statistical analysis are the same for morphometric studies as for any other scientific investigations.[2] If the goal of the research is to determine neuroprotective efficacy, a two-way mixed model ANOVA with the neurodegenerative agent and the neuroprotective drug as the two independent ("between group") factors will probably be appropriate. Selection of treatment levels may be dictated by available information on minimally effective or lethal doses. Enough dose levels (5 or more for the protective drug, perhaps 2–3 for the neurodegenerative agent) should be included to characterize the shape of the dose-response relationship. Subjects should be randomly assigned to treatment groups, and if the experiment cannot be conducted on all subjects treated as a single set, it should be arranged as identical, replicated blocks. This means that all treatment combinations (neurodegenerative dose/neuroprotective dose pairings) should be repeated several times on blocks of subjects assigned randomly to treatment groups and replicates. This randomized assignment protects against systematic bias that may occur with variation in such things as accuracy of dose preparation, intensity of staining between repeated batches of tissue sections, seasonal or other periodic hormonal fluctuations, etc. The randomization is also necessary to meet the assumption that all observations are independent that underlies the theory of analysis of variance procedures. Anatomical measurements made at several different locations should be treated as repeated ("within group") measures, since they are intercorrelated.

Balanced designs with equal numbers of animals per group are preferable to unbalanced designs with missing observations. With two group factors, it is desirable to use a complete factorial design; that is, subgroups of each group of subjects assigned to each level of variable 1 should be present and randomly assigned to each level of variable 2. These complete factorial designs are easier to interpret in the presence of interactions between the variables, which cannot be evaluated in partial factorial designs. Thus this type of design would provide comprehensive information to the drug developer about the efficacy of neuroprotective agents, which may vary with the degree of the neurodegenerative insult.

Attention must be paid to the selection of the dependent variables to be measured so that they represent unbiased estimates of means that are "biologically meaningful," *i.e.*, ones that reflect the neurodegenerative process to be protected against. This is a question both of choosing appropriate staining procedures for the sections that have been sampled, and then obtaining measurements from the stained material.

### *Stereological Considerations*

The theoretical underpinnings of the choice of appropriate parameters to measure is within the field of stereology.[1,3-5] The basic principles of stereology address the measurement of structural parameters such as volume density ($V_v$) and surface density ($S_v$). These parameters are independent of any assumptions as to the shape of the objects being measured (the stereologist, like the topologist, is someone who cannot tell the difference between a doughnut and a coffee cup!). As a practical matter, the implication is that the fractional area ($A_a$) of an irregularly shaped structure of interest (such as mitochondria) can be directly measured. After outlining the "mitochondrial phase" of the section manually (or as the computer defines it from relative optical density measurements), the ratio of mitochondrial area to section area (measured as number of pixels in each phase) is an unbiased estimate of the value of $A_a$. Mathematically, this ratio is also an unbiased estimate of $V_v$, the ratio of mitochondrial volume to tissue volume (or perikaryal volume, if extracellular space is excluded) (Weibel, p. 26[1]). We do not have to make any assumptions about the average size or shape of mitochondria.

As pointed out by Weibel, stereological "structure parameters" such as the volume density ($V_v$) or the surface density ($S_v$) sometimes conceal a lot of information: they reflect the average proportion over the entire volume of interest. For example, a decrease in volume density may occur when the same number of objects is present, if the size of each object is reduced. Alternately, a decrease in volume density may also reflect a reduction in number of objects with no change in their size. Stereological "structure parameters" such as $V_v$ cannot distinguish between these alternatives. In some cases, an alternate stereological approach ("particle parameters") to compute $N_v$, the numerical density of particles in a given volume, can be employed. Certain of these approaches require assumptions about the shape and size of the particles being counted, such as synapses[6] while others provide unbiased estimates of particle number, regardless of their shape or size.[5]

## METHODS

### *General Histological Procedures*

For optimal results in brain tissue with most of the methods, it is desirable to perfuse the subject through the aorta with an appropriate fixative to minimize postmortem deterioration or artifacts. Routine 3.75% formaldehyde suffices for most procedures, although 1–3% paraformaldehyde mixed with 0.1–4% gluteraldehyde can be substituted to improve membrane preservation for electron microscopic studies.

For histochemical light microscopic work, sections can be readily prepared using a vibrating microtome to cut the cooled (but unfrozen) brain tissue. This avoids the creation of freezing artifacts, especially troublesome for ultrastructural studies, due to formation of inter- and intracellular ice crystals. It also limits the potential loss of antigens (particularly ethanol-soluble ones) during the preparation of paraffin- or plastic-embedded tissue blocks.

For temporary storage of sections of rat or mouse brain, it is convenient to use 24-well culture dishes containing buffered 1% formaldehyde (silver degeneration stain) or simply 0.1 M buffer (all other stains) which are readily stacked in a refrigerator at 4°C. After sectioning, a sequence of experiments can be undertaken with the aim of minimizing the required storage period prior to staining. Staining baskets can be made by drilling 24 holes in a solid block of plastic and fastening nylon window-screening material to one side with cyanoacrylate adhesive.

### *Evaluating Protection against Acute Neurodegenerative Processes*

The procedures available for histological evaluation of neurodegeneration can be roughly divided into those especially useful for detecting relatively rapid, acute damage to neurons and their processes versus procedures capable of detecting slower, more subtle changes in structure that may be produced by continual, chronic, gradual neurodegenerative processes. Only the former procedures will be discussed here, since it is desirable to test neuroprotective agents against models that cause rapid, reproducible damage such as acute neurotoxicants or ischemia models.

#### *Silver Impregnation of Degenerating Processes*

Vibratome, frozen, or paraffin sections can be utilized in silver staining procedures designed to impregnate only axon terminals or neuronal cell bodies that are dead or dying. Although a number of techniques are available,[7–12] the procedure outlined by Nadler and Evenson[13] is simple and can provide excellent results. The neurotoxicity of trimethyltin[14,15] has been studied with silver degeneration-selective methods (FIG. 1) applied up to several months postexposure.[16,17] We have also used this method recently to study the neurotoxicity of the "excitotoxic" seafood contaminant domoic acid,[18] as illustrated in FIGURE 2. The methods should be equally suitable for determining the efficacy of neuroprotective agents in blocking this type of neural damage.

#### *Immunohistochemistry of Neurotoxicity Biomarkers*

Immunohistochemical staining is a highly flexible and useful technique by which nearly any antigenic chemical component of the tissue section can be local-

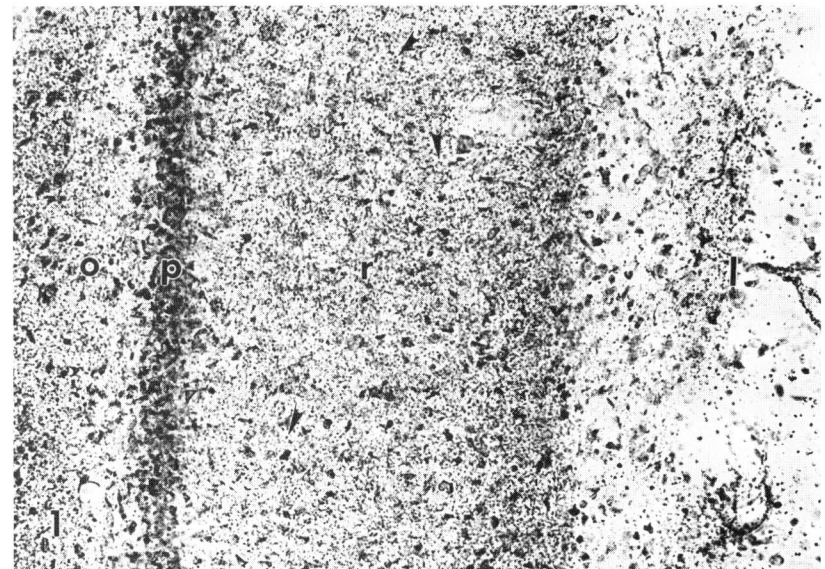

**FIGURE 1.** Silver-stained 40 micron vibratome section illustrating degenerating axon terminals in the hippocampal CA1 stratum radiatum (r) and stratum oriens (o) subfields of a rat one month after 4.5 mg/kg TMT. *Arrowheads* point to several of the many individual silver grains. Note the sparse number of stratum pyramidale (p) cells, although the remaining neurons are viable (*i.e.*, not dark like the dead neurons of FIG. 2). Presumably, dead neurons that populated CA1 stratum pyramidale closer to the onset of the TMT lesion have been phagocytized by this time. Note also that the stratum lacunosum (l) is relatively spared.

ized. The same method[19,20] can be used to visualize a variety of antigens, although sometimes adjustments of the fixation approach may have to be made to accommodate an individual antigen. Some progress has been made in identifying specific proteins or fluorescent DNA labels that may selectively mark only cells undergoing an acute apoptotic or necrotic process.[21] More widespread use has been made of markers such as c-fos/c-jun protein immunoreactivities,[22-24] which indicate acute cellular metabolic activity in some but not all neuronal populations, and heat shock protein (HSP-72 and others) antibodies[25,26] which may label neurons responding acutely to a neurotoxic exposure.

Although these markers cannot be interpreted as indicating dead or dying neurons, they do serve the potentially valuable purpose of marking neuroanatomical regions of acute cellular activation. The neuroanatomy may then aid in understanding the mechanisms by which certain types of neurotoxins may propagate damage throughout the brain. Immunohistochemical markers such as glial fibrillary acidic protein (GFAP), though found only in nonneuronal astrocytic cells, can nevertheless be considered biomarkers of acute neurotoxicity. The presence of increased GFAP with cytoplasmic and/or nuclear enlargement (FIG. 3) may signal either the presence of a gliosis that was "reactive" to prior neuronal damage or perhaps an alteration of the normally cooperative role of astrocytes in neuronal ammonia/

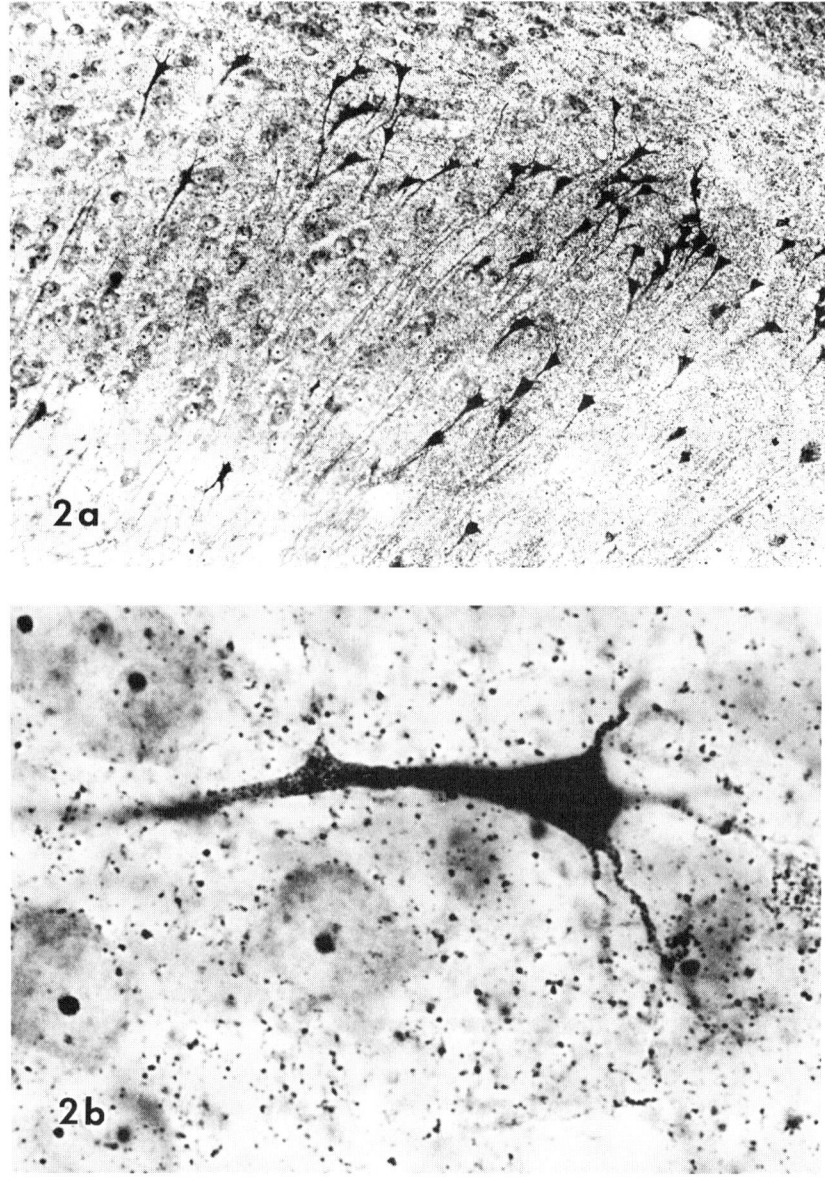

FIGURE 2. (a) Silver degeneration stains (40 micron vibratome section) distinguish necrotic *(dark black)* from viable *(lighter-shaded,* with prominent nuclei and nucleoli) neurons between CA1 and subiculum subfields of the hippocampus of a cynomolgus monkey treated one week earlier with 4 mg/kg i.v. of the convulsant neurotoxicant domoic acid, a seafood contaminant. (b) Higher magnification micrograph of one necrotic and several viable neurons.

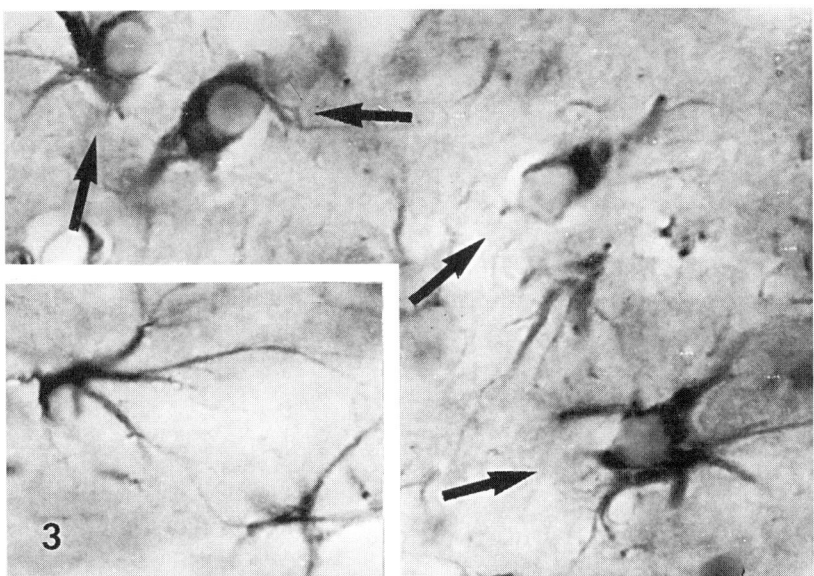

**FIGURE 3.** Immunohistochemical labeling of GFAP-positive astrocytes near the hippocampal CA1 s. pyramidale. *Arrows* point to the greatly swollen nuclei of 4 adjacent astrocytes illustrating Alzheimer's type II gliosis in a rat treated one month earlier with TMT. *Inset* shows the appearance of control astrocytes at the same magnification.

glutamate/GABA metabolism.[18] Macrophage cell surface markers for microglia (for example, as applied to ibogaine neurotoxicity[27]) may also be of use as neurotoxicological biomarkers. Caution must be taken for each individual model of neurotoxic damage to determine whether the prior presence of the desired immunohistochemical marker is indeed predictive of that damage. If so, the efficacy of neuroprotective agents can be determined based on their success in preventing the occurrence of (apoptosis), heat shock, gliosis, etc. as indicated by the immunohistochemical biomarkers.

*Instrumentation Requirements for Morphometry*

The silver impregnation procedures result in deposits of black, reduced silver which are selectively retained in degenerating (membrane-damaged) neurons. If the cell bodies are damaged, a high-contrast image of distinctly separated neurons can usually be obtained (see FIG. 2). If axonal damage is present, its appearance is like a dusting of individual silver grains or small groups of grains across the region innervated by the damaged axons (FIG. 1). High-contrast images of the cell bodies can be acquired by a frame grabber board installed in a personal computer or workstation, and then the digital version of the image can be measured by software that computes its optical density (''darkness' in terms of generally 256 grey-level quanta). The number of objects present that are at least as dark or darker than a desired level, meet a size criteria or a "form factor" describing its shape, or match other criteria can be selected, measured, and counted automatically. Analysis of relatively small, individual silver grains can be conducted in a similar fashion, and offers the advantage that the density of a degenerating pathway from disparate neurons converging in a given terminal zone may reflect an integration of the toxicity to a large group of cells otherwise difficult to count. These systems generally deal with images of a single microscopic plane through a sample and offer contrast enhancement, edge erosion, and several other image processing options to precondition the image prior to measurement. Immunostained tissues can be analyzed very similarly to the silver impregnated degenerating neurons described above, although they may not offer quite the degree of contrast.

A common problem encountered is that the edges of the object(s) to be measured and/or counted are out of the limited plane of focus of the standard light microscope. A reasonable solution can sometimes be obtained from the edge enhancement or other image processing algorithms or using metal-intensified diaminobenzidine procedures to enhance contrast. The increased use of various confocal microscopy approaches is also likely to help solve edge detection or focus problems. In the absence of sufficient depth of field as provided by confocal microscopy, the exact threshold setting chosen will markedly effect the number of objects detected. For this reason, a systematic approach for each section must be employed to avoid biasing the results. For example, the average density (in greyscale levels) of 5 target silver grains and 5 nearby background densities from different parts of the digitized field-of-view of a section can be determined. Setting the threshold level halfway between their means provides a systematic and unbiased approach to counting grains.

*Example: Trimethyltin Treatment Causes Increased Axon Terminal Degeneration in Aged Rats*

Trimethyltin (TMT) is a neurotoxic chemical with human workplace exposure potential that was formerly used as an ingredient for such things as barnacle repellent paints used in shipyards. It has been demonstrated to damage CA1 pyramidal neurons in the hippocampus, to increase hippocampal content of glial fibrillary acidic protein (GFAP), to alter glutamate metabolism, and to impair passive avoidance retention.[16,17,28–32] Therefore the effects of TMT in a young animal resemble, in some respects, the effects of spontaneous aging.

Quantitative silver grain measurement was used to evaluate the degree of neurotoxicity of a relatively low dose of TMT administered to rats of selected ages. The hypothesis was that older rodents' hippocampi would be more susceptible to TMT neurodegeneration than young rodents, and that we could relate this neurotoxic susceptibility to age. Several previous studies have suggested that the aged rat may be more sensitive to neurotoxic exposure than the young adult rat.[17,33,34] However, none of these studies employed a silver degeneration-selective method to quantitatively evaluate the severity of damage from neurotoxins administered at a broad range of ages.

Our example evaluates the neurohistological effects of TMT by a silver-staining procedure specific for neuronal and terminal degeneration,[13,20] followed by measurement of the density of silver grains labeling the degenerating axon terminals in the CA1 stratum radiatum.

All experimental subjects were male Fischer 344 rats which were barrier raised in individual cages at NCTR. Prior to experimentation, they were removed from the barrier facility and acclimatized to the animal room outside the barrier in the same caging, for at least two weeks. Lighting in both facilities was on for 12 hours and off for 12 hours. The experiment was conducted as an 8-group design (n = 16). Animals of four different age cohorts (6, 12, 18 and 24 months) were obtained on the same date, and half of each age group received a single injection of TMT chloride (Aldrich Chemical Co., 4.5 mg/kg i.p.) while the other half were saline-dosed controls. Animals were then allowed to return to their home cages for one month. A suitable dose and survival time for the purposes of this study had been determined on the basis of previous research.[17]

To evaluate the nature and presence of brain damage, rats from each of the eight age and treatment groups were anesthetized with 60 mg/kg nembutal and perfused with 50 ml of 0.9% saline in 0.1 M, pH 7.4 potassium phosphate buffer followed immediately by 450 ml of 4% formaldehyde in the same buffer. Perfusate was delivered through the ascending aorta using a peristaltic pump at a flow rate of 35 ml/min. Brains were removed and stored overnight in the perfusate, then sectioned at 50 $\mu$m on a Vibratome. Sections for the modified Fink-Heimer degeneration stain[13,17,20] were stored in the formaldehyde perfusate until processing within the week. This method impregnates degenerating axon terminals, dendrites, and cell bodies. Sections were processed in a staining basket with multiple wells. This allowed processing, *as a batch,* single hippocampal sections chosen from each of the rats assigned to one of the eight experimental groups. Because of possible qualitative variations of staining between branches, we always included a sample from each and every subject of a replicate in a block or batch to be stained. If necessary, then the entire block can be repeated to optimize the staining as desired without having to resort to comparing animals' tissues processed in different batches.

Microscopic images of the resulting silver-impregnated degenerating axon terminals appearing in the medial portion of the CA1 s. radiatum subfield (see FIG. 1) were then digitized as described above and the density of silver grains per unit area was plotted as a function of age (FIG. 4). A two-way analysis of variance revealed significant effects of TMT treatment ($F(1,15) = 89.6, p < 0.0001$), as well as age ($F(3,15) = 13.9, p < 0.01$). As hypothesized, the effects of TMT were considerably larger in the older rats, as indicated by a significant interaction between age and the effects of TMT ($F(3,15) = 11.1, p < 0.01$). Because of the relatively small sample size, additional blocks of subjects are being prepared and evaluated to expand this example.

## SUMMARY

The application of quantitative morphometric methods to neurotoxicology is a relatively recent endeavor, and appropriate techniques are still evolving. How-

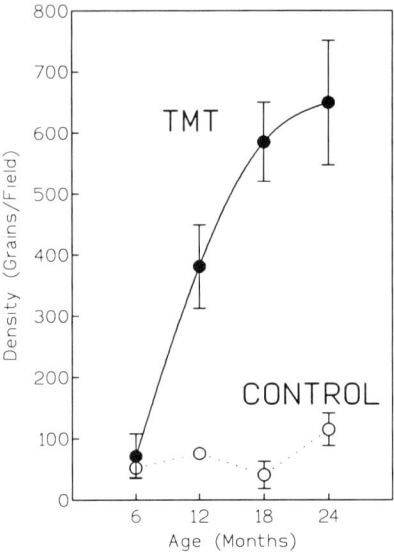

**FIGURE 4.** Graph indicating the number of grains per visual field (means ± SEM) counted in CA1 stratum radiatum in different age rats given 4.5 mg/kg TMT i.p. The effects of TMT were not statistically detectable in six-month-old rats, but were significant ($p < 0.05$) at twelve months, and highly significant ($p < 0.01$) at eighteen and twenty-four months.

ever, such methods are essential for subsequent use of neurohistological data in mathematical representations of the risk of exposure to neurotoxicants.[35-39] It can be predicted that the same methods will also be of great utility in studies of the efficacy of neuroprotective drugs. When the neuropathological conditions to be prevented or reversed are best monitored by neurohistology, quantitative morphometry should be considered as the most direct means to demonstrate the efficacy of a neuroprotective agent. Initially, a decision to choose the most appropriate histological procedure must be made. The rationale for such decisions with regard to several common histochemical techniques was discussed. The appropriate stereological and statistical considerations to be addressed by the sampling strategy were also presented. It is anticipated that quantitative morphometric methods will play an increasingly important role in the evaluation of the efficacy and toxicity of neuroactive compounds.

## ACKNOWLEDGMENTS

The author would like to thank Mr. Robert Rountree and Ms. Shelly Lensing for help with data collection and analysis and Drs. Kettie Terry and Sherry Ferguson for very helpful comments on the manuscript. He would also like to thank his collaborators in the Division of Neurotoxicology: Drs. William Slikker, Jr.,

Syed Ali, Merle Paule, Larry Schmued, Zbigniew Binienda, Florence Caputo, Jennifer Sandberg and John Bowyer.

## REFERENCES

1. WEIBEL, E. R. 1979. Stereological Methods: Practical Methods for Biological Morphometry. Academic Press. London.
2. WINER, B. J. 1971. Statistical Principles in Experimental Design. 2nd Edit. 127–201. McGraw-Hill. New York.
3. RUSS, J. C. 1986. Practical Stereology. Plenum Press. New York.
4. REITH, A. & T. M. MAYHEW, Eds. 1988. Stereology and Morphometry in Electron Microscopy: Some Problems and Their Solutions. Hemisphere Publications. New York.
5. STERIO, D. C. 1984. The unbiased estimation of number and sizes of arbitrary particles using the disector. J. Microsc. **134:** 127–136.
6. COLLONIER, M. & C. BEAULIEU. 1985. An empirical assessment of stereological formulae applied to the counting of synaptic disks in the cerebral cortex. J. Comp. Neurol. **231:** 175–179.
7. NAUTA, J. H. 1954. Silver impregnation of degenerating axons in the central nervous system: a modified technique. Stain Technol. **27:** 91–93.
8. FINK, R. P. & L. HEIMER. 1967. Two methods for selective impregnation of degenerating axons and their synaptic endings in the central nervous system. Brain Res. **4:** 369–374.
9. DE OLMOS, J. S. 1969. A cupric-silver method for impregnantion of terminal axon degeneration and its further use in staining granular argyrophilic neurons. Brain Behav. Evol. **2:** 210–237.
10. GALLYAS, F., J. R. WOLFF, H. BOTTCHER & L. ZABORSZKY. 1980. A reliable method for demonstrating axonal degeneration shortly after axotomy. Stain. Technol. **55:** 291–297.
11. GALLYAS, F., J. R. WOLFF, H. BOTTCHER & L. ZABORSZKY. 1980. A reliable and sensitive method to localize terminal degeneration and lysosomes in the central nervous system. Stain Technol. **55:** 299–306.
12. GALLYAS, F., F. H. GULDNER, G. ZOLTAY & J. R. WOLFF. 1990. Golgi-like demonstration of "dark" neurons with an argyrophil III method for experimental neuropathology. Acta Neuropathol. **79:** 620–628.
13. NADLER, J. V. & D. A. EVENSON. 1983. Use of excitatory amino acids to make axon sparing lesions of the hypothalamus. Methods Enzymol. **103:** 393–400.
14. CHANG, L. W., T. M. TIEMEYER, G. R. WENGER & D. E. MCMILLAN. 1982. Neuropathology of mouse hippocampus in acute trimethyltin intoxication. Neurobehav. Toxicol. Teratol. **4:** 149–156.
15. MILLER, D. B. & J. P. O'CALLAGHAN. 1984. Biochemical, functional, and morphological indicators of neurotoxicity: effects of acute administration of trimethyltin to the developing rat. J. Pharmacol. Exp. Ther. **231:** 744–751.
16. BALABAN, C. D., J. P. O'CALLAGHAN & M. L. BILLINGSLEY. 1988. Trimethyltin-induced neuronal damage in the rat brain: comparative studies using silver degeneration stains: immunocytochemistry and immunoassay for neuronotypic and gliotypic proteins. Neuroscience **26:** 337–361.
17. MATTHEWS, J. C. & A. C. SCALLET. 1991. Nutrition, neurotoxicants, and age-related neurodegeneration. Neurotoxicology **12:** 547–558.
18. SCALLET, A. C., Z. BINIENDA. F., A. CAPUTO, S. HALL, M. G. PAULE, R. L. ROUNTREE, L. SCHMUED, T. SOBOTKA & W. SLIKKER, JR. 1993. Domoic acid-treated cynomolgus monkeys *(M. fascicularis)*: effects of dose on hippocampal neuronal and terminal degeneration. Brain Res. **627:** 307–313.
19. STERNBERGER, L. A., P. H. HARDY, JR., J. J. CUCULIS & H. G. MEYER. 1970. The unlabeled antibody enzyme method of immunohistochemistry. J. Histochem. Cytochem. **13:** 315–333.

20. SCALLET, A. C., G. W. LIPE, S. F. ALI, R. R. HOLSON, C. H. FRITH & W. SLIKKER, JR. 1988. Neuropathological evaluation by combined immunohistochemistry and degeneration-specific methods: application of methylenedioxymethamphetamine. Neurotoxicology **9:** 529–538.
21. JOHNSON, E. M., JR., & T. L. DECKWERTH. 1993. Molecular mechanisms of developmental neuronal death. Annu. Rev. Neurosci. **16:** 31–46.
22. MORGAN, J. I., D. R. COHEN, J. L. HEMPSTEAD & T. CURRAN. 1987. Mapping patterns of c-fos expression in the central nervous system after seizure. Science **237:** 192–197.
23. ZAWIA, N. H. & G. J. HARRY. 1993. Trimethyltin-induced c-fos expression: adolescent vs. neonatal rat hippocampus. Toxicol. Appl. Pharmacol. **121:** 99–102.
24. DRAGUNOW, M., D. YOUNG, P. HUGHES, G. MACGIBBON, P. LAWLOR, K. SINGLETON, E. SIRIMANNE, E. BEILHARZ & P. GLUCKMAN. 1993. Is c-jun involved in nerve cell death following status epilepticus and hypoxic-ischemic brain injury? Mol. Brain Res. **18:** 347–352.
25. SHIMOSAKA, S., Y. T. SO & R. P. SIMON. 1992. Distribution of HSP-72 induction and neuronal death following limbic seizures. Neurosci. Lett. **138:** 202–206.
26. LI, Y., M. CHOPP, J. H. GARCIA, Y. YOSHIDA, Z. G. ZHANG & S. R. LEVINE. 1992. Distribution of the 72-kd heat-shock protein as a function of transient focal ischemia in rats. Stroke **23:** 1292–1298.
27. O'HEARN, E., D. B. LONG & M. E. MOLLIVER. 1993. Ibogaine induces glial activation in parasaggital zones of the cerebellum. NeuroReport **4:** 299–302.
28. DYER, R. S., W. J. WALSH, H. S. SWARTZWELDER & M. J. WAYNER. 1982. Neurotoxicology of the alkyltins. Neurobehav. Toxicol. Teratol. **4:** 125–278.
29. DYER, R. S., T. J. WALSH, W. F. WONDERLIN & M. BERCEGEAY. 1982. The trimethyltin syndrome in rats. Neurobehav. Toxicol. Teratol. **4:** 127–133.
30. HIKAL, A. H., G. W. LIPE, W. SLIKKER, JR., A. C. SCALLET & G. D. NEWPORT. 1988. Determination of amino acids in different regions of the rat brain. Application to the acute effects of tetrahydrocannabinol (THC) and trimethyltin (TMT). Life Sci. **42:** 2029–2035.
31. REUHL, K. R. 1987. Neuropathology of organometalic compounds: review of selected literature. *In* Neurotoxicants and Neurobiological Function. A. H. Tilson & S. B. Sparber, Eds. 118–136. John Wiley and Sons. New York.
32. SLOVITER, R. S., C. VON KNEBEL DOEBERITZ, T. J. WALSH & D. W. DEMPSTER. 1986. On the role of seizure activity in the hippocampal damage produced by trimethyltin. Brain Res. **367:** 169–182.
33. RAO, V. L. R. & C. R. K. MURPHY. 1988. Age-dependent variation in the sensitivity of rat brain glutamine synthetase to $L$-methionine-DL-sulfoxime. Int. J. Dev. Neurosci. **6:** 425–430.
34. WOZNIAK, D. F., G. R. STEWART, J. P. MILLER & J. W. OLNEY. 1991. Age-related sensitivity to kainate neurotoxicity. Exp. Neurol. **114:** 250–253.
35. MCMILLAN, D. E. 1987. Risk assessment for neurobehavioral toxicity. Environ. Health Perspect. **76:** 155–161.
36. GAYLOR, D. W. & W. SLIKKER, JR. 1990. Risk assessment for neurotoxic effects. Neurotoxicology **11:** 211–218.
37. SLIKKER, W., JR. & D. W. GAYLOR. 1990. Biologically-based dose-response model for neurotoxicity risk assessment. Korean J. Toxicol. **6:** 205–213.
38. SLIKKER, W., JR. 1991. Biomarkers of neurotoxicity: an overview. Biomed. Environ. Sci. **4:** 192–196.
39. SCALLET, A. C. & W. SLIKKER, JR. 1992. Biomarkers of developmental neurotoxicity. *In* Risk Assessment of Prenatally-Induced Adverse Health Effects. D. Neubert, R. J. Kavlock, H-J. Merker & J. Klein, Eds. 63–78. Springer-Verlag. Berlin, Heidelberg.

# Discussion

D. K. J. E. von Lubitz (*National Institute of Diabetes and Digestive and Kidney Diseases, NIH, Bethesda, MD*): It is very encouraging that quantitative (morphologic) analysis is being used again. Silver staining helped to determine that striatal neurons become damaged long before the CA4 sector following a brief ischemia (Crain et al., 1988), and quantitative electron microscopy (EM) revealed as early as 1983, that synapses in the CA1 striatum are severely deranged already 10 min after ischemia (von Lubitz and Diemer, 1983).

S. Goldin (*Cambridge NeuroScience*): Lamotragine (LTG), you stated, is maximally neuroprotective at 10-times the anticonvulsant dose. Is this also true for BW619C89?

J. H. Swan (*Wellcome Research Laboratories, Beckenham, UK*): No. BW619C89 is weaker as an anticonvulsant. The maximal neuroprotectant dose of BW619C89 of approximately 20 mg/kg is 2 times the anticonvulsant dose.

A. Scallet (*National Center for Toxicological Research, FDA, Jefferson, AR*): Would kyneurenate itself be expected to be neuroprotective in the spontaneously hypertensive rat (SHR), since it may not cross the blood-brain barrier effectively?

Swan: Kyneurenate is known to protect infarct volume in the normotensive rat following ip administration. Its lack of effect in the SHR is probably due to the inherent cerebrovascular differences between normotensive and SH rats.

Scallet: Does BW619C89 effect blood pressure or body temperature in control animals or ischemic animals?

Swan: BW619C89 has no effect on body temperature in either control or ischemic animals. In anesthetized animals, BW619C89 has a transient effect on blood pressure and heart rate, but recovery to control levels is quick. However, in conscious rats, BW619C89 has no adverse cardiovascular effects. Moreover, in humans BW619C89 has no significant effects on these cardiovascular parameters.

G. C. Palmer (*Fisons Pharmaceuticals, Rochester, NY*): Do you use only a middle cerebral artery (MCA) infarct or do you use unilateral carotid clamping in conjection with your model? I believe you get a larger infarct with the MCA plus unilateral carotid clamping.

Swan: I use only the MCA infarct. It is true that some investigators claim larger, more consistent infarcts using both.

W. Slikker (*National Center for Toxicological Research, FDA, Jefferson, AR*): What criteria can be used to validate animal models of neurotoxicological insult?

Scallet: One criteria would be that the measure be reflective of the actual neuronal damage. That is, either a direct measure of structural damage or an indirect (neurochemical, behavioral) measure that has been shown to correlate highly with structural damage. Another criteria would be that the endpoint be measurable and subject to standard procedures of experimental design and statistical analysis. If there is a good strong cross-correlation between measures obtained from a set of several models, the validation will be more generally acceptable.

Candidate animal models for cross-validation would certainly include MCA occlusion (MCAO), kainate or other know dose-determined lesion models, percussion head-injury models, mitochondrial neurotoxicants and others.

Z. BINIENDA (*National Center for Toxicological Research, FDA, Jefferson, AR*): There is no single ideal animal model that could be directly extrapolated to human. None of the models addresses all the particular factors of the multifactorial neurotoxicological insult. The set of endpoints that would be similar to human should be considered.

PALMER: Your rat data indicate at 50% infarct reduction after iv calcitonin gene-related peptide (CGRP) in the MCA model. Why do you feel you need to go to intrathecal administration—is the blood-brain barrier compromised during MCA? Thus, CGRP would be readily available to the brain.

J. HOLLAND (*Atkinson Morley's Hospital, London*): From the clinical standpoint, systemic dosing of CGRP produces too many side effects. There is also a question as to whether CGRP receptors are found on tiny arterioles and capillaries which act to increase cerebral blood flow.

ANONYMOUS: Have you looked at behavioral effects following fetal hypoxia in rats at any age later than one month?

BINIENDA: Yes, we tested them in the complex maze with water reinforcement at postnatal day 50, however, without any positive results. I think we need to find more sensitive tests (*e.g.*, passive avoidance) and also perform them at later ages.

SLIKKER: What endpoints are most important for assessment of neurological damage (*i.e.*, models for assessment of neuroprotective agents)?

BINIENDA: There is a set of endpoints (histopathological, behavioral, neurochemical, electrophysiological) that should be addressed in the models. It is hard to say what endpoints are more or less important, but it seems that neurobehavior is an important endpoint if it is sensitive enough.

SWAN: In the MCAO model, which has been used in the evaluation of efficacy of BW619C89, we assessed reduction of infarct volume and attenuation of neurological deficit. I believe these two parameters to be of major importance when investigating a neuroprotective agent. Clinicians look for improvement of neurological deficit as a marker for efficacy. So if such an improvement can be illustrated in animal models, I believe this to be a most important endpoint.

SCALLET: A variety of endpoints must be used. It is important, as Dr. Swan's data demonstrate, to monitor the volume of effected tissue following a controlled insult such as MCAO. However, it is also important to monitor the severity of tissue damage *within* the damaged region. Thus, are cells killed outright within this area? What percentage are killed? Are the remainder impaired as indicated by Golgi methods, etc.?

GOLDIN: Is the bell-shaped dose-response curve for neuroprotection observed with LTG due to hypotensive effects at high doses? Is the contrast with the dose-response profile of BW619C89 explainable in terms of the channel selectivity profiles of the two compounds?

SWAN: The differences are unrelated to ion channel selectivity. LTG only reduces infarct volume and neurological score at one dose of 20 mg/kg. At high intravenous doses, lamotrigine is profoundly hypotensive which may contribute to the bell-shaped dose-response curve. In contrast, BW619C89 only produces a

## DISCUSSION

transient hypotension in anesthetized animals (Graham, S. H., J. Chen, J. Lan, *et al.,* J. Pharm. Exp. Ther., 1994, *269:* 854–859).

ANONYMOUS: Have you applied the silver degeneration stain technique to the fetal model of hypoxia? This is of major interest, since brain regions most vulnerable following global mild fetal hypoxia have not been characterized.

BINIENDA: Yes, we tried to stain brain sections (cortex, hippocampus) three days after the hypoxic insult and did not observe neuronal damage. The problem is to find an appropriate time window for this type of analysis so damage has time to develop and dead cells will not be removed by the macrophages.

ANONYMOUS: What is the minimum animal model pharmacology one would need before one would test a compound clinically for neuroprotection?

BINIENDA: Animal models only address certain aspects of this problem. As there may not be a single, ideal neuroprotective drug, there may not be a single, ideal animal model to investigate the multifactional process of hypoxic brain damage.

# Brain Injury and Inflammation

## A Putative Role of TNFα

BABAK ARVIN,[a] LEWIS F. NEVILLE,[b] FRANK C. BARONE,[a]
AND GIORA Z. FEUERSTEIN[a,c]

[a] *Department of Cardiovascular Pharmacology*
*SmithKline Beecham Pharmaceuticals*
*King of Prussia, Pennsylvania 19046*
*and*
[b] *Department of Surgery*
*Jefferson Medical College*
*Philadelphia, Pennsylvania 19107*

## INTRODUCTION

The response to tissue injury in the periphery is manifested by the rapid production of a wide array of inflammatory mediators that initiate inflammatory processes. A key mediator of this response is tumor necrosis factor-α (TNFα), which acts as a pleiotropic peptide to elicit the production of other cytokines (*e.g.*, interleukin (IL)-1β, IL-6, IL-8), endothelial cell adhesion molecules (*e.g.*, endothelial leukocyte adhesion molecule 1 (ELAM-1), intercellular adhesion molecule 1 (ICAM-1), VCAM-1) and to upregulate surface adhesion ligands on neutrophils and monocytes (*e.g.*, very late activation antigen 4 (VLA-4), leukocyte function-associated antigen 1 (LFA-1), and Mac-1 integrins: for reviews see Refs. 1–3). The resultant activation of cytokine-adhesion molecule interaction promotes neutrophil adherence to activated endothelium and tissue infiltration. Ensuing tissue damage occurs as a direct consequence of the transendothelial migration of neutrophils and their generation of oxygen radicals and cytotoxic enzymes into surrounding tissue.[4] The ability of neutralizing anti-TNFα monoclonal antibodies to prevent this inflammatory cascade in the periphery, suggests a key role for TNFα in inflammation.[5]

The inflammatory response of the brain to injury (*e.g.*, following a loss in blood supply as in ischemia) parallels the systemic reactions described above.[6] Thus, infiltration and activation of polymorphonuclear leukocytes (PMNs) into the infarct occurs within 6–12 hours after the insult,[7–10] which persists for several days and declines 2–4 weeks later. These findings have been demonstrated in experimental models of stroke[11–13] and head injury[14,15] and in the human ischemic brain.[16]

The responses of the brain to ischemia can be characterized by immediate membrane channel dysfunction leading to an increase in intracellular $Na^+$, $Ca^{++}$ and $Cl^-$ ions and accumulation of extracellular $K^+$ together with depletion of

---

[c] Author for correspondence.

oxygen, glucose and cellular acidosis. The depolarized state leads to a sequelae of biochemical changes including $Ca^{++}$-dependent and -independent transmitter release (notably glutamate) into the extracellular fluid and intracellular modification of enzymes. Clearly, at this early stage, the introduction of $Na^+$ and $Ca^{++}$ ion channel blockers[17] and glutamate receptor antagonists[18] can be beneficial. Nevertheless, the "lag-time" for patient drug administration following a stroke clearly limits the therapeutic exploitation of such treatment paradigms.

This review will discuss the concept that TNFα is involved in the latter stages of brain injury, in particular of that seen following ischemia. New insights into the role of TNFα under these conditions could provide a new therapeutic arsenal to combat stroke.

## Evidence for CNS Production of TNFα

Recently, the presence of TNFα has been reported in different cellular elements of the central nervous system (CNS), including microglia, astrocytes and neurons.[19] Furthermore, radio-ligand binding studies have shown the existence of high-affinity TNFα receptors within the CNS.[20] Evidence for a biological role of TNFα within the CNS has been derived from its ability to stimulate the proliferation of astrocytes[21] and neuronal progenitor cells.[22-24] Additionally, TNFα has been shown to modulate benzodiazepine binding sites in cultured astrocytes,[25] and TNFα immunoreactivity has been localized in striatal neurones following surgical injury to the hippocampus.[26] Furthermore, elevated levels of locally produced TNFα have been reported in certain CNS diseases such as meningococcal meningitis,[27,28] HIV infection,[29,30] Alzheimer's disease,[31] multiple-sclerosis,[32,33] and experimentally-induced brain injury (TABLE 1). Therefore, these findings strongly suggest the involvement of TNFα in numerous physiological and pathological processes within the CNS.

## Involvement of TNFα in Brain Injury

There are few reports linking the role of TNFα to brain injury. Indirect evidence for a putative role of TNFα in neuronal excitotoxicity is derived from findings using a proconvulsive dose of the excitotoxin kainic acid. In these studies, intraperitoneal administration of kainic acid induced TNFα mRNA expression in the hippocampus, cerebral cortex, thalamus, and hypothalamus.[34] However, a peptide expression was not evaluated in these studies. Our group recently evaluated the effect of middle cerebral artery occlusion (MCAO) on TNFα mRNA accumulation and peptide localization within the CNS.[35] In this study, an induction of TNFα mRNA was observed in the ischemic cortex 1–3 hr following the insult. This increase in TNFα mRNA peaked by 12 hr and persisted for 5 days. Furthermore, TNFα peptide was localized within nerve fibres 6–12 hr post-MCAO, indicating a possible key role of neuronally derived TNFα in promoting the infiltration of inflammatory cells following ischemia. The time course of TNFα peptide expression and leukocyte recruitment would suggest that TNFα may play a key role as

TABLE 1. Role of TNFα in Brain Injury[a]

| Model | Observations | Reference |
|---|---|---|
| Trauma | | |
| Rat, closed head injury, TNFα cytotoxicity assay | TNFα activity increased in the contused hemisphere (peak at 4 hr) | Shohami, E. et al. 1994[15] |
| Rat, fluid percussion brain trauma, Northern blots | early increase in TNFα mRNA expression in injured brain | Fan, K. et al. 1993[14] |
| Human, severe head injury, ELISA on serum TNF | serum TNFα levels increased after severe head injury | Goodman, J.C. et al. 1990[63] |
| Rat, fluid percussion trauma, ELISA | TNFα levels elevated (at 3 hr, 8 hr), returned to basal at 18 hr | Toulmond, T.V. et al. 1993[64] |
| Mice, injection of saline with charcoal into hippocampus, immunohistochemistry | within 6 days TNFα was observed in neurons in striatum & thalamus | Thelingerian, J.L. et al. 1993[65] |
| Neurotoxicity | | |
| Rat, LPS injection, ip, RT-PCR | TNFα mRNA was induced (+60 min) in the pituitary & hypothalamus, but not in striatum or hippocampus | Gatti, S. et al. 1993[66] |
| Rat, kainic acid, ip, RT-PCR | TNFα mRNA was increased (+2 hr +4 hr) in cortex, hippocampus, striatum, thalamus & hypothalamus | Minami, M. et al. 1991[34] |
| Rat, LPS, iv, icv, TNFα bioassay | LPS (iv) increased blood TNFα, LPS (icv) increased blood and CSF TNFα. | Siren, A.L. et al. 1992[67] |
| Ischemia | | |
| Rat (SHR), PMCAO, Northern blots, immunohistochemistry, histology | TNFα mRNA increased in ischemic cortex (+1 hr to 5 days post-MCAO), TNFα immunohistochemistry demonstrated in neurons after MCAO | Liu, T. et al. 1994[36] |
| Rat (SHR), MCAO with reperfusion, Northern blots | increase TNFα mRNA from 1–24 h after ischemia | Wang, X.K. et al. 1994[45] |

[a] CSF = colony-stimulating factor; ELISA = enzyme-linked immunosorbent assay; LPS = lipopolysaccharide; PMCAO = permanent middle cerebral artery occlusion; RT-PCR = reverse transcription–polymerase chain reaction; SHR = spontaneously hypertensive rats.

a primary "trigger" for the early infiltration of PMNs as measured by myeloperoxidase activity (FIG. 1). That is, the rapid and sustained induction of TNFα (within an hour following ischemia) elicits the production of other cytokines (e.g., IL-1β, IL-6), and also chemokines,[36] which promote neutrophil infiltration into the infarct area. Additional evidence for this scenario is derived from studies in which focal administration of TNFα into rat cortex produced significant PMN accumulation in capillaries and adherence in small blood vessels within 24 hr after microinjection.[35]

*Role of PMNs in Brain Injury*

A pivitol link in the development of ischemic injury is the accumulation of PMNs. This is strongly reinforced by the use of highly specific antileukocytic

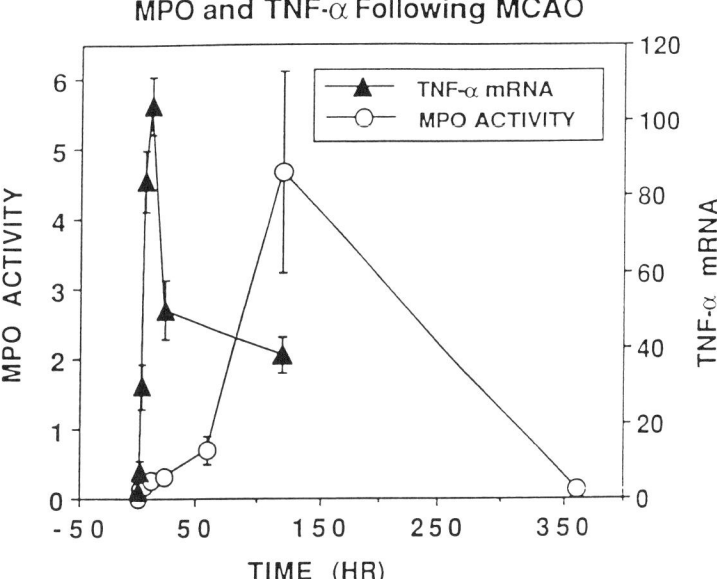

**FIGURE 1.** Time course for myeloperoxidase (MPO) activity (units/gm wet weight; *left axis; open circles*) in ischemic cortex following permanent middle cerebral artery occlusion (PMCAO). MPO activity is an index of the influx of leukocytes following PMCAO as described in Ref. 62. Also plotted for comparative purpose is the time course for TNFα mRNA expression in ischemic cortex following PMCAO (percent radioactivity of macrophage standard reference after correction for loading differences on Northern blots; *right axis; solid triangles*). TNFα protein was identified in ischemic cortical neurons using immunohistochemical techniques as described in Ref. 36.

antibodies, which effectively "buffer" neutrophils and provide protection against ischemia. For example, in a rat MCAO model followed by reperfusion, anti-neutrophil antiserum[37] or monoclonal antibodies[38] attenuated the ischemia-induced infarct. Similar protective effects were reported following the administration of mechloroethamine and vinblastine in dog and rat models of ischemia, respectively.[39,40] Moreover, in rat global cerebral ischemia either vinblastine-induced neutropenia[41] or antineutrophil serum[42] is neuroprotective. In summary, it would appear that depletion of leukocytes can afford protection against experimentally-induced ischemic brain injury. However, the clinical implementation of this approach may not be appropriate.

### *Role of Adhesion Molecules in Brain Injury*

Based on the accumulation and adherence of PMNs to capillaries in cerebral ischemia, it is likely, in parallel with the systemic response to inflammation, that adhesion molecule upregulation occurs both on the endothelial and on the PMN side. In support of this notion, it has been shown that glial cells respond to TNFα (and IL-1β) by expressing ELAM-1, ICAM-1 and VCAM-1.[43] Also, integrin upregulation has been reported in PMNs in response to TNFα.[44] However, although evidence is quite compelling for leukocyte migration and adherence into ischemic tissue, identification of the specific adhesion molecule on brain capillaries in this process has not been clearly defined. Recent studies from our laboratory using the rat MCAO model of ischemia showed an early (1–3 hr) expression of ICAM-1 mRNA which persisted for 24 hrs, and early upregulation of ELAM-1 mRNA (6 hr) which persisted for 5 days.[45] Furthermore, in a primate model of transient focal cerebral ischemia, both ICAM-1 and P-selectin were upregulated following the insult.[46]

Thus, it seems that there are at least three main steps required for leukosequestration following brain injury. First, the generation of TNFα and presumably related cytokines (*e.g.*, IL-1β). Second, the production of a chemotactic gradient to promote neutrophil infiltration into inflamed foci. Third, the co-ordinated expression of endothelial and leukocyte adhesion molecules.

### *Potential TNFα-Directed Therapeutic Strategies for Prevention of Brain Injury*

It would appear that cytokines, in particular TNF and chemokines, play major roles in the development of brain inflammation following ischemia. Moreover, the accumulation of PMNs in ischemic tissue appears to contribute in a major way to brain injury. Hence, effective pharmacological strategies to prevent such damage are likely to focus on inhibition of PMN accumulation and/or inhibition of cytokine synthesis as discussed below.

#### *Inhibition of TNFα Synthesis*

*Effect at Transcriptional Level.* One of the ways which the cellular production of TNFα can be controlled is at the level of transcription. Therefore, TNFα mRNA synthesis inhibitors could be useful drugs for the treatment of brain injury. Such drugs include phosphodiesterase IV inhibitors such as rolipram, which is a specific TNFα synthesis inhibitor in vitro.[47] Other novel classes of drugs could include highly specific protein kinase C (PKC) inhibitors such as calphostin C, which has been shown to potently inhibit lipopolysaccharide (LPS)-stimulated TNF production from human monocytes *in vitro*.[48]

*Effect at Translational Level.* TNFα production can also be controlled at the level of translation.[1] Thus drugs that can hamper translation by dissociating mRNAs from ribosomes could be useful in preventing ischemic injury. Such drugs include pyridinyl imidazoles,[49] which have been found to be potent translational inhibitors of TNF and IL-1 independent of cyclic adenosine monophosphate (cAMP) elevating mechanisms.[50]

*Inhibition of TNFα Action*

This approach would include drugs that neutralize TNFα, such as anti-TNFα monoclonal antibodies (mAbs) or soluble TNFα receptors. Better types of drugs could be derived from the development of TNFα receptor antagonists which currently remain elusive.

*Interference with Adhesion of Leukocytes*

A possible therapeutic paradigm to prevent brain inflammation could be through the use of highly specific antibodies against adhesion molecules. Two examples where this strategy has been evaluated in experimental models include monoclonal antibodies directed against ICAM and CD11/CD18 (integrin) adhesion molecules. Both these treatments afforded protection in animal models of ischemia.[51–54] The recent availability of recombinantly expressed soluble ICAM-1 and ELAM-1 fragments, also might represent a future therapeutic strategy to prevent neutrophil accumulation in cerebral ischemia.

## SUMMARY

This review has focused on the role of inflammatory cells and cytokines, in particular TNF, in the pathophysiology underlying stroke. The pattern of events following an ischemic insult (*i.e.*, time course of appearance of inflammatory mediators and histopathological findings) parallel those reported in the periphery following tissue injury. TNFα produced centrally in the brain would appear to be critical in mediating tissue injury as well as orchestrating the production of other key inflammatory and procoagulant mediators (*e.g.*, chemokines, adhesion molecules and platelet activating factor) required for fulminant brain injury. However, it should be noted that although TNFα may play a pivotal role in tissue damage underlying ischemia, the accumulating evidence also indicates that TNFα is very important in the repair and regeneration of injured tissue. TNFα has been shown to act synergistically with IL-1β to stimulate the production of nerve growth factor (NGF) from astrocytes in culture.[55] In turn, NGF and other similar growth factors (*e.g.*, basic fibroblast growth factor and insulin-like growth factor) have been shown to be protective in numerous neurotoxic models *in vitro* and *in vivo*.[56–60] Moreover, in cultured hippocampal, cortical and septal neurones, TNFα prevented neuronal death following both metabolic (glucose deprivation) and excitotoxic (via application of glutamate, $N$-methyl-D-aspartate (NMDA)) and $\alpha$-amino-3-hydroxy-5-methylisoxazole-4-proprionic acid (AMPA) challenge.[19] The mechanism by which growth factors afford neuroprotection is unclear, but could involve their ability to stabilize intracellular $Ca^{++}$[19] and/or quench free radicals.[61]

## CONCLUSION

Based on the above information, TNFα inhibition may prevent brain injury and inflammation following stroke. However, such treatment paradigms may also inhibit the TNFα-dependent healing processes initiated in the CNS following an ischemic episode. This situation is somewhat analogous to sepsis and septic shock, in which low, but not high doses of TNF are thought to be beneficial in mounting a successful immune response. The development of drugs to target TNFα in brain injury is only beginning and will depend on establishing the methodology to accurately quantify and localize tissue cytokine levels.

## REFERENCES

1. TRACEY, K. J. & A. CERAMI. 1993. Tumor necrosis factor, other cytokines and disease. Annu. Rev. Cell Biol. **9:** 317–343.
2. POBER, J. S. & R. S. COTRAN. 1990. Cytokines and endothelial cell biology. Physiol. Rev. **70:** 427–451.
3. SPRINGER T. A. 1990. Adhesion receptors of the immune system. Nature **346:** 425–434.
4. HALLENBECK, J. M. & A. J. DUTKA. 1990. Background review and current concepts of reperfusion injury. Arch. Neurol. **47:** 1245–1254.
5. FONG, Y., K. J. TRACEY, L. L. MOLDAWER, D. G. HESSE, K. B. MANOGUE, J. S. KENNEY, A. T. LEE, G. C. KUO, A. C. ALLISON, S. F. LOWRY & A. CERAMI. 1989. Antibodies to cachectin/tumor necrosis factor reduce interleukin 1β and interleukin 6 appearance during lethal bacteremia. J. Exp. Med. **170:** 1627–1633.
6. KOCHANEK, P. M. & J. M. HALLENBECK. 1992. Polymorphonuclear leukocytes and monocytes/macrophages in the pathogenesis of cerebral ischemia and stroke. Stroke **23:** 1367–1379.
7. DERESKI, M. O., M. CHOPP, R. A. KNIGHT, H. CHEN & J. H. GARCIA. 1992. Focal cerebral ischemia in the rat: temporal profile or neutrophil responses. Neurosci. Res. Commun. **11:**179–186.
8. CLARK, R. K., E. V. LEE, C. J. FISH, R. F. WHITE, W. J. PRICE, Z. L. JONAK, G. Z. FEUERSTEIN & F. C. BARONE. 1993. Development of tissue damage, inflammation and resolution following stroke: an immunohistochemical and quantitative planimetric study. Brain Res. Bull. **31:** 565–572.
9. CLARK, R. K., E. V. LEE, R. F. WHITE, Z. L. JONAK, G. Z. FEUERSTEIN & F. C. BARONE. 1994. Reperfusion following focal stroke hastens inflammation and resolution of ischemic injury. Brain Res. Bull. **35:** 387–392.
10. BARONE, F. C., L. M. HILLEGASS, M. N. TZIMAS, D. B. SCHMIDT, J. J. FOLEY, R. F. WHITE, W. J. PRICE, G. Z. FEUERSTEIN, R. K. CLARK, D. E. GRISWOLD & H. M. SARAU. 1995. Changes in myeloperoxidase activity and leukotriene B4 receptor binding reflect leukocyte influx in cerebral focal stroke. Mol. Chem. Neuropathol. **24:** 13–30.
11. BARONE, F. C., D. B. SCHMIDT, W. J. PRICE, R. F. WHITE, G. Z. FEUERSTEIN, R. K. CLARK, E. V. LEE, D. E. GRISWOLD & H. M. SARAU. 1992. Reperfusion increases neutrophils and LTB₄ receptor binding in rat focal ischemia. Stroke **23:** 1337–1348.
12. GARCIA, J. H. & Y. KAMIJYO. 1974. Cerebral infarction: evolution of histopathological changes after occlusion of a middle cerebral artery in primates. J. Neuropathol. Exp. Neurol. **33:** 409–421.
13. HALLENBECK, J. M., A. J. DUTKA, T. TANISHIMA, P. M. KOCHANEK, K. K. KUMMAROO, C. B. THOMPSON, T. P. OBRENOVITCH & T. J. CONTRERSA. 1986. Polymorphonuclear leukocyte accumulation in brain regions with low blood flow during the early postischemic period. Stroke **17:** 246–253.
14. FAN, K., P. R. YOUNG, F. C. BARONE, G. Z. FEUERSTEIN, T. A. GENNARELLI, D. H. SMITH & T. K. MCINTOSH. 1993. Experimental traumatic brain injury induces expression of tumor necrosis factor-α mRNA in the rat brain. Eleventh Annual Neurotrauma Society Meeting, Washington, DC, 1993. (Abstract).
15. SHOHAMI, E., M. NOVIKOV, R. BASS, A. YAMIN & R. GALLILY. 1994. Closed head injury triggers early production of TNFα and IL-6 by brain tissue. J. Cereb. Blood Flow Metab. **14:** 615–619.

16. POZZILLI, C., G. L. LENZI, C. ARGENTINO, A. CAROLEI, M. RASURA, A. SIGNOR, L. BOZZAO & P. POZZILI. 1985. Imaging of leukocytic infiltration in human cerebral infarcts. Stroke **16:** 251–255.
17. FEUERSTEIN, G. Z., J. HUNTER & F. C. BARONE. 1992. Calcium channel blockers and neuroprotection. *In* Emerging Strategies in Neuroprotection. H. Lal & P. J. Marango, Eds. 129–150. Brikhauser. Boston.
18. MELDRUM, B. 1990. Protection against ischemic neuronal damage by drugs using an excitatory neurotransmission. Cerebrovasc. Brain Metab. Rev. **2:** 27–57.
19. CHENG, B., S. CHRISTAKOS & M. P. MATTSON. 1994. Tumor necrosis factors protect neurons against metabolic-excitotoxic insults and promote maintenance of calcium homeostasis. Neuron **12:** 139–153.
20. SMITH, R. A. & C. BAGLIONI. 1992. Characterization of TNF receptors. Immunol. Ser. **56:** 149–160.
21. SELMAJ, K. W., M. FAROOQ, W. T. NORTON, C. S. RAINE & C. F. BROSNAN. 1990. Proliferation of astrocytes *in vitro* in response to cytokines. A primary role for tumor necrosis factor. J. Immunol. **144:** 129–135.
22. BAZAN, J. F. 1991. Neuropoietic cytokines in the hematopoietic fold. Neuron **7:** 197–208.
23. MERRILL, J. E. 1992. Tumor necrosis factor alpha, interleukin 1 and related cytokines in brain development: normal and pathologic. Dev. Neurosci. **14:** 1–10.
24. MEHLER, M. F., R. ROZENTAL, M. DOUGHERTY, D. C. SPRAY & J. A. KESSLER. 1993. Cytokine regulation of neuronal differentiation of hippocampal progenitor cells. Nature **362:** 62–65.
25. BOURDIOL, F., S. TOULMOND, A. SERRANO, J. BENVIDES & B. SCATTON. 1991. Increase in $\omega 3$ (peripheral type benzodiazepine) binding sites in the rat cortex and striatum after local injection of interleukin-1, tumour necrosis factor-$\alpha$ and lipopolysaccharide. Brain Res **543:** 194–200.
26. TCHELINGERIAN, J.-L., J. QUINONERO, J. BOOSS & C. JACQUE. 1993. Localization of TNF$\alpha$ and IL-1$\alpha$ immunoreactivites in striatal neurons after surgical injury to hippocampus. Neuron **10:** 213–224.
27. LEIST, T. P., K, FREI, S. KAM-HANSEN, R. M. ZINKERNAGEL & A. FONTANA. 1988. Tumor necrosis factor $\alpha$ in cerebrospinal fluid during bacterial, but not viral, meningitis: evaluation in murine model infections and in patients. J. Exp. Med. **167:** 1743–1748.
28. WAAGE, A., A. HOLSTENSEN, R. SHALABY, P. BRANDTZAEG, P. KIERULF, & T. ESPEVICK. 1989. Local production of tumor necrosis factor $\alpha$, interleukin-1 and interleukin-6 in meningococcal meningitis: relation to the inflammatory response. J. Exp. Med. **170:** 1859–1867.
29. GRIMALDI, L. M. E., G. V. MARTINO, D. M. FRANCIOTTA, R. BRUSTIA, A. COSTAGNO, R. PRISTERA & A. LAZZARIN. 1991. Elevated alpha-tumor necrosis factor levels in spinal fluid from HIV-1 infected patients with central nervous system involvement. Ann. Neurol. **29:** 21–25.
30. MERRILL, J. E. & I. S. Y. CHEN. 1991. HIV-1 macrophages, glial cells, and cytokines in AIDS nervous system brain. J. Exp. Med. **5:** 2391–2397.
31. FILLIT, H., W. DING, L. BUEE, J. KALMAN, L. ALTSTIEL, B. LAWLOR & G. WOLFKLEIN. 1991. Elevated circulating tumor necrosis factor levels in Alzheimer's disease. Neurosci. Lett. **131:** 318–320.
32. HOFMAN, F. M., D. R. HINTON, K. JOHNSON & J. E. MERRILL. 1989. Tumor necrosis factor identified in multiple sclerosis brain. J. Exp. Med. **170:**607–612.
33. SHARIEF, M. K. & E. J. THOMSON. 1992. *In vivo* relationship of tumor necrosis factor-alpha to blood brain barrier damage in patients with active multiple sclerosis. J. Neuroimmunol. **38:** 27–34.
34. MINAMI, M., Y. KURAISHI & M. SATOH. 1991. Effects of kainic acid on messenger RNA levels of IL-1$\beta$, IL-6, TNF$\alpha$ and LIF in the rat brain. Biochem. Biophys. Res. Commun. **176:** 593–598.
35. LIU, T., P. R. YOUNG, P. C. MCDONNELL, R. F. WHITE, F. C. BARONE & G. Z.

FEUERSTEIN. 1993. Cytokine-induced neutrophil chemoattractant mRNA expressed in cerebral ischemia. Neurosci. Lett. **164:** 125–128.
36. LIU, T., R. K. CLARK, P. C. MCDONNELL, P. R. YOUNG, R. F. WHITE, F. C. BARONE & G. Z. FEUERSTEIN. 1994. Tumor necrosis factor-$\alpha$ expression in ischemic neurons. Stroke **25:** 1481–1488.
37. CHEN, H., M. CHOPP & G. BODZIN. 1992. Neutropenia reduces the volume of cerebral infarct after transient middle cerebral artery occlusion in the rat. Neurosci. Res. Commun. **11:** 93–99.
38. SHIGA, Y., H. ONNODERA, K. KOGURE, Y. YAMASAKI, Y. YASHIMA, H. SYOZUHARA & F. SENDO. 1991. Neutrophil as a mediator of ischemic edema formation in the brain. Neurosci. Lett. **125:** 110–112.
39. DUTKA, A. J., P. M. KOCHANEK & J. M. HALLENBECK. 1989. Influence of granulocytopenia on canine cerebral ischemia induced by an embolism. Stroke **20:** 390–395.
40. VASTHARE, U. S., L. A. HEINEL, R. H. ROSENWASSER & R. F. TUMA. 1990. Leukocyte involvement in cerebral ischemia and reperfusion injury. Surg. Neurol. **33:** 261–265.
41. HEINEL, L. A., S. RUBIN, R. H. ROSENWASSER, U. S. VASTHARE & R. F. TUMA. 1994. Leukocyte involvement in cerebral infarct generation after ischemia and reperfusion. Brain Res. Bull. **34:** 137–141.
42. GROGAARD, B., L. SHURER, B. GERDIN & K. E. ARFORS. 1989. Delayed hypoperfusion after incomplete forbrain ischemia in the rat. The role of polymorphonuclear leukocytes. J. Cereb. Blood Flow Metab. **9:** 500–505.
43. ARTHUR, A. A., W. D. LYMAN, M. P. GUIDA, T. M. CALDERON & J. W. BERMAN. 1992. Tumor necrosis factor $\alpha$ induces adhesion molecule expression in human fetal astrocytes. J. Exp. Med. **176:** 1631–1636.
44. ALOISI, F., G. BORSELLINO, P. SAMOGGIA, U. TESTA & C. CHELUCCI. 1992. Astrocyte cultures from human embryonic brain: characterization and modulation of surface molecules by inflammatory cytokines. J. Neurosci. Res. **32:** 494–506.
45. WANG, X. K., T-L. YUE, F. C. BARONE & G. Z. FEUERSTEIN. 1995. Demonstration of increased endothelial-leukocyte adhesion molecule-1 mRNA expression in rat focal ischemic cortex using quantitative reverse transcription and polymerase chain reaction. Stroke. In press.
46. OKADA, Y., B. R. COPELAND, E. MORI, M. M. TUNG, W. S. THOMAS & G. J. DEL ZOPPA. 1994. P-selectin and intercellular adhesion molecule-1 expression after focal brain ischemia and reperfusion. Stroke **25:** 202–211.
47. SEMMLER, J. H., H. WACHTEL & S. ENDRES. 1993. The specific type IV phosphodiesterase inhibitor rolipram suppresses tumor necrosis factor-$\alpha$ production by human mononuclear cells. Int. J Immunopharmacol. **15:** 409–413.
48. PROBHAKAR, U., D. LIPSHUTZ, M. PULLEN, H. TURCHIN, S. KASSIS & P. NAMBI. 1993. Protein kinase C regulates TNF-alpha production by human monocytes. Eur. Cytokine Network **4**(1): 31–37.
49. YOUNG, P., P. MCDONNELL, D. DUNNINGTON, A. HAND, J. LAYDON & J. LEE. 1993. Pyridinyl imidazoles inhibit IL-1 and TNF production at the protein level. Agents Actions **39:** C67–C69.
50. KASSIS, S. & U. PRABHAKAR. 1993. Inhibition of interleukin-1 (IL-1) and tumor necrosis factor (TNF) production by pryridinyl imidazole compounds is independent of cAMP elevating mechanisms. Agents Actions **39:** C64–C66.
51. CLARK, W. M., K. P. MADDEN, R. ROTHLEIN & J. A. ZIVIN. 1991. Reduction of central nervous system ischemic injury by monoclonal antibody to intercellular adhesion molecule. J. Neurosurg. **75:** 623–627.
52. ZHANG, R. L., M. CHOPP, Y. LI, C. ZALOGA, N. JIANG, M. JONE, M. MIYASAKA & P. WARD. 1994. Anti-ICAM-1 antibody reduces ischemic cell damage after transient middle cerebral artery occlusion in the rat. Neurology **44:** 1747–1751.
53. CHEN, H., M. CHOPP, R. L. ZHANG, G. BODZIN, Q. CHEN, R. J. RUSCHE & R. F. TODD III. 1994. Anti-CD11b monoclonal antibody reduces ischemic cell damage after transient focal cerebral ischemia in rat. Ann. Neurol. **35:** 458–463.
54. CHOPP, M., R. L. ZHANG, H. CHEN, Y. LI, N. JIANG & J. R. RUSCHE. 1994. Post

ischemic administration of an anti-MAC-1 antibody reduces ischemic cell damage after transient middle cerebral artery occlusion in the rat. Stroke 25: 869–876.
55. GADIENT, R. A., K. C. CRON & U. OTTEN. 1990. Interleukin-1 beta and tumor necrosis factor-alpha synergistically stimulate nerve growth factor (NGF) release from cultured rat astrocytes. Neurosci. Lett. 117(3): 335–340.
56. HEFTI, F., J. HARTIKKA & B. KNUSEL. 1989. Function of neurotrophic factors in the adult and aging brain and their possible use in the treatment of neurodegenerative diseases. Neurobiol. Aging 10: 515–523.
57. MATTSON, M. P., Y. ZHANG & S. BOSE. 1993a. Growth factors prevent mitochrondrial dysfunction, loss of calcium homeostasis and cell injury, but not ATP depletion in hippocampal neurons deprived of glucose. Exp. Neurol. 121: 1–13.
58. SHIGENO, T., T. MIMA, K. TAKAKURA, D. I. GRAHAM, G. KATO, Y. HASHIMOTO & S. FURUKAWA. 1991. Amelioration of delayed neuronal death in hippocampus by nerve growth factor. J. Neurosci. 11: 2914–2919.
59. GLUCKMAN, P., N. KEMPT, J. GUAN, C. MALLARD, E. SIRIMANNE, M. DRAGUNOW, M. KLEMPT, K. SINGH, C. WILLIAMS & K. NIKOLICS. 1992. A role of IGF-1 in the rescue of CNS neurons following hypoxic-ischemic injury. Biochem. Biophys. Res. Commun. 182: 593–599.
60. NOZAKI, K., S. P. FINKLESTEIN & M. F. BEAL. 1993. Basic fibroblast growth factor protects against hypoxia-ischemia and NMDA neurotoxicity in neonatal rats. J. Cereb. Blood Flow Metab. 13: 221–228.
61. ZHANG, Y., T. TATSUNO, J. M. CARNEY & M. P. MATTSON. 1993. Basic FGF, NGF, and IGFs protect hippocampal and cortical neurons against iron-induced degeneration. J. Cereb. Blood Flow Metab. 13: 378–388.
62. BARONE, F. C., L. M. HILLEGASS, W. J. PRICE, R. F. WHITE, E. V. LEE, G. Z. FEUERSTEIN, H. M. SARAU, R. K. CLARK & D. E. GRISWOLD. 1991. Polymorphonuclear leukocyte infiltration into cerebral focal ischemic tissue: myeloperoxidase activity assay and histologic verificaiton. J. Neurosci. Res. 29: 336–345.
63. GOODMAN, J. C., C. S. ROBERTSON, R. G. GROSSMAN & R. K. NARAYAN. 1990. Elevation of tumor necrosis factor in head injury. J. Neuroimmunol. 30: 2–3.
64. TOULMOND, T. V., A. SERRANO, J. BENAVIDES & F. ZAVALA. 1993. Increase in IL-6 and TNF levels in rat brain following traumatic lesion. Influence of pre- and posttraumatic treatment with Ro54866, a peripheral-type (p site) ligand. J. Neuroimmunol. 42: 177–185.
65. THELINGERIAN, J. L., J. QUINONERO, J. BOOSS & C. JACQUE. 1993. Immunoreactivities in striatal neurons after surgical injury to the hippocampus. Neuron 10: 213–224.
66. GATTI, S. & T. BARTAI. 1993. Induction of tumor necrosis factor-alpha mRNA in the brain after peripheral endotoxin treatment: comparison with interleukin-1 family and interleukin-6. Brain Res. 624: 291–294.
67. SIREN, A. L., E. HELDMAN, D. DORON, P. G. LYSKO, T. L. YUE, T. LIU, G. Z. FEUERSTEIN & J. HALLENECK. 1992. Release of proinflammatory and prothrombotic mediators in the brain and peripheral circulation in spontaneously hypertensive and normotensive Wistar-Kyoto rats. Stroke 23: 1643–1651.

# Comparison of Glutamine-Enhanced Glutamate Release from Slices and Primary Cultures of Rat Brain

JOHN F. BOWYER,[a,d] GEORGE W. LIPE,[a]
JOHN C. MATTHEWS,[c] ANDREW C. SCALLET,[a] AND
DAVID L. DAVIES[b]

*[a] Division of Neurotoxicology*
*National Center for Toxicological Research*
*Jefferson, Arkansas 72079-9502*
*[b] Department of Anatomy*
*University of Arkansas Medical Sciences*
*Little Rock, Arkansas 72205*
*[c] Department of Pharmacology*
*University of Mississippi School of Pharmacy*
*University, Mississippi 38677*

## INTRODUCTION

Though extracellular levels of glutamate are normally highly regulated, elevated glutamate levels are known to occur in a variety of pathological conditions such as hypoxia, hypoglycemia, and seizure.[1] The increased extracellular levels of glutamate are strongly implicated in the cellular damage that results from such conditions.[2,1,3,4] Previously, attention was directed toward the effect of exogenous glutamine on the $K^+$-evoked release of glutamate from synaptosomes and brain slices.[5–8] Spontaneous release of glutamate, and concomitant NMDA receptor-mediated dopamine (DA) release, evoked by 1 mM of exogenous glutamine has been demonstrated in striatal slices[9] but has not been thoroughly investigated.

Elevated extracellular glutamine could cause elevation of extracellular glutamate by a number of possible mechanisms. Elevated extracellular glutamine could enhance glutamine uptake and, thereby, elevate neuronal and glial cytosolic glutamine. Glutamine can serve as a biochemical precursor of glutamate in presynaptic glutamatergic terminals,[10,6,7] and increased cytosolic glutamine could, therefore, result in increased production of glutamate in these compartments. In glial cells glutamate is converted to glutamine by the action of glutamine synthetase.[11,12] Elevated cytosolic glutamine in glia could inhibit this reaction and indirectly inhibit glial glutamate uptake. Alternatively, extracellular glutaminase present in striatal slices could be a contributing source to the production of glutamate from glutamine.[13]

Extracellular central nervous system (CNS) glutamine levels may normally be

---

[d] Author to whom correspondence should be addressed.

in the 100 µM range or less. However, millimolar concentrations of glutamine have been observed *in vivo* in brain after hepatic failure[14] or portocaval anastomosis.[15] Elevated CNS extracellular glutamine levels may also occur as a result of the action of neurotoxic compounds such as trimethyltin, since regional total tissue content has been observed to increase.[16-18] The studies presented herein were conducted to further elucidate mechanism(s) by which glutamine potentiates glutamate release.

## MATERIALS AND METHODS

### Preparation of Striatal Slices for Superfusion

Unanesthetized male Sprague-Dawley rats weighing 250 to 350 g were decapitated, and striata, hippocampus or brain stem with midbrain were obtained by dissection on ice. Slices, approximately 350 µm thick, from the three brain regions were then prepared using a McIlwain tissue chopper. The striatal and hippocampal slices were incubated at 35°C for 10 min with intermittent aeration in a Krebs-Ringer bicarbonate buffer (K-R buffer) (115 mM NaCl, 1.5 mM KCl, 1.5 mM $K_2HPO_4$, 1.5 mM $MgSO_4$, 10 mM D-glucose, 25 mM $NaHCO_3$, 1.25 mM $CaCl_2$, and 0.1 mM L-ascorbate, pH 7.4, aerated with 95% $O_2$ 5% $CO_2$). When either $Ca^{++}$ or $Mg^{++}$ was omitted from buffer the NaCl concentration was increased to maintain isotonicity. This buffer, with added reagents, was the standard solution for all superfusions and incubations for both the brain slices and primary cultures. [$^3$H]dopamine ([$^3$H]DA) (30 to 36 Ci/mmol; 25 nM final concentration) was then added to the striatal slices while [$^3$H]norepinephrine ([$^3$H]NE) (15 Ci/mmol; 25 nM final concentration) was added to the hippocampal slices. The slices were incubated for an additional 25 min at 35°C. Brain stem slices were prepared (caudal to the pons, $-11.0$, to $-14.0$ mm from the bregma), and incubated for superfusion in a manner identical to the other brain regions with the exception that [$^3$H]catecholamines were omitted.

After incubation the slices were placed (2 brain stem, 3 striatal or 5 hippocampal per chamber) in the superfusion chambers. The weights of the slices in the superfusion chambers were estimated by weighing the unused slices. The apparatus and methods used to superfuse the slices were similar to those described previously.[9] The slices were superfused at a flow rate of 0.8 ml/min at 35°C for 30 min. Test substances were added to the superfusion medium, and 30 min thereafter glutamine (100–1000 µM) was added to the superfusion medium. In all instances the test substances were present during the 30-min glutamine exposure period.

### Determination of Glutamate, [$^3$H]NE and [$^3$H]DA Release and Statistical Evaluations

The levels of amino acids in the superfusate exiting the slices were determined from 200 ul aliquots of the 4-ml fractions collected for 5 min every 5 min starting 5 min prior to glutamine exposure and continuing until 30 min after the initiation of glutamine exposure. The remainder of each fraction was used to determine the fractional release of [³H]catecholamines. At the end of superfusion the slices were immediately removed from the superfusion chambers, frozen on dry ice, and stored at −70°C for later analysis of amino acids and [³H]catecholamines. Values for the release of [³H]DA and [³H]NE or their [³H]metabolites are expressed as the percent of total ³H stores released during each 5-min interval.

The amino acids in the superfusate fractions were determined by derivatization with o-phthaldialdehyde and separation by high-performance liquid chromatography (HPLC) with electrochemical detection using methods similar to Zielke[19] as modified from Lindroth and Mopper.[20] To insure that most of the glutamate and other amino acids detected in the buffers exposed to either slice or primary glial cultures originated from these tissues, amino acids levels were determined in the media exposed to culture or superfusion conditions in which neither slices nor primary cultures were present. The preparation of the superfused slices for determining tissue amino acids levels was similar to that described by Zielke.[19]

### Preparations of Striatal Cultures

Primary astrocyte-enriched cultures were prepared using methods previously described by Davies and Cox.[21] Briefly, the corpora striata of 3-day-old Sprague-Dawley rats were dissected and dissociated by repeated pipetting in a sterile 0.2% trypsin/phosphate-buffered saline (PBS) solution. After incubation for 20 min at 37°C, the suspension was mixed with an equal volume of Dulbecco's modified Eagle's medium (DMEM; Gibco) fortified with 10% fetal bovine serum (FBS:-Hyclone) and triturated. The resultant cell suspension was centrifuged, and the pellet resuspended in DMEM/10% FBS containing penicillin G (25 units/ml), streptomycin (25 $\mu$g/ml) and Fungizone® (Gibco, 1 $\mu$g/ml). The suspension was sieved through 48-$\mu$m Nitex mesh and cells were plated into 24-well tissue culture plates (Corning) at a density equivalent to one striatum per 30 cm². Cultures were incubated at 37°C in a 5% $CO_2$ humidified atmosphere. The nutrient medium was replaced 24 hr after plating and at 2-day intervals thereafter.

### Immunocytochemistry

Cell types present in these primary cultures at 9 days *in vitro* (DIV) were identified by immunocytochemical localization of glial fibrillary acidic protein (GFAP) and neurofilament protein (NFP), respectively. Immunocytochemical procedures were modifications of the unlabeled antibody method of Sternberger et al.[22] Antibodies were purchased from Dako Corp. (Santa Barbara, CA). Control for immunolocalization of GFAP and NFP was the substitution of primary antibodies with normal serum.

### Determination of Amino Acids in the K-R Buffer Perfusate from Primary Cultures

After primary striatal cultures were maintained for 8 DIV, the cultures were rinsed twice with K-R buffer and then 600 $\mu$l of K-R buffer containing the test reagents at 37°C was added. After 30 min exposure amino acids in this perfusate were determined as described above for the superfusates. Incubations were terminated by placing the cultures on ice and samples (300 $\mu$l) of the perfusate were withdrawn and immediately frozen on dry ice and stored at $-70°C$ for subsequent analysis of amino acid content. The remaining 300 $\mu$l of perfusate was then removed from each culture, and the cells were immediately frozen on dry ice for later determination of protein levels[23] and in some instances amino acid content.

Student $t$ test, or, when appropriate, analysis of variance (ANOVA), was used to analyze the various treatments. With data that showed significant differences when analyzed by ANOVA, Duncan's post-hoc tests were used to determine significant differences between individual groups.

## RESULTS

### Glutamate and [³H]Catecholamine from Brain Slices

Glutamine, in the absence of $Mg^{++}$, produced concentration-dependent increases in the release of glutamate and tritium ([³H]DA and [³H]metabolites) from striatal slices, and glutamate and tritium ([³H]NE and [³H]metabolites) from hippocampal slices (FIG. 1). $Mg^{++}$ was omitted to greatly potentiate N-methyl-D-aspartate (NMDA) receptor-mediated dopamine release.[24] Although not shown, either 1.25 mM $Mg^{++}$ or 2.5 $\mu$M MK-801 (a noncompetitive NMDA antagonist) blocked the 1-mM glutamine-enhanced release of catecholamines, but not the glutamate release, from hippocampal and striatal slices. The DA release produced by exposure to 250, 500 or 1000 $\mu$M glutamine was equivalent to the DA release produced by 30, 60 or 100 $\mu$M of exogenous glutamate, respectively.[9]

Neither 2 $\mu$M tetrodotoxin, 100 $\mu$M kainate, 2 $\mu$M quinpriole (DA $D_2$ agonist), nor 5 $\mu$M sulpiride (DA $D_2$ antagonist) affected the glutamine-enhanced glutamate release from striatal slices with 1.25 mM $Ca^{++}$ and 1.5 mM $Mg^{++}$ present (data not shown). The magnitude of the glutamine-enhanced glutamate release was greater in the brain stem than in the forebrain regions (FIG. 2). The release was inhibited to approximately the same extent in all three regions by removal of $Ca^{++}$ for 60 min (FIG. 2) but was not reduced by a 60-min exposure to buffer containing 0.1 mM $Ca^{++}$.

FIGURE 3 shows that in striatal slices, the $Ca^{++}$ antagonist $Cd^{++}$ also reduces the glutamine-enhanced glutamate release. Taurine is concentrated and localized within the striatum,[25] and has been reported to affect DA release[26] and to protect against cellular damage.[27] However, taurine did not significantly reduce glutamine-enhanced glutamate release. Both mechanical compression (M.C.) of striatal slices produced by the blunt end of forceps to create damage, but not penetrate the slices, and a 30-min exposure to 2 mM kynurenate, an antagonist to the glycine binding site on glutamate receptors and an intermediate in the metabolism of kynurenine[28] significantly potentiated the glutamine-enhanced glutamate release in striatal slices (FIG. 3) and hippocampal and brain stem slices (data not shown). The most potent stimulator of glutamate release (3-fold) in brain slices was a 20-min superfusion with hypotonic ($-115$ mM NaCl) K-R buffer 30 min prior to

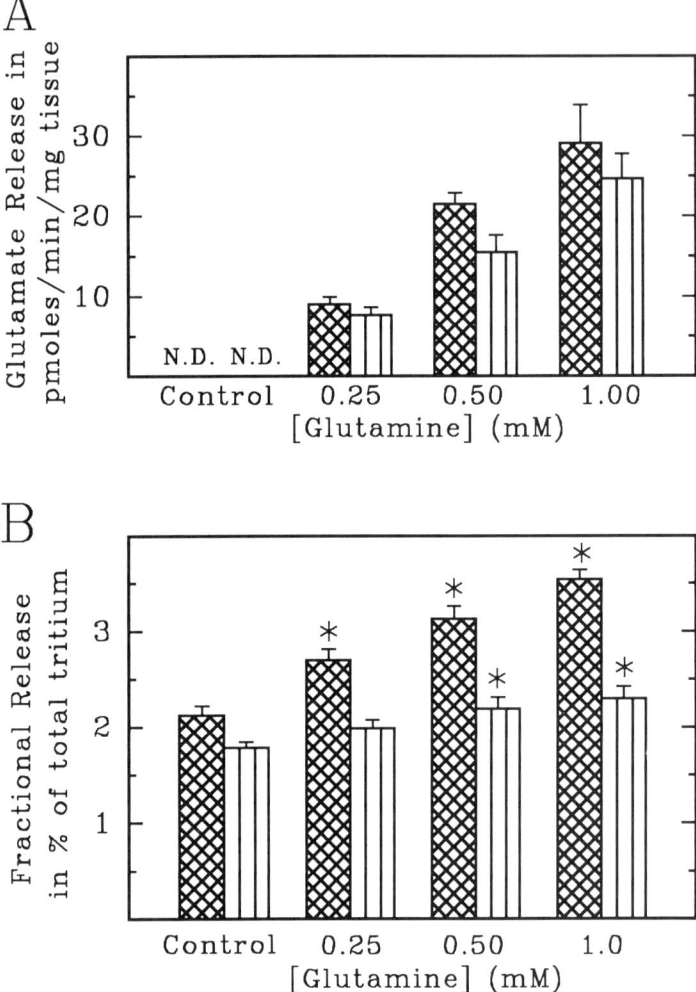

**FIGURE 1.** Glutamine-enhanced release of glutamate and tritium from brain slices. Within 15 min after the addition of glutamine to the superfusion buffer (no $Mg^{++}$ present) an increase was obtained in (**A**) the glutamate efflux from either striatal *(crosshatched bars)* or hippocampal *(striped bars)* slices, and (**B**) the tritium release from either striatal slices labeled with [$^3$H]DA or hippocampal slices labeled with [$^3$H]NE. Five to 15 pairs of slices were used to generate the mean ± SE depicted by each bar. * Tritium release was significantly greater than control ($p < 0.05$).

glutamine exposure (data not shown). Finally, neither 0 nor 10 mM, instead of 1.5 mM, $PO_4^-$ affected glutamine-enhanced glutamate release (data not shown).

*In vitro* exposure to glutamine increased the glutamate and gamma-aminobutyric acid (GABA) content of striatal slices but did not significantly alter the levels of aspartate, glycine or taurine (TABLE 1). Superfusion of striatal slices with 2

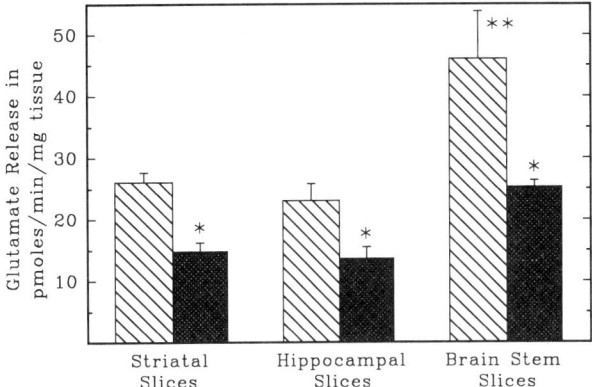

**FIGURE 2.** Effects of $Ca^{++}$ removal on glutamine-enhanced glutamate release from brain slices. The presence *(hatched bars)* or absence *(filled bars)* of 1.25 mM $Ca^{++}$ during superfusion was used to test for $Ca^{++}$ effects on glutamate release from brain slices at 25 to 30 min after 500 μM glutamine exposure. Four to 8 pairs of slices were used to generate the mean ± SE depicted. * Glutamate release was significantly ($p < 0.025$) reduced in the absence of $Ca^{++}$. ** Glutamate release was significantly ($p < 0.025$) greater in brain stem slices when compared with striatal or hippocampal slices.

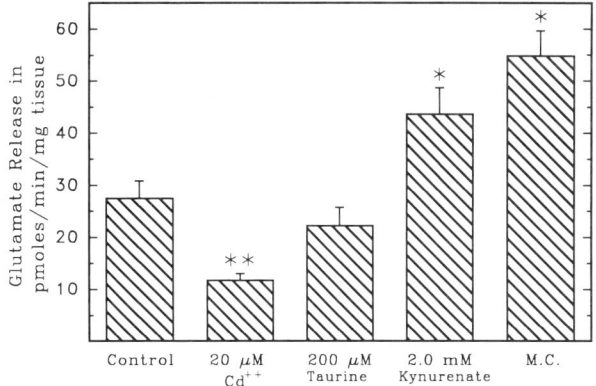

**FIGURE 3.** The effects of various treatments on glutamine-enhanced glutamate release from striatal slices. Slices were exposed to either $Cd^{++}$, taurine, or kynurenate 30 min prior to and during glutamine exposure, or the slices were compression damaged (M.C.) at the time they were placed in the superfusion chamber. Four to 8 pairs of slices were used to generate the mean ± SE depicted. * Glutamate release was significantly ($p < 0.025$) increased over control. ** Glutamate release was significantly ($p < 0.025$) decreased from control.

TABLE 1. Levels (Mean ± S.E. in $\mu$ moles/mg Slice) of Several Amino Acids within Brain Slices after Superfusion in K-R Buffer[a]

| Type of Slice | [Glutamine] Present during Superfusion | Aspartate | Glutamate | Glycine | Taurine | GABA | n |
|---|---|---|---|---|---|---|---|
| Striatal | — | 1.84 ± .08 | 3.57 ± .22 | 0.51 ± .04 | 0.95 ± .12 | 0.66 ± .09 | 6 |
| Striatal | 250 $\mu$M | 2.01 ± .56 | 6.23 ± .41* | 0.43 ± .08 | 1.07 ± .16 | 0.98 ± .15* | 5 |
| Straital | 500 $\mu$M | 2.04 ± .14 | 5.78 ± .32* | 0.56 ± .13 | 1.20 ± .08 | 1.02 ± .04* | 6 |
| Striatal | 500 $\mu$M + 2 mM kynurenate | 2.06 ± .09 | 6.84 ± .58* | 0.58 ± .08 | 1.56 ± .13 | 1.19 ± .15* | 5 |
| Striatal | 500 $\mu$M + damage[b] | 2.43 ± .12 | 5.63 ± .18* | 0.50 ± .05 | 0.94 ± .10 | 0.76 ± .16 | 6 |
| Striatal | 500 $\mu$M (no $Ca^{++}$) | 1.62 ± .13** | 4.95 ± .45* | 0.51 ± .04 | 0.93 ± .12 | 0.99 ± .11* | 8 |
| Hippocampal | 250 $\mu$M | 1.77 ± .10 | 5.99 ± .31 | 0.61 ± .08 | 1.07 ± .11 | 1.06 ± .12 | 8 |
| Hippocampal | 500 $\mu$M | 1.64 ± .09 | 5.32 ± .23 | 0.45 ± .05 | 1.15 ± .13 | 1.19 ± .11 | 6 |
| Brain stem | 500 $\mu$M | 1.15 ± .06 | 1.82 ± .24 | 1.28 ± .08 | N.Q. | 0.75 ± .05 | 5 |

[a] GABA = gamma-aminobutyric acid; N.Q. = not quantitatively determined (levels were below 0.10 $\mu$ moles/mg slice).
[b] Damage to slices was produced by the blunt end of forceps just prior to superfusion.
* Significantly increased by glutamine ($p < 0.02$).
** Significantly decreased by $Ca^{++}$ removal ($p < 0.02$).

mM kynurenate tended to increase the levels of glutamate and taurine in the slice but this increase was not statistically significant. Removal of $Ca^{++}$ decreased the aspartate and glutamate levels within striatal slices; however, only the decrease in aspartate was significant ($p < 0.05$).

## Glutamate and Taurine Release from Cultured Glia

In parallel experiments, the effects of glutamine on glia were assessed in primary cultures of rat striatum. In the primary cultures, immunolocalization of GFAP indicated that astrocytes were predominant, while phase contrast microscopy revealed a subpopulation of phase bright process-bearing cells presumed to be oligodendrocytes. Immunostaining for neurofilament protein was negative; therefore, the cultures were considered to be virtually free of neurons.

To assess the effects of glutamine on glutamate release in these cultures, the cultures were incubated for 30 min in K-R buffer containing exogenous glutamine. Exposure to glutamine produced a concentration-dependent increase in glutamate content of the perfusate. Statistically significant increases were found at concentrations of 250 $\mu$M and greater (FIG. 4).

As previously observed by Kimelberg et al.,[28] osmotic stress and $K^+$ depolarization increased glutamate and taurine levels in the perfusate following exposure to either stimuli for 30 min (FIG. 5). However, glutamate but not taurine levels in the perfusate were potentiated by the addition of 500 $\mu$M glutamine in the presence of osmotic stress and $K^+$ depolarization. Furthermore, glutamine enhanced the release of glutamate evoked by depolarization to a greater extent than osmotic stress. Exposure of the primary cultures to either methamphetamine (METH) or kainate, each at 100 $\mu$M, did not affect taurine release; whereas, kynurenate (1 or 2 mM) slightly elevated taurine release (FIG. 6). Kainate, METH and kynurenate, in the absence of glutamine, did not significantly increase glutamate levels in the perfusate. In the presence of 500 $\mu$M glutamine kynurenate significantly

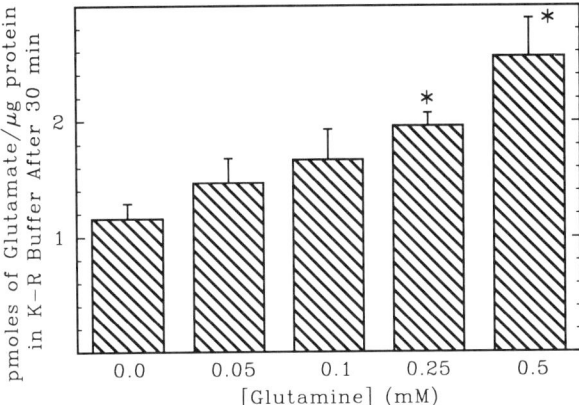

FIGURE 4. Glutamine-enhanced glutamate release from rat primary striatal cultures. Exposure of primary striatal cultures to K-R buffer containing graded concentrations of glutamine produced a concentration-dependent increase in glutamate release. Data represent the mean ± SE of 4 to 8 cultures. * Glutamate levels significantly elevated by glutamine ($p < 0.02$).

increased glutamate levels above those produced by glutamine alone (FIG. 6). The inclusion of glutamine in the buffer was less effective with kainate (no change) or METH (slight increase).

## DISCUSSION

There are several pathological conditions in which extracellular glutamine levels could be elevated in brain.[15,14,16,17] If elevation of extracellular glutamine causes elevated glutamate levels, the potential for cellular damage will be enhanced.[1] Therefore, it is important to identify the mechanism(s) by which glutamine enhances glutamate release. The studies reported here compare glutamine-enhanced glutamate release from brain slices and virtually neuron-free primary striatal cultures. The results of these studies lead us to conclude that glial cells represent an important source of extracellular glutamate under conditions where extracellular glutamine is elevated.

The concentration of $Ca^{++}$ necessary to support glutamine-enhanced glutamate release was found to be below that shown by many investigators to be necessary to support the vesicular release of glutamate. Tetrodotoxin, which inhibits the $Ca^{++}$-dependent synaptosomal release of glutamate,[29] did not affect glutamine-enhanced glutamate release from striatal slices.[8] The release of glutamate from nerve terminals in striatal slices and from synaptosomes has been reported to be regulated by DA $D_2$ receptors.[30,31] However, glutamine-enhanced glutamate release was not affected by a DA $D_2$ agonist or antagonist (FIG. 3). Together, these results indicate that, unlike the release of glutamate evoked by $K^+$ depolarization, when nondepolarizing conditions (4.5 mM $K^+$) are used, the glutamine-enhanced glutamate release is probably not from vesicular stores of neuronal origin.

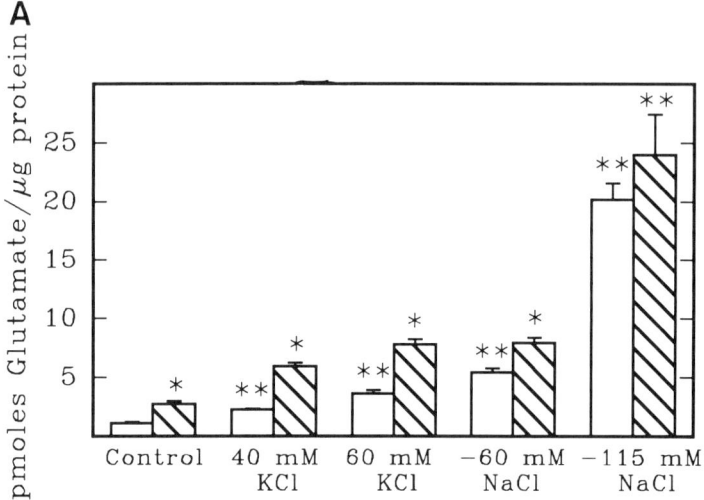
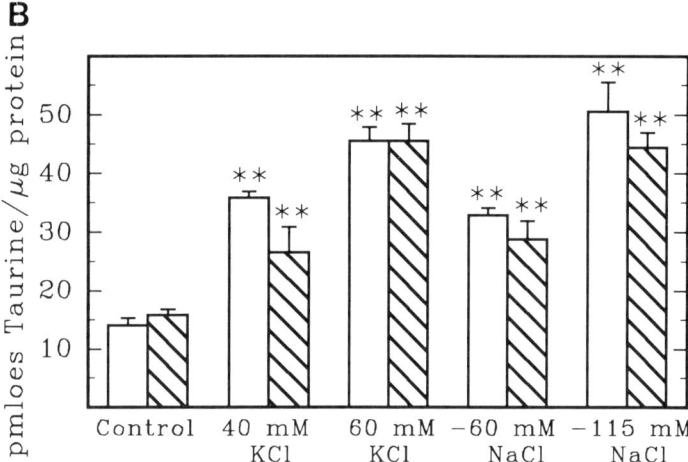

**FIGURE 5.** The effects of osmotic stress and K$^+$ depolarization on **(A)** glutamate and **(B)** taurine release from primary striatal cultures. Exposure of primary striatal cultures to either osmotic stress or depolarization produced an increase in the glutamate and taurine release after 30 min of incubation in the presence *(crosshatched bars)* and absence *(open bars)* of 500 µM glutamine. Data represent the mean ± SE of 4 to 8 cultures. * Glutamate levels were significantly elevated by 500 µM glutamine over those observed for the same condition without glutamine ($p < 0.02$). ** Ionic composition of the K-R buffer significantly increased glutamate and taurine release above controls ($p < 0.02$).

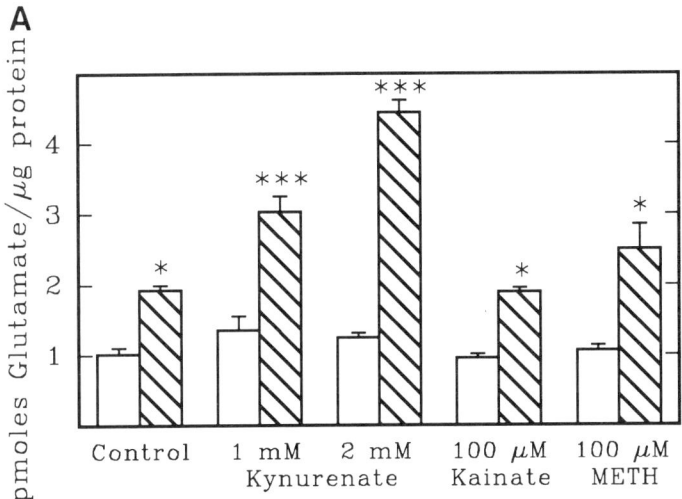

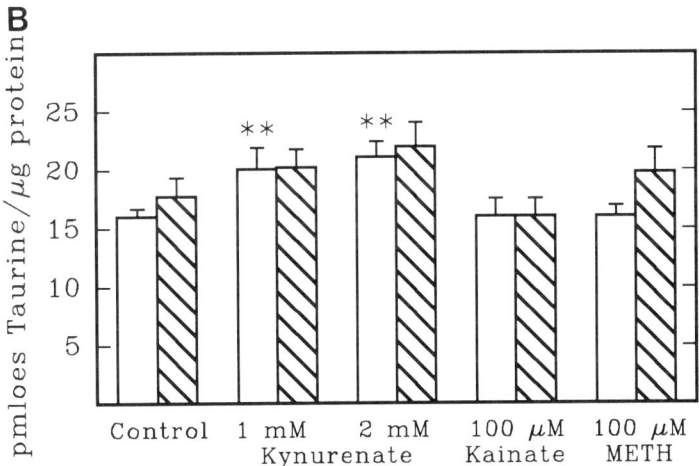

FIGURE 6. Effects of kynurenate, kainate and METH on (A) glutamate and (B) taurine release in primary striatal cultures. The effects of exposing primary striatal cultures for 30 min to various compounds in the presence *(crosshatched bars)* and absence *(open bars)* of 500 µM glutamine on glutamate release are shown. Data represent the mean ± SE of 4 to 8 cultures. * Glutamate levels were significantly elevated by 500 µM glutamine over those observed for the same condition without glutamine ($p < 0.02$). ** Kynurenate significantly increased taurine levels above controls ($p < 0.02$). *** Kynurenate significantly increased glutamate levels above 500 µM glutamine ($p < 0.02$).

The magnitudes of glutamine-enhanced glutamate release is greatest from brain stem slices, and less from either striatum or hippocampus slices (FIG. 2), which does not correlate with the content of glutamatergic terminals in these tissues.[32] Also, alpha-ketoglutarate and not glutamine may be the primary source of glutamate in terminals of cultured granule cells.[33] For these reasons, it is unlikely that vesicular stores of glutamate in nerve terminals are the source of glutamine-enhanced glutamate release from the slices.

Although nonvesicular glutamate release from neuronal terminals could be a primary source of glutamine-enhanced glutamate release in brain slices, there are several mechanisms by which glial cells may be producing this effect. Elevated extracellular glutamine, through enhancement of uptake processes, would be expected to produce increases in glutamine concentrations in glial cytosol. The substrate increase might then stimulate glutaminase activity to convert glutamine to glutamate.[34-36] This process has been demonstrated to occur with astrocytes.[13] In addition, elevated glial concentrations of glutamine would also be expected to produce end-product inhibition of glutamine synthetase. Reduced conversion of glutamate to glutamine within glia would elevate glutamate levels in glial cytosol, and thus, inhibit its further uptake and increase its release. Both of these actions would serve to elevate extracellular glutamate.

The action of glutaminase to convert glutamine to glutamate may be an important process in the glutamine-enhanced elevation of extracellular glutamate in brain slices and primary striatal cultures. Extracellular glutaminase released from damaged glia or neurons is probably not the major contributor to glutamine-enhanced glutamate release from striatal slices and primary cultures for at least three reasons. First, extracellular glutaminase would be sensitive to phosphate concentrations in the buffer superfusing brain slices. Altering the phosphate concentration of the medium had no effect (Results). Second, kynurenate potentiated glutamine-enhanced glutamate release (FIGS. 3 and 6). The mechanisms by which kynurenate increases the conversion of glutamine to glutamate are not clear, but kynurenate should not affect the enzymatic activity of extracellular glutaminase. The final reason is that prolonged withdrawal from $Ca^{++}$ is necessary to inhibit glutamine-enhanced glutamate release from slices. This indicates that a depletion of intracellular $Ca^{++}$ is necessary for this inhibition. Extracellular glutaminase should not be sensitive to intracellular calcium levels.

Reducing the concentration of extracellular $Ca^{++}$ on slices versus cultures produced the only major disparity between the responses observed from brain slices versus striatal cultures. $Ca^{++}$ removal from slices produced decreases in glutamate release in the presence of glutamine (FIG. 2), while in cultured glia a significant increase in the glutamate release was observed (results not shown). Taurine release was also potentiated to the same extent as glutamate in the cultures. Therefore, the mechanisms by which $Ca^{++}$ removal potentiates glutamate release in cultures may not be the same as that produced by either kynurenate or $K^+$ depolarization (FIGS. 5 and 6).

Driscoll et al.[37] have observed that mitochondria containing glutaminase, released from primary mesencephalic cultures, may produce neurotoxic levels of glutamate after 3 hrs exposure in Dulbecco's modified Eagle's medium containing 4 mM glutamine. Their results are not inconsistent with what we observed with primary striatal cultures. However, differences in the present study such as the lower glutamine concentrations, shorter time course of glutamine exposure and buffer composition differences make direct comparisons difficult. Furthermore, although superfusion of striatal slices with glutamine produces only moderate increases in the glutamate released into the superfusion buffer, a prominent NMDA receptor-mediated DA release is evoked by the glutamine exposure.[9] The magnitude of the NMDA receptor-mediated release of DA indicates that glutamate levels around dopaminergic terminals increase by approximately 100 $\mu$M in the presence of 1 mM exogenous glutamine. The time course and magnitude of such a glutamate increase are difficult to envision as being the result of free mitochondria in slice preparations.

In conclusion, the results of this study indicate that a primary source of increased glutamate release from brain slices produced by exogenous glutamine may be glia. Additional studies are necessary to determine whether, under normal physiological conditions, increases in extracellular glutamine result in increased glutamate levels mediated by glial activity, and if more potent and specific drugs can be found to modulate the glutamine-enhanced glutamate release.

## SUMMARY

Increased extracellular glutamate has been associated with a wide range of effects including production of neurotoxicity. Glutamine has previously been shown to cause increased release of glutamate from a variety of preparations. Extracellular central nervous system (CNS) glutamine levels are known to increase with neurotoxin exposures, hepatic failure, renal failure, head trauma or stroke. However, the action of glutamine to enhance the release of glutamate under nondepolarizing conditions has not been well studied. Since glutamine-mediated increases in extracellular glutamate are potentially of significance in cellular damage as a result of CNS insult, further examination of this phenomenon is important.

Striatal and hippocampal slices or virtually neuron-free primary striatal glial cultures were employed in studies to further elucidate the mechanism(s) of glutamine-enhanced glutamate release. Elevated extracellular glutamine caused increased glutamate release in all three preparations. In hippocampal and striatal slices elevated glutamine caused an enhancement of $N$-methyl-D-aspartate (NMDA) receptor-mediated [$^3$H]catecholamine release equivalent to that produced by high concentrations (up to 100 $\mu$M) of exogenous glutamate. In both striatal slices and primary cultures kynurenate increased glutamate release in the presence of 500 $\mu$M glutamine, while kainate either had no effect or decreased glutamate levels in the presence of glutamine. Since several presynaptic modulators of release did not affect the glutamate release produced by glutamine in slices, vesicular release of glutamate from nerve terminals was probably not involved in the effects of the exogenous glutamine. The similarities between striatal slices and primary striatal cultures indicate that enzymatic conversion of glutamine to glutamate within glia may be an important factor in the glutamine-mediated elevation of extracellular glutamate levels.

## REFERENCES

1. ROTHMAN, S. M. & J. W. OLNEY. 1987. TINS. **10**: 299–302.
2. OLNEY, J. W. 1969. Science **164**: 719–720.
3. CHOI, C. W. 1991. J. Neurobiol. **23**: 1261–1276.
4. LOPACHIN, R. M. & M. ASCHNER. 1983. Toxicol & Appl. Pharmacol. **118**: 141–158.
5. BENJAMIN, A. M. & J. H. QUASTEL. 1972. Biochem J. **128**: 631–646.
6. HAMBERGER, A., G. H. CHIANG, E. S. NYLEN, S. W. SCHEFF & C. W. COTTMAN. 1979. Brain Res. **168**: 513–530.
7. WARD, H. K. & H. F. BRADFORD. 1979. J. Neurochem. **33**: 339–342.
8. SZERB, J. C. & P. O. O'REGAN. 1985. J. Neurochem. **44**: 1724–1731.
9. BOWYER, J. F., A. C. SCALLET, R. R. HOLSON, G. W. LIPE, W. SLIKKER, JR. & S. F. ALI. 1991. J. Pharmacol. Exp. Ther. **257**: 262–270.
10. BENJAMIN, A. M. & J. H. QUASTEL. 1974. J. Neurochem. **23**: 457–464.
11. HERTZ, L. 1979. Prog. Neurobiol. **13**: 277–323.
12. SHANK, R. P. & M. H. APRISON. 1981. LIFE SCI. **28**: 837–842.
13. ZIELKE, R. H., J. T. TILDON, C. L. ZIELKE, P. J. BAAB & M. E. LANDRY. 1989. Neurochem. Res. **14**: 327–332.
14. LAVOIE, J., J. F. GIGUERE, G. P. LAYRARGUES & R. F. BUTTERWORTH. 1987. J. Neurochem. **49**: 692–697.
15. BUTTERWORTH, R. F. & J. F. GIGUERE. 1984. *In* Advances in Hepatic Encephalopathy and Urea Cycle Diseases. G. Kleinberger, P. Ferenci, P. Riederer & H. Thaler, Eds. 394–401. Karger. Basel, Switzerland.
16. HIKAL, A. H., W. SLIKKER, JR., S. F. ALI & A. C. SCALLET. 1988. Life Sci. **42**: 125–130.
17. LIPE, G. W., S. F. ALI, G. D. NEWPORT, A. C. SCALLET & W. SLIKKER, JR. 1991. Pharmacol & Toxicol. **68**: 450–455.
18. MATTHEWS, J. C. & A. C. SCALLET. 1991. Neurotoxicology **12**: 547–558.
19. ZIELKE, R. H. 1985. J. Chromatogr. **347**: 320–324.
20. LINDROTH, P. & K. MOPPER. 1979. Anal. Chem. **51**: 1667–1674.
21. DAVIES, D. L. & W. E. COX. 1991. Brain Res. **547**: 53–61.
22. STERNBERGER, L. A., P. H. HARDY, JR., J. J. CUCULIS & H. J. MEYER. 1970. J. Histochem. Cytochem. **18**: 315–333.
23. LOWRY, O. H., N. J. ROSEBROUGH, A. L. FARR & R. J. RANDALL. 1951. J. Biol. Chem. **193**: 265–275.
24. COLLINGRIDGE, G. L. & R. A. J. LESTER. 1989. Pharmacol Rev. **40**: 143–210.
25. DELLA CORTE, L., D. J. CLARKE, J. P. BOLAM & A. D. SMITH. 1987. *In* The Biology of Taurine: Methods and Mechanisms. R. J. Huxtable, F. Franconi & A. Giotti, Eds. 285–294. Plenum Press. New York.
26. KONTRO, P. 1987. *In* The Biology of Taurine: Methods and Mechanisms. R. Huxtable, F. Franconi & A. Giotti, Eds. 347–355. Plenum Press. New York.
27. AZUMA, J., T. HAMAGUCHI, H. OHTA, K. TAKIHARA, N. AWATA, A. SAWAMURA, H. HARADA, Y. TANAKA & S. KISHIMOTO. 1987. *In* The Biology of Taurine: Methods and Mechanisms. R. J. Huxtable, F. Franconi & A. Giotti, Eds. 167–179. Plenum Press. New York.
28. KIMELBERG, H. K., S. K. GODERIE, S. HIGMAN, S. PANG & R. A. WANIEWSKI. 1990. J. Neurosci. **10**: 1583–1591.
29. TIBBS, R., A. P. BARRIE, F. J. E. VAN MIEGHEM, H. T. MCMAHON & D. G. NICHOLLS. 1989. J. Neurochem. **53**: 1693–1699.
30. ROWLAND, G. J. & P. J. ROBERTS. 1980. Eur. J. Pharmacol. **62**: 241–242.
31. MAURA, G., A. GIARDI & M. RAITERI. 1989. J. Pharmacol Exp. Ther. **247**: 680–684.
32. OTTERSEN, O. P. & J. STORM-MATHISEN. 1984. *In* Handbook of Chemical Neuroanatomy. A. Bjorklund, T. Hokfelt & M. J. Kuhar, Eds. Vol. 3, Chap. 5. Elsevier Science. B.V. Canada.
33. PENG, L. A., A. SCHOUSBOE & L. HERTZ. 1991. Neurochem. Res. **16**: 29–34.
34. NIMMO, G. A. & K. F. TIPTON. 1981. Eur. J. Biochem. **117**: 57–64.

35. KVAMME, E., G. SVENNEBY, L. HERTZ & A. SCHOUSBOE. 1982. Neurochem. Res. **7:** 761–770.
36. KVAMME, E., G. SVENNEBY & I. A. TORGNER. 1983. Neurochem. Res. **8:** 25–38.
37. DRISCOLL, B. F., G. E. DEIBLER, M. J. LAW, & A. M. CRANE. 1993. J. Neurochem. **61:** 1795–1800.

# Effect of Hypocapnia on Extracellular Glutamate and Glycine Concentrations during the Periischemic Period in Rabbit Hippocampus[a]

KYU TAEK CHOI,[b,e] JUNG KIL CHUNG,[b] CHUN SIK KWAK,[c] AND HAE KYU KIM[d]

[b] Department of Anesthesiology
[c] Department of Biochemistry
Keimyung University School of Medicine
Taegu 700-310, Korea
[d] Department of Anesthesiology
Pusan National University School of Medicine
Pusan, Korea

## INTRODUCTION

The clinical management of patients in coma after cardiac arrest involves the restoration of adequate cardiopulmonary function to prevent further cerebral injury. Over the years, many therapeutic approaches have been devised to alleviate the dismal outcome of cerebral ischemia. One of these modalities is the idea of regulating $PaCO_2$ to reduce ischemic brain damage. Manipulation of the arterial carbon dioxide tension ($PaCO_2$) is a potent means by which changes in cerebral blood flow (CBF) can be affected. There are many reports that support the beneficial effect of hyperventilation.[1] One of the underlying mechanisms of the beneficial effect of hyperventilation would be the improvement of intracellular acidic environment.[2] However, numerous studies demonstrated that hyperventilation after traumatic brain injury is deleterious. Possible disadvantages include cerebral vasoconstriction to such an extent that cerebral ischemia ensues with only a transient effect on the cerebrospinal fluid (CSF) pH with loss of $HCO_3^-$ buffer from the CSF. Prolonged hyperventilation provided a relative ischemia in brain tissue and promoted production of brain lactate.[3] Accordingly, as long as hyperventilation has a cerebral protective action, there should be other mechanisms in addition to the above-mentioned ones. Glutamate is a known neurotoxin when present in

---

[a] This study was supported by a research grant from the Keimyung Medical Science Institute, 1993.
[e] Address for correspondence: Kyu Taek Choi, Department of Anesthesiology, Asan Medical Center, 388-1 Poongnapdong, Songpagu, Seoul 138-040, Korea.

excessive concentrations and may produce neuronal destruction. Under anoxic or ischemic conditions, synaptically released excitatory transmitters, most likely glutamate, accumulate until they reach a neurotoxic level. Also, neurotransmitter release is enhanced by anoxia. If we can demonstrate that hypocapnia during the periischemic period lowers the extracellular glutamate concentration, we can explain a part of the protective mechanism to be the ability of hypocapnia to attenuate the increased release of glutamate. We used the well-established rabbit model of global ischemia[4] and evaluated the changes produced by a 3-h period of hypocapnia.

## MATERIALS AND METHODS

Six New Zealand white rabbits weighing 2.24 ± 0.21 (mean ± SD) kg were anesthetized in a plexiglas box with 5% halothane in oxygen. After intubation of the trachea with a 3.5 mm uncuffed wire reinforced endotracheal tube, anesthesia was maintained with 1.2% halothane in oxygen, and the animals were mechanically ventilated with animal ventilator to maintain normocapnia (animal ventilator, Harvard Appartus, USA; $PaCO_2$ = 35–45 mmHg). Body temperature was servo controlled and maintained at 37.5°C. After infiltration with 0.25% bupivacinae, a catheter (PE-90) was inserted into the femoral artery for measurement of arterial blood pressure and sampling for the arterial blood gases. The femoral vein was also cannulated for the administration of drugs during inflation of the neck tourniquet. An ear vein catheter was inserted for the administration of fluids (0.9% saline) and drugs. All rabbits were initially hydrated with 0.9% saline solution (40 ml·$kg^{-1}$) administered over a one-hour period. This was followed by a maintenance infusion at 4 ml·$kg^{-1}$·$h^{-1}$ throughout the study. The rabbit's head was positioned in a stereotactic frame (David Kopf, USA), and a pneumatic tourniquet (8 inches in length, Zimmer, USA) was secured loosely around the neck. After infiltration with 0.25% bupivacaine, the cranium was exposed and burr holes were made bilaterally over the dorsal hippocampus (4 mm posterior and 4 mm lateral to the bregma) for the insertion of microdialysis probes (CMA-10, Carnegie Medicin, Sweden). Biparietal needle electrodes were placed into the scalp for continuous recording of the electroencephalogram (EEG). Monitored variables included mean arterial pressure, heart, rate, arterial blood gases, hematocrit, blood glucose concentration, esophageal temperature, and the EEG. Following the completion of these surgical preparations, the inspired halothane concentration was decreased to 1%.

Recovery rates for each microdialysis probe were determined using $10^{-2}$ M dextrose solution *in vitro* prior to their insertion into the brain. The dura over the dorsal hippocampus were then incised, and microdialysis probes of concentric design (fiber length = 4 mm, diameter = 0.25 mm) were inserted vertically to a depth of 6 mm using micromanipulators (David Kopf, USA). The probes were perfused with artificial cerebrospinal fluid (147 mM NaCl, 2.3 mM $CaCl_2$, 0.9 mM $MgCl_2$, 4.0 mM KCl) at a rate of 2 µL·$min^{-1}$. After implantation into the brain, the probes were perfused for at least 1 hour prior to collecting baseline samples of brain tissue microdialysate.

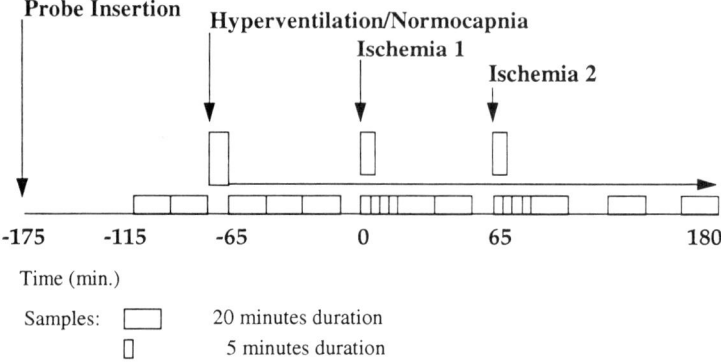

**FIGURE 1.** Time course of experiment showing ischemic periods and dialysate collection.

was allowed to hyperventilate to the level of $PaCO_2$ 25–35 mmHG 60 min prior to the onset of ischemia. $PaCO_2$ was maintained throughout the study. Group 2 (n = 3) was a normal control group that maintained normocapnia.

Global cerebral ischemia was induced by lowering the mean arterial blood pressure to less than 50 mmHg by using bolus doses (10 mg) of trimethapan, and the application of positive end-expiratory airway pressure.

The neck tourniquet was then inflated to a pressure of 20 psi for 7.5 minutes. A tendency to hypertension during the first three minutes of ischemia was treated with additional doses of trimethapan as needed to keep mean arterial pressure below 50 mmHg. Global cerebral ischemia was verified in each rabbit by observation of an isoelectric EEG within 30 seconds after tourniquet inflation. Immediately after deflation of the tourniquet, a bolus dose and then infusion of phenylephrine was done to restore the mean arterial pressure to 75 mmHg. After one hour of recirculation, a second identical period of global ischemia was instituted.

At the end of the study period, the microdialysis probes were removed and the recovery rate for each microdialysis probe was again determined using $10^{-2}$ M dextrose solution *in vitro*. To verify the position of probes, 5 ml of Evans blue dye (2%) was administered intravenously. After the animal was euthanized, the brain was removed and sectioned coronally to see the staining of the dye along the tracks of the probes.

Samples of microdialysate were collected as follows from the dorsal hippocampus. Two baseline samples (each of 20 minutes' duration) were collected 60 minutes after insertion into the brain. After collection of baseline samples manipulation of ventilation was started. Three samples (20 minutes' duration) were collected in all groups before the onset of the first ischemia.

Global cerebral ischemia was induced as described and every five minutes samples were taken (two ischemia samples, followed by two immediate reperfusion samples). Two samples (20 minutes' duration) were collected before the onset of the second ischemia. For the second ischemia this process was repeated. Finally, three reperfusion samples (each 20 minutes' duration) were collected at 80, 120 and 160 minutes after the onset of the first ischemia (FIG. 1).

All samples were collected on ice and immediately frozen and stored at $-25°C$ until their analysis for amino acid content by high-performance liquid chromatography (HPLC).

The dialysate from the dorsal hippocampus was analyzed for glutamate and glycine concentrations using HPLC with ophthaldehyde derivatization on a reversed-phase C-18 column. Derivatives were detected fluorometrically and peak areas were integrated and quantified based on linear calibration with known amino acid standards. This method has been shown to be sensitive to low picomolar range concentrations of glutamate.

The means and SEMs for the concentrations of glutamate and glycine were calculated for each time period. Data for amino acid concentrations were corrected using *in vitro* recovery rates for dextrose and analyzed by 2-way analysis of variance (ANOVA; groups vs time). Physiological data were tabulated and compared using the ANOVA test at each point. Differences with $p < 0.05$ were considered statistically significant.

## RESULTS

Physiologic data are shown in TABLE. 1 Other than the intended differences in $PaCO_2$ and pH, there were no other significant differences in physiologic variables between the groups. As intended, $PaCO_2$ decreased from the mean value of $39.7 \pm 3.2$ mmHg to $31 \pm 2.2$ mmHg in the hyperventilation group. These differences in $PaCO_2$ persisted throughout the study (FIG. 2). *In vitro* mean recovery rate of microdialysis catheters for dextrose was $28 \pm 5\%$.

Prior to the onset of ischemia, stable concentrations of extracellular glutamate and glycine were documented (from t = 595 to $-2$-minutes). In the control group the hippocampal extracellular concentrations of glutamate and glycine were significantly elevated during each episode of ischemia (FIGS. 3 and 4); these levels returned to baseline within 10 minutes after reperfusion. In contrast, in the hyperventilation group hippocampal glutamate and glycine concentrations increased during ischemia, but they were not statistically significant. Two-way ANOVA for the periischemic periods ($t = 15,80$) revealed lower glutamate values for the hyperventilated animals ($p = 0.06$). A similar analysis of periischemic glycine concentrations revealed significantly lower values in the hyperventilated group ($t = 10,15,75,80: p = 0.03$) as compared to normal controls.

## DISCUSSION

Considerable evidence has now accumulated from both neuronal cultures and *in vivo* experiments that excitatory amino acids play an important role in the evolution of ischemic brain damage. It appears that these excitatory amino acids are released into the brain's extracellular space during normal neurotransmission as well as in response to a variety of insults including hypoxia and ischemia.[4-7] Acutely, glutamate, acting at postsynaptic N-methyl-D-aspartate (NMDA) receptors, activates associated ion channels resulting in a massive influx of $Na^+$ and

TABLE 1. Summary of Physiologic Data

| Variable | Control (n = 3) | Hyperventilation (n = 3) | Variable | Control (n = 3) | Hyperventilation (n = 3) |
|---|---|---|---|---|---|
| | pH | | | Mean Arterial Pressure | |
| Initial | 7.35 ± 0.02 | 7.36 ± 0.05 | Initial | 69 ± 3 | 72 ± 8 |
| Hyperventilation | 7.33 ± 0.02 | 7.45 ± 0.05* | Hyperventilation | 70 ± 3 | 72 ± 4 |
| 10 min after ischemia | 7.28 ± 0.02 | 7.46 ± 0.04* | 10 min after ischemia | 86 ± 9 | 80 ± 13 |
| 75 min after ischemia | 7.29 ± 0.03 | 7.38 ± 0.03* | 75 min after ischemia | 81 ± 8 | 68 ± 12 |
| 120 min after ischemia | 7.36 ± 0.02 | 7.45 ± 0.01* | 120 min after ischemia | 67 ± 2 | 80 ± 3 |
| 160 min after ischemia | 7.36 ± 0.01 | 7.49 ± 0.02* | 160 min after ischemia | 67 ± 2 | 76 ± 7 |
| | $PaCO_2$ | | | Heart Rate | |
| Initial | 38.8 ± 1.3 | 39.7 ± 3.2 | Initial | 235 ± 10 | 257 ± 2 |
| Hyperventilation | 38.6 ± 1.6 | 31 ± 2.2* | Hyperventilation | 255 ± 5 | 266 ± 6 |
| 10 min after ischemia | 41.1 ± 2.2 | 23.3 ± 1.9* | 10 min after ischemia | 229 ± 6 | 223 ± 9 |
| 75 min after ischemia | 40.5 ± 2 | 27.6 ± 0.5* | 75 min after ischemia | 219 ± 5 | 197 ± 3 |
| 120 min after ischemia | 39.7 ± 1.2 | 27.1 ± 1.6* | 120 min after ischemia | 241 ± 8 | 217 ± 12 |
| 160 min after ischemia | 39.3 ± 0.8 | 27 ± 1* | 160 min after ischemia | 247 ± 8 | 235 ± 20 |
| | $PaO_2$ | | | Esophageal Temperature | |
| Initial | 371 ± 49 | 429 ± 23 | Initial | 38.5 ± 0.1 | 37.6 ± 0.4 |
| Hyperventilation | 444 ± 22 | 467 ± 7 | Hyperventilation | 38.4 ± 0.1 | 38.2 ± 0.3 |
| 10 min after ischemia | 446 ± 32 | 490 ± 8 | 10 min after ischemia | 38.4 ± 0.1 | 37.8 ± 0.2 |
| 75 min after ischemia | 468 ± 40 | 506 ± 9 | 75 min after ischemia | 38.4 ± 0.1 | 37.6 ± 0.1 |
| 120 min after ischemia | 460 ± 37 | 501 ± 23 | 120 min after ischemia | 38.4 ± 0.1 | 37.7 ± 0.4 |
| 160 min after ischemia | 440 ± 46 | 462 ± 16 | 160 min after ischemia | 38.5 ± 0.1 | 37.8 ± 0.5 |
| | B.E. | | | Blood Glucose | |
| Initial | −3 ± 0.7 | −2.1 ± 2.9 | Initial | 140 ± 13 | 172 ± 51 |
| Hyperventilation | −4 ± 1.1 | −0.7 ± 1.5 | Hyperventilation | 129 ± 17 | 130 ± 24 |
| 10 min after ischemia | −6.2 ± 1.1 | −4.7 ± 1.4 | 10 min after ischemia | 139 ± 14 | 135 ± 27 |
| 75 min after ischemia | −6.1 ± 1.4 | −6.5 ± 1.8 | 75 min after ischemia | 130 ± 14 | 99 ± 11 |
| 120 min after ischemia | −2 ± 1.4 | −2.7 ± 1.5 | 120 min after ischemia | 122 ± 13 | 88 ± 13 |
| 160 min after ischemia | −1.6 ± 0.7 | −0.8 ± 1.7 | 160 min after ischemia | 113 ± 13 | 85 ± 10 |
| | Hematocrit | | | | |
| Hyperventilation | 30.2 ± 1.2 | 32 ± 2.1 | | | |
| 160 min after ischemia | 30.1 ± 0.9 | 32 ± 2.5 | | | |

* $p < 0.05$ from control.

$Cl^-$ ions and $H_2O$.[8] This influx of water can lead to an acute osmotic lysis of the neuron. Delayed neuronal damage is thought to be secondary to the glutamate-induced calcium influx.[9] An excessive rise in intracellular $Ca^{++}$ results in overactivation of lipases, proteases, and endonucleases which may be detrimental to cellular homeostasis.[4,5] Electron microscopy has demonstrated that the neuropathological state produced by glutamate is characterized by rapid cellular swelling and is most marked near dendrosomal components of the neurons that contain the excitatory amino acid receptors.[10]

Glycine has a facilitatory effect on glutamate's neurotoxic action. Activation of the NMDA receptor by glutamate was recently shown to require the presence of glycine at a strychnine-insensitive binding site.[11,12] Thus, any intervention that results in reduction of such elevated levels may be expected to lessen ischemic injury. To prevent further ischemic neuronal damage, it would be better to block the initial step in this cascade of events.

Glutamate is normally released by $Ca^{++}$-dependent exocytosis,[13] but adenosine triphosphate (ATP) is also required and the release is therefore arrested within a few minutes after start of ischemia.[14] Two transport pathways are integral to

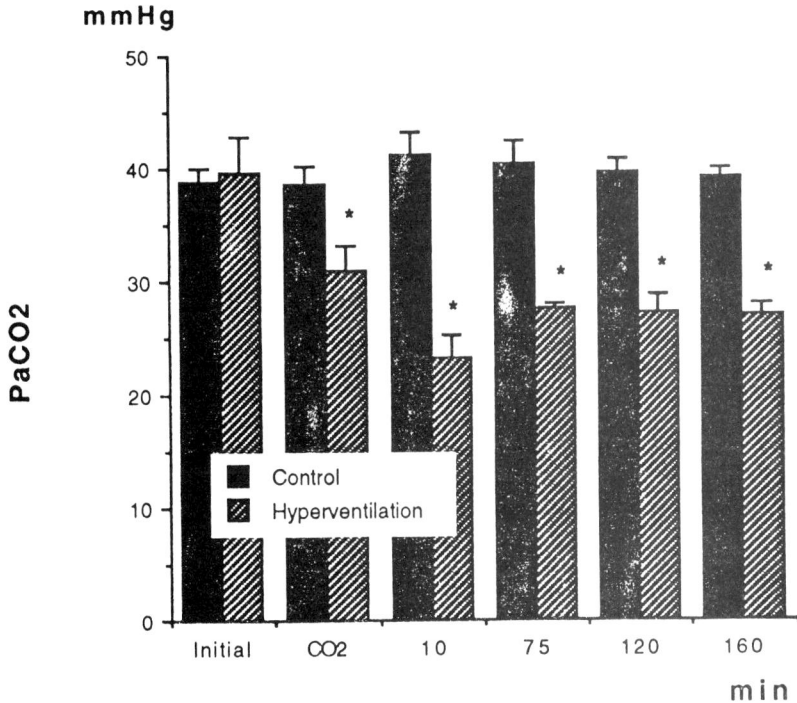

**FIGURE 2.** $PaCO_2$ changes during the study. * $p < 0.05$ between groups.

the ability to function as a neurotransmitter: first, a powerful uptake carrier located in both neurons and glia and capable of lowering the extracellular glutamate concentration to about 1 $\mu$M; second, a more specific transporter capable of packaging glutamate into a subpopulation of synaptic vesicles for subsequent exocytosis.

Since there are several glutamate pools, the question arises from which compartment(s) glutamate is released during ischemia: (presynaptic) cytoplasm, vesicles, neuronal soma, astrocytes, etc. Because the vesicular release of glutamate is inhibited when ATP levels fall after a few minutes anoxia, it seems likely that much of the glutamate released into the extracellular space during anoxia is $Ca^{++}$-independent, nonvesicular release.[15]

During ischemia, the extracellular $K^+$ concentration in the brain, $[K^+]o$, increases steeply to 60–80 mM.[16,17] A rise in $[K^+]o$ will release more glutamate into the extracellular space in two ways. First, it will depolarize neurons, increasing vesicular release of glutamate (if this is not already inhibited by a fall in ATP levels; see below); second, it will promote the release of glutamate by reversal of the plasma membrane glutamate uptake carrier. Several factors lead to failure of glutamate uptake in the pathologic conditions described above. First, a rise in $[K^+]o$ inhibits uptake directly because it hinders the loss of counter-transported

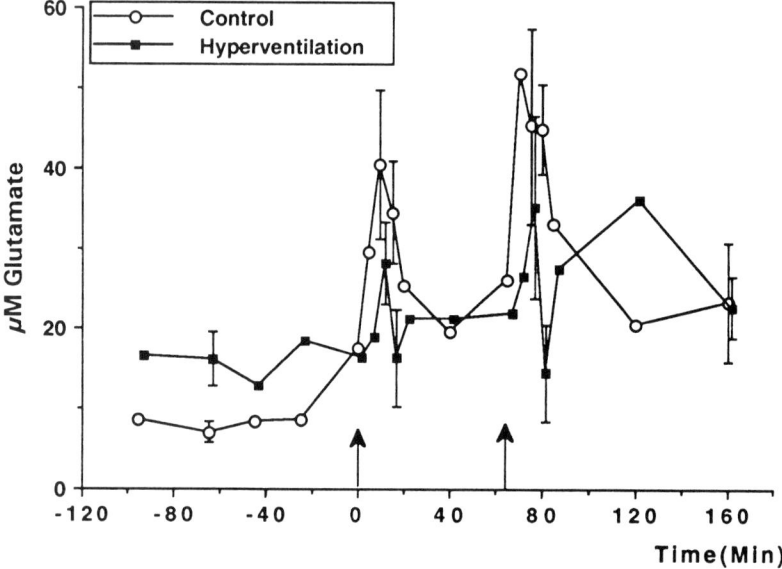

**FIGURE 3.** Ischemia-induced glutamate increase (mean ± SEM). *Arrows* indicate onset of ischemia.

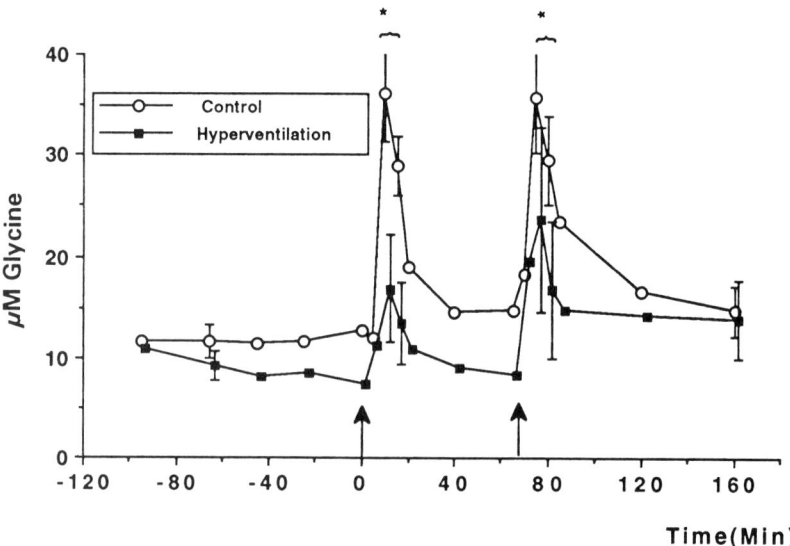

**FIGURE 4.** Ischemia-induced glycine increase (mean ± SEM). *Arrows* indicate ischemic episodes. * $p < 0.05$ between groups.

$K^+$ from the carrier. Second, depolarization of the cell by the raised $[K^+]o$ inhibits uptake. Third, arachidonic acid released by the high glutamate concentration inhibits uptake. Finally, a decrease in $[Na^+]o$, which can result from low ATP levels inhibiting the $Na^+$ pump or from a large $Na^+$ influx through glutamate- and voltage-gated $Na^+$ channels, also inhibits uptake.[18] The combination of these factors is sufficient to reduce the rate of uptake to less than 10% of its normal magnitude.[19] The resulting from glutamate concentration will depolarize neurons further and thus release more $K^+$.[19] This is a positive feedback system that tends to lead to a larger rise in extracellular glutamate concentration. Thus, blocking the increase of $[K^+]o$ can be a part of the cerebral protective measures during ischemia. Hypocapnia causes respiratory alkalosis, which in turn induces an intracellular shift of $K^+$ to compensate for the decreased concentration of $H^+$ in extracellular fluid (ECF), and thus $[K^+]o$ decreases.[20] If hyperventilation in the periischemic period can also attenuate the increase of $[K^+]o$, the increased levels of glutamate in extracellular fluid would be prevented. We did not measure $[K^+]o$. However, it would be possible to assume that $[K^+]o$ is already reduced by hyperventilation and that $[K^+]o$ during the ischemia might be lower than $[K^+]o$ without hyperventilation. The main finding of this study was that hypocapnia during the periischemic period attenuated the increase of glutamate and glycine concentrations following transient global ischemia. Thus, our results might support such an assumption.

In addition to discussion concerning the absolute concentration of $[K^+]o$ during ischemia, ion channels that modulate $K^+$ currents have received much attentions.[21] Electrophysiological studies have shown that $K^+$-channel openers could protect neurons against ischemic injury.[22,23] Intracellular recordings show that a brief anoxic episode in the CA3 region of hippocampal slices induces a transient hyperpolarization due to the activation of $K^+$ currents, followed by a depolarization resulting in glutamate release.[24,25] In the first minutes, anoxic depolarization is sensitive to tetrodotoxin, reduced by the application of the $K^+$-channel openers, and enhanced by the blocker. The release of glutamate evoked by a 6–8-min period of ischemia was reduced by 25–40% in the presence of $K^+$-channel openers, lemakalim, RP52891 and galanin. Hyperpolarization resulting from the opening of the $K^+$ ATP channel by the openers could temporarily protect neurons against the dramatic depolarization subsequent to ischemia and delay cytosolic glutamate release.[26] It is uncertain that hyperventilation during ischemia has an association with activation of the potassium channel. Hypercapnia leads to hyperpolarization of nerve cells. However, the hyperpolarization in hypercapnia is accompanied by increased membrane resistance indicating a mechanism of hyperpolarization different from the one causing hyperpolarization during anoxia (which activates the $K^+$ channel).[27] This requires further investigation.

Clearly, there are other mechanisms by which hypocapnia may have a protective effect on neuronal injury. The potential beneficial effects of hyperventilation include a reduction in CBF with the consequent reduction in cerebral blood volume and intracranial pressure.[28,29] Hypocapnia may induce a redistribution of CBF from normal areas (with preserved $CO_2$ reactivity) to injured areas with abnormal $CO_2$ reactivity ("inverse steal" phenomenon).[30]

On the contrary, cerebral arteriolar diameter in experimental animals was found to be decreased shortly after institution of hyperventilation, but returned to baseline within 24 hours and increased slightly over baseline after that period.[31]

Thus, we can assume that prolonged hyperventilation cannot guarantee persistent reduction of intracranial pressure (ICP). Severe hyperventilation can result in a reduction in CBF that is sufficient to produce cerebral ischemia, particularly if $PaCO_2$ is rapidly decreased below approximately 20 mmHg. If $PaCO_2$ is allowed to go below 20 mmHg, cerebral vasoconstriction may be so intense as to impede oxygen delivery, thus exacerbating the existing cerebral ischemia and its deleterious effects.

Recently, animals treated with sustained hyperventilation ($PaCO_2$ = 20 mmHg) produced the highest lactate concentration that have been reported.[3] It has been reported that moderate hypocapnia ($PaCO_2$ ~25–30 mmHg) contrary to severe hypocapnia ($PaCO_2$ <25 mmHg) produces a better outcome in head-injured patients.[32,33] According to clinical experience, active hyperventilation during the recording of an EEG enhances epileptiform activity; therefore, hypocapnia may influence seizure activity.[34]

Cerebral metabolic acidosis is often found after cerebral ischemia and is correlated with poor outcome.[35] As $CO_2$ freely passes the blood-brain barrier, hyperventilation should diminish cerebral $CO_2$ thereby increasing the pH of extracellular fluid and counteract acidosis.[36,2]

When respiratory alkalosis is induced by hyperventilation, normalization of CSF acid-base balance is attained rapidly within 8–12 hr after deviation of normal pH.[37] This limits potential beneficial effect of hyperventilation.

It is apparent that the potential for both beneficial and detrimental effects exists. Therefore, the aim of this study was to elucidate the possible association of excitatory amino acids, GLU and GLY, with the favorable action of hyperventilation in brain ischemia.

In our study, hyperventilation attenuated the increase of glutamate level in periischemic periods, even if it did not reach statistical significant ($p$ = 0.06). Another interesting finding of this study was the periischemic glycine levels were lower in the hyperventilation group. Since glycine facilitates the actions of glutamate at the NMDA receptor,[38,11,39,40] this provides a possible explanation for hypocapnia's beneficial effect on neurologic outcome. Attenuation of glutamate's actions may prevent neuronal injury.

In conclusion, preexisting hypocapnia was associated with decreased periischemic concentrations of glutamate in brain tissue collected from an *in vivo* model of global cerebral ischemia. Glycine levels were decreased also during the periischemic period and this may account, in part, for previous reports of cerebral protective action associated with hyperventilation.

## SUMMARY

Glutamate (GLU) is a neurotransmitter. Massive release of GLU and glycine (GLY) into the brain's extracellular space may be triggered by ischemia, and may result in acute neuronal lysis or delayed neuronal death. The aim of this study was to evaluate the possible relationship between hyperventilation and the level of GLU and GLY during brain ischemia.

Rabbits were anesthetized with halothane and oxygen. Group 1 was allowed to hyperventilate ($PaCO_2$ 25–35 mmHg). $PaCO_2$ was maintained throughout the study. Group 2 was a normal control group that maintained normocapnia. Two global cerebral ischemic episodes were produced. Microdialysate was collected during the periischemic and reperfusion periods from the dorsal hippocampus. GLU and GLY concentrations were determined using high-performance liquid chromatography.

In the control group, GLU and GLY were significantly elevated during each episode of ischemia; these levels returned to baseline within 10 minutes after reperfusion. In contrast, in the hyperventilation group GLU and GLY concentrations increased during ischemia, but they were not statistically significant. Two way ANOVA for the periischemic periods ($t = 15,80; p = 0.06$) revealed lower GLU values for the hyperventilated animals. A similar analysis for periischemic GLY concentrations revealed significantly lower values in the hyperventilated group ($t = 10,15,75,80: p = 0.03$) as compared to normal controls.

We were able to demonstrate that hypocapnia during periischemic period lowered extracellular GLU and GLY concentrations. These results can explain a part of the protective action of hypocapnia during cerebral ischemia.

## REFERENCES

1. TODD, M. M., C. TOMMASINO & H. M. SHAPIRO. 1985. Cerebrovascular effects of prolonged hypocarbia and hypercarbia after experimental global ischemia in cats. Crit. Care Med. **13:** 720–723.
2. VANICKY, I., M. MARSALA, J. MURAR & J. MARSALA. 1992. Prolonged postischemic hyperventilation reduces acute neuronal damage after 15 min of cardiac arrest in the dog. Neurosci. Lett. **135:** 167–170.
3. YOSHIDA, K. & A. MARMAROU. 1991. Effects of tromethamine and hyperventilation on brain injury in cat. J. Neurosurg. **74:** 87–96.
4. SIEJO, B. K. 1992. Pathophysiology and treatment of focal cerebral ischemia. Part I. Pathophysiology. J. Neurosurg. **77:** 169–184.
5. SIEJO, B. K. 1992. Pathophysiology and treatment of focal cerebral ischemia. Part II. Mechanism of damage and treatment. J. Neurosurg. **77:** 337–354.
6. ZIVIN, J. A. & D. W. CHOI. 1991. Stroke therapy. Sci. Am. **265:** 56–63.
7. BENVENISTE, H., M. B. JORGENSEN, M. SANDBERG, T. CHRISTENSEN, H. HAGBERG & N. H. DIEMER. 1989. Ischemic damage in hippocampal CA1 is dependent on glutamate release and intact innervation from CA3. J. Cereb. Blood Flow Metab. **9:** 629–639.
8. CHOI, D. W., J-Y. KOH & S. PETERS. 1988. Pharmacology of glutamate neurotoxicity in cortical cell culture: attenuation of NMDA antagonists. J. Neurosci. **8:** 185–196.
9. ROTHMAN, S. M., J. H. THURSTON & R. E. HAUHART. 1987. Delayed neurotoxicity of excitatory amino acids *in vitro*. Neuroscience **22:** 471–480.
10. ROTHMAN, S. M. & J. W. OLNEY. 1986. Glutamate and the pathophysiology of hypoxic-ischemic brain damage. Ann. Neurol. **19:** 105–111.
11. FOSTER, A. C. & J. A. KEMPT. 1989. Glycine maintains excitement. Nature **338:** 337–378.
12. KLOOG, Y., H. LAMDANI-ITKIN & M. SOKOLOVSHY. 1990. The glycine site of the *N*-methyl-D-aspartate receptor channel: differences between the binding of HA-966 and of 7-chlorokynurenic acid. J. Neurochem. **54:** 1576–1583.

13. NICHOLLS, D. 1989. Release of glutamate, aspartate and gamma-aminobutyric acid from isolated nerve terminals. J. Neurochem. **52:** 331–341.
14. SIEJO, B. K. 1988. Mechanisms of ischemic brain damage. Crit. Care Med. **16:** 954–963.
15. SÁNCHEZ-PRIETO, J. & P. GONZÁLEZ. 1988. Occurrence of a large $Ca^{2+}$-independent release of glutamate during anoxia in isolated nerve terminals (synaptosomes). J. Neurochem. **50:** 1322–1324.
16. HANSEN, A. J. 1985. Effect of anoxia on ion distribution in the brain. Physiol. Rev. **65:** 101–148.
17. HANSEN, A. J., J. HOUNSGAARD & H. JAHNSEN. 1982. Anoxia increases potassium conductance in hippocampal nerve cells. Acta Physiol. Scand. **115:** 301–310.
18. SZATKOWSKI, M., B. BARBOUR & D. ATTWELL. 1990. Non-vesicular release of glutamate from glial cells by reversed electrogenic glutamate uptake. Nature **348:** 443–446.
19. NICHOLLS, D. & D. ATTWELL. 1991. The release and uptake of excitatory amino acids. TIPS Special Reports 68–74.
20. FLEMMA, R. J. & W. G. YOUNG. 1964. The metabolic effects of mechanical ventilation and respiratory alkalosis in postoperative patients. Surgery **56:** 36–43.
21. COOK, N. S. 1988. The pharmacology of potassium channels and their therapeutic potential. TIPS **9:** 21–28.
22. ABELE, A. E. & R. J. MILLER. 1990. Potassium channel activators abolish excitotoxicity in cultured hippocampal pyramidal neurons. Neurosci. Lett. **115:** 195–200.
23. HAMILTON, T. C., S. W. WEIR & A. H. WESTON. 1986. Comparison of the effects of BRL 34915 and verapamil on electrical and mechanical activity in rat portal vein. Br. J. Pharmacol. **88:** 103–111.
24. BEN-ARI, Y. 1990. Galanin and glibenclamide modulate the anoxic release of glutamate in rat CA3 hippocampal neurons. Eur. J. Neurosci. **2:** 62–68.
25. FUJIWARA, N., H. HIGASHI, K. SHIMOJI & M. YOSHIMURA. 1987. Effects of hypoxia on rat hippocampal neurons *in vitro*. J. Physiol. **384:** 131–151.
26. ZINI, S., M. P. ROISIN, C. ARMENGAUD & A. Y. BEN. 1993. Effect of potassium channel modulators on the release of glutamate induced by ischaemic-like conditions in rat hippocampal slices. Neurosci. Lett. **153:** 202–205.
27. CASPERS, H. & E. J. SPECKMANN. 1972. Cerebral pO2, pCO2 and pH: changed during convulsive activity and their significance for spontaneous arrest of seizures. Epilepsia **13:** 699–725.
28. MAIESE, K. & J. J. CARONNA. 1988. Coma following cardiac arrest: a review of the clinical features, management, and prognosis. J. Intensive Care Med. **3:** 153–163.
29. SOLOWAY, M., W. NADEL, M. S. ALBIN & R. J. WHITE. 1968. The effect of hyperventilation on subsequent cerebral infarction. Anesthesiology **29:** 975–980.
30. ARTRU, A. A. & H. G. MERRIMAN. 1989. Hypocapnia added to hypertension to reverse EEG changes during carotid endarterectomy. Anesthesiology **70:** 1016–1018.
31. MUIZELAAR, J. P., H. G. POEL & Z. C. LI. 1988. Pial arteriolar vessel diameter and $CO_2$ reactivity during prolonged hyperventilation in the rabbit. J. Neurosurg. **69:** 923–927.
32. GORDON, E. & M. ROSSANDA. 1970. Further studies on cerebrospinal fluid acid-base status in patients with brain lesions. Acta Anaesthesiol. Scand. **14:** 97–109.
33. MUIZELAAR, J. P., A. MARMAROU & J. D. WARD. 1991. Adverse effects of prolonged hyperventilation in patients with severe head injury: a randomized clinical trial. J. Neurosurg. **75:** 731–739.
34. CHATER, S. N. & K. H. SIMPSON. 1988. Effect of passive hyperventilation on seizure duration in patients undergoing electroconvulsive therapy. Br. J. Anaesth. **60:** 70–73.
35. LJUNGREN, B., K. MORBERG & B. K. SIEJO. 1974. Influence of tissue acidosis upon restitution of brain energy metabolism following total ischemia. Brain Res. **77:** 173.
36. MARUKI, Y., R. C. KOEHLER, S. M. ELEFF & R. J. TRAYSTMAN. 1993. Intracellular pH during reperfusion influences evoked potential recovery after complete cerebral ischemia. Stroke **24:** 697–793.
37. CHRISTENSEN, M. S. 1974. Acid-base changes in cerebrospinal fluid and blood, and blood volume changes following prolonged hyperventilation. Br. J. Anaesth. **46:** 348.
38. FORSYTHE, I. D., G. L. WESTBROOK & M. L. MAYER. 1988. Modulation of excitatory

synaptic transmission by glycine and zinc in cultures of mouse hippocampal neurons. J. Neurosci. **8:** 3733–3741.
39. KLECKNER, N. & R. DINGLEDINE. 1988. Requirement for glycine in activation of NMDA-receptors expressed in *Xenopus* oocytes. Science **241:** 835–837.
40. LARSON, A. A. & A. J. BEITZ. 1988. Glycine potentiates strychnine-induced convulsions: role of NMDA receptors. J. Neurosci. **8:** 3822–3826.

# Discussion

C. WILLIAMS (*University of Aukland, New Zealand*): Do astrocytes die? You postulated that glial failure leads to accumulation of excitatory amino acids (EAAs). Do you know what causes the glia to fail, since they are very resistant to hypoxic ischemic injury?

R. BULLOCK (*Medical College of Virginia*): We have no data to indicate whether the astrocytes die. We *speculate* that the ultrastructural swelling of astrocytes which we see in head injured patients is due to uptake of $K^+$ and glutamate. This would eventually become saturated, or would fail when swelling is very marked, or the cells would burst.

J. F. BOWYER (*National Center for Toxicological Research, FDA, Jefferson, AR*): Will circulatory levels of glutamate, which could enter the brain after destruction of the blood-brain barrier, cause significant increases in brain glutamate levels?

BULLOCK: Probably not, because 1) circulating levels in plasma are $\pm 27$ $\mu$mol—which is most likely well below the neurotoxic level, and 2) in brain, astrocytes and presynaptic astrocytic processes have potent glutamate uptake systems, with $>1:10,000$ concentrating ability, and they remove glutamate from extracellular fluid (ECF) (Nichols et al., TIPS, 1990).

S. JONAS (*New York University*): You showed close-to-normal glutamate and aspartate levels in subdural hematoma. Were these acute or chronic subdural hematomas?

BULLOCK: All were acute subdural hematomas. Only when a secondary ischemic insult was present, did ECF glutamate and aspartate rise to high levels ($>5$-fold increase).

G. C. PALMER (*Fisons Pharmaceuticals, Rochester, NY*): From a clinical standpoint do you think treatment of neonatal hypoxia with excitatory amino acid antagonists might be disruptive to the long-term development of the nervous system in view of the role of NMDA receptors in plasticity of the CNS?

WILLIAMS: MK801 was indeed toxic at high doses in our studies but we did not test many doses. Excitatory amino acid antagonists most likely would be harmful if given on a chronic basis to the developing animal.

U. TUOR (*Hospital for Sick Children, Toronto*): Your group has demonstrated that repetitive insults with relatively short time intervals between them result in exacerbation of brain damage. Have you tried extending the time between the ischemic episodes to determine if you could actually reduce ischemic damage?

WILLIAMS: We have observed an exacerbation of damage when the injuries are repeated at 1-h intervals and to a lesser degree at 5-h intervals. We have not completed studies at longer time intervals that may in fact be protective.

C. C. CHIUEH (*National Institute of Mental Health, NIH, Bethesda, MD*): We recently demonstrated that hypothermia decreases the *in vivo* generation of cytotoxic hydroxyl free radicals in the striatum (Chiueh, et al. Ann. N.Y. Acad. Sci., in press). Would you comment on a possible use of hypothermic procedures in rescuing brain neurones from ischemia/reperfusion injury in both preclinical and clinical situations?

## DISCUSSION

BULLOCK: This is a rapidly expanding area of investigation. Numerous animal studies and four controlled "phase II"-type clinical studies in head trauma patients support cautious optimism that this mechanism may become clinically useful. A seven-center phase III study of moderate hypothermia (32–33°C) for 48 h after severe head trauma is in progress (NIH funded).

# Neuroprotective Effects of Free Radical Scavengers and Energy Repletion in Animal Models of Neurodegenerative Disease

JÖRG B. SCHULZ AND M. FLINT BEAL[a]

*Neurochemistry Laboratory and Neurology Service*
*Massachusetts General Hospital*
*and*
*Harvard Medical School*
*Boston, Massachusetts 02114*

## INTRODUCTION

The pathogenesis of nerve cell death in neurodegenerative diseases is unknown. Neurodegenerative illnesses are characterized by gradually evolving, slow, relentless neuronal death, not accompanied by an intense tissue reaction or inflammatory response. There is selective loss of certain defined groups of neurons which may be related either anatomically or physiologically. The diseases are exemplified by Alzheimer's disease (AD), Parkinson's disease (PD), Huntington's disease (HD), amyotrophic lateral sclerosis (ALS) and cerebellar degenerations. Each of these illnesses has a characteristic pattern of pathology, but there is occasional overlap, *e.g.,* that seen with the parkinsonism-dementia-ALS complex of Guam in which pathologic features of PD, AD and ALS can occur in various combinations. In addition striatonigral and cerebellar degeneration are part of multiple system atrophy. This raises the possibility that some common underlying mechanisms may play a role in these disorders.

### *Excitotoxicity, Bioenergetic Defects, and Oxidative Stress in Neurodegenerative Diseases*

Excitotoxicity, mitochondrial dysfunction and free radical-induced oxidative damage have been implicated in the pathogenesis in several different neurodegenerative diseases, such as ALS, PD, AD and HD.[1-3] How can a neurotoxic action of glutamate result in an insidious slowly evolving process of neuronal loss occurring over many years? One possibility is that a progressive impairment of energy metabolism may secondarily result in slow excitotoxic neuronal death.[4-6] Several studies have reported decreased glucose metabolism and abnormalities in mitochondrial electron transport enzymes in neurodegenerative diseases (reviewed in

---

[a] Address for correspondence: Dr. M. Flint Beal, Warren 408, Neurology Service, Massachusetts General Hospital, Boston, MA 02114

Refs. 4–7), which may be exacerbated by a decline in mitochondrial function which occurs with normal aging.[8]

The role of oxidative stress in neurologic diseases is an independent area of intense investigation.[1] Oxidative stress refers to the cytotoxic effects of oxygen radicals such as superoxide anion ($\cdot O_2^-$), hydroxyl radical ($\cdot OH$) and hydrogen peroxide ($H_2O_2$). An accumulation of oxidative damage may contribute to the delayed onset and progressive nature of neurodegenerative diseases. Recent evidence has suggested that excitotoxicity and oxidative stress may be sequential and interactive mechanisms leading to neuronal degeneration.[1] A link between excitotoxicity and oxidative stress has been investigated *in vitro*. An initial study showed that several free radical scavengers could attenuate kainate toxicity in cultured cerebellar neurons.[9] More direct evidence linking excitotoxicity to oxidative stress was recently reported in studies of cultured cerebellar neurons.[10] These studies used electron paramagnetic resonance to provide direct evidence that *N*-methyl-D-aspartate (NMDA) receptor activation leads to the generation of superoxide radicals.

### *Animal Models of Neurodegenerative Diseases*

Much of the interest in the association of neurodegeneration with mitochondrial dysfunction and oxidative damage emerged from studies of 1-methyl-4-phenyl-1,2,3,6-tetrahydropyridine (MPTP)-induced parkinsonism.[11] MPTP is converted to 1-methyl-4-phenylpyridinium ion ($MPP^+$) by monamine oxidase B (MAO-B). $MPP^+$ is selectively taken up by high-affinity dopamine and noradrenaline uptake systems at catecholaminergic terminals and is subsequently accumulated in millimolar concentrations within mitochondria of dopaminergic neurons. There it disrupts oxidative phosphorylation by inhibiting complex I of the mitochondrial electron transport chain by binding near or at the rotenone binding site.[12] The interruption of oxidative phosphorylation results in decreased levels of adenosine triphosphate (ATP).[13,14] A consequence is partial neuronal depolarization and secondary activation of voltage-dependent NMDA receptors, which may result in excitotoxic neuronal cell death.[5] Consistent with this hypothesis we and others found that administration of NMDA antagonists attenuated the neurotoxic effects of MPTP in mice[15] and $MPP^+$ in rats,[14,16] although this result is controversial.[17,18] NMDA antagonists were effective in attenuating MPTP neurotoxicity in primates.[19,20] The close relationship between mitochondrial dysfunction and oxidative damage is apparent with $MPP^+$ toxicity, since $MPP^+$ induces superoxide formation,[21] increases lipid peroxidation,[21] produces hydrogen peroxide and hydroxyl radicals,[22,23] and with prolonged exposure irreversibly inhibits complex I by a mechanism that may be due to oxidative damage to complex I.[24]

Evidence supporting a role of mitochondrial dysfunction in the pathogenesis of HD is the observation that 3-nitropropionic acid (3-NP) produces selective basal ganglia lesions and delayed dystonia when accidentally ingested in humans.[25] 3-NP is an irreversible inhibitor of succinate dehydrogenase that inhibits both the Krebs cycle and complex II of the mitochondrial electron transport chain. In rats administration of this mitochondrial toxin results in age-dependent striatal excitotoxic lesions as a consequence of an impairment of mitochondrial energy metabolism.[26,27] Chronic administration of 3-NP over 1 month produces selective striatal lesions that replicate many of the characteristic histologic and neurochemical features of HD.[27] The histologic alterations mimic the profile of neuronal degeneration observed in HD and suggest that the genetic abnormality of HD may be associated with a defect in mitochondrial energy metabolism. Striatal lesions produced by local administration of 3-NP, however, were not attenuated with NMDA antagonists.[27] In contrast, striatal lesions produced by malonate, a reversible succinate dehydrogenase inhibitor, were blocked by the noncompetitive NMDA antagonist MK-801,[28] by the competitive NMDA antagonist LY274614, and by the glutamate release inhibitor lamotrigine.[29] We found that 3-NP produced a more severe and prolonged ATP depletion than malonate. A more severe energy compromise leads to glutamate release and neuronal death mediated by both NMDA and non-NMDA receptors, whereas a mild energy compromise leads to selective NMDA receptor-mediated neuronal death.[30] We suspect this explains why striatal lesions produced by local injections of malonate are protected by NMDA antagonists, whereas those produced by local injection of 3-NP are not.

The histopathology and neurochemistry of striatal lesions produced by malonate strongly resemble those which occur in HD. Neuronal loss and gliosis are accompanied by a relative sparing of somatostatin[27] and the reduced form of nicotinamide-adenine dinucleotide phosphate (NADPH) diaphorase neurons.[29] *In vivo* water-suppressed proton chemical shift magnetic resonance imaging showed a focal and age-dependent increase in lactate after striatal infusions of malonate.[29]

3-Acetylpyridine (3-AP), a nicotinamide antagonist, is a potent neurotoxin when administered to laboratory animals by single intraperitoneal injections. Systemic administration of 3-AP produces a selective pattern of neuronal vulnerability, with preferential involvement of the inferior olive and substantia nigra. It has therefore been proposed that 3-AP may be model of olivopontocerebellar atrophy with associated parkinsonism,[31] which is a common feature of multiple system atrophy. We recently showed that striatal injections of 3-AP produce age-dependent lesions, which are attenuated by competitive and noncompetitive NMDA antagonists.[32] Consistent with an NMDA receptor-mediated excitotoxic effect, histologic studies showed that 3-AP lesions result in relative sparing of NADPH-diaphorase neurons.[32]

### *Neuroprotective Effects of Free Radical Scavengers*

Free radical spin traps are compounds which react with free radicals to form more stable adducts.[33] They can therefore serve as free radical scavengers. They are effective in attenuating both age-related oxidative damage to proteins[34] and ischemic lesions *in vivo*.[35-37]

We therefore examined whether pretreatment of rats with the free radical spin trap N-*tert*-butyl-$\alpha$-(2-sulfophenyl)-nitrone (S-PBN) can attenuate striatal lesions produced by stereotaxic injections of inhibitors of energy metabolism: $MPP^+$, malonate, and 3-AP.[38] Lesion volumes were determined using the triphenyltetra-

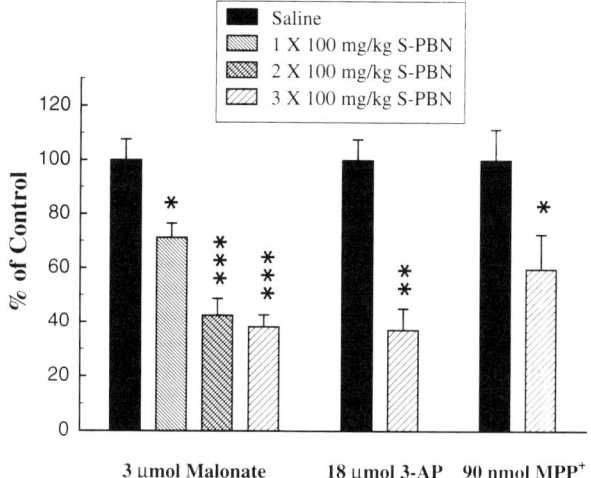

**FIGURE 1.** Effects of treatment with 1, 2 or 3 doses of S-PBN (100 mg/kg each) on striatal lesions produced by malonate and effects of pretreatment with S-PBN (100 mg/kg 1 h before and 2 h and 5 h after striatal injection) on striatal lesions produced by 3-AP, MPP$^+$. * $p$ <0.05, ** $p$ <0.01, *** $p$ <0.001.

zolium chloride monohydrate (TTC) method.[39] As shown in FIGURE 1 S-PBN significantly attenuated lesions produced by 3-AP, MPP$^+$, and malonate. The protective effect against 3-AP was slightly greater than that seen with either MPP$^+$ or malonate. Further studies examining the effects of 1, 2 or 3 injections of S-PBN (100 mg/kg i.p.) showed that its neuroprotective effects against malonate were dose dependent with a maximal protection of 62% (FIG. 1).

We also examined whether pretreatment with S-PBN can attenuate striatal excitotoxic lesions produced by the direct acting excitatory amino acid receptor agonists $N$-methyl-D-aspartate (NMDA), $\alpha$-amino-3-hydroxy-5-methylisoxazole-4-proprionic acid (AMPA) and kainic acid (KA).[38] S-PBN significantly attenuated excitotoxic lesions produced by AMPA, KA, and NMDA.

To assess whether administration of S-PBN is associated with attenuation of free radical generation we used the salicylate method to detect hydroxyl (·OH) radicals.[40] The reaction of salicylate with ·OH radicals results in the formation of 2,3 and 2,5 dihydroxybenzoic acid (DHBA), of which 2,3 DHBA is thought to be the more specific marker.[41] One hour after intrastriatal administration of 18 $\mu$mol 3-AP and 3 $\mu$mol malonate there were significant increases in both of 2,3 DHBA/salicylate and 2,5 DHBA/salicylate ratios. The increase in 2,3 DHBA was significantly attenuated by pretreating with S-PBN, consistent with a free radical scavenging effect.

Furthermore, we examined whether pretreatment with S-PBN had effects on striatal ATP concentrations following malonate injections.[42] ATP was significantly reduced in the lesioned striatum, but ATP concentrations in the lesioned and unlesioned striatum were not altered by S-PBN treatment. Using water-sup-

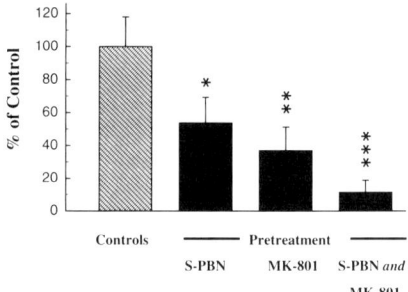

**FIGURE 2.** Effects of pretreatment with S-PBN (3 × 100 mg/kg i.p.), MK-801 (2 × 4 mg/kg i.p.) or their combination on striatal malonate or 3-AP lesions. The combination produced additive neuroprotective effects ($p < 0.05$). * $p < 0.05$, ** $p < 0.01$, *** $p < 0.001$ as compared to controls.

pressed proton chemical shift magnetic resonance imaging in real time,[26] the lactate concentration in the lesioned striatum was significantly increased 3 h after intrastriatal malonate injections. S-PBN pretreatment had no influence on this increased lactate production. Therefore, it is unlikely that S-PBN has any direct effects on oxidative phosphorylation.

We used electrophysiologic studies to examine whether S-PBN has effects on excitatory amino acid receptors *in vivo*. Electrodes were placed in the striatum and the spontaneous activity of multiple units was recorded. The mean spontaneous firing rate in the striatum was unchanged following treatment with S-PBN; however, the NMDA antagonist MK-801 produced a rapid and profound decrease in firing rate.

Since excitotoxicity and oxidative stress may produce neuronal injury by sequential interactive mechanisms, a combination of an excitatory amino acid antagonist and a free radical scavenger may be more efficacious than either compound alone. We therefore examined whether treatment with S-PBN in combination with MK-801 had additive effects in lesions produced by striatal malonate injection. The combination of S-PBN and MK-801 treatment showed a significantly better protection than MK-801 pretreatment alone ($p < 0.05$) (FIG. 2).

### *Neuroprotective Effects of Energy Repletion*

If the mechanism of excitoxic lesions produced by specific inhibitors of the mitochondrial electron transport chain, *e.g.*, malonate, is truly a consequence of energy depletion, then agents which bypass or ameliorate the energy defect should attenuate the lesions. Coenzyme $Q_{10}$ ($CoQ_{10}$) is an essential component of the electron transport chain, where it serves as an electron donor and acceptor. It also improves membrane fluidity and acts as an antioxidant.[43] Administration of $CoQ_{10}$ results in increased activity of the mitochondrial electron transfer system *in vivo* and *in vitro*[44,45] and protects against ischemia in the heart.[46]

We examined the effects of oral treatment with $CoQ_{10}$ on lesions produced by malonate. Rats received oral $CoQ_{10}$ at doses of 100, 200, and 400 mg/kg for 10 days prior to intrastriatal injection of malonate. Pretreatment with $CoQ_{10}$ dose-dependently attenuated lesions produced by malonate.

Nicotinamide is a cofactor of the electron transport chain and has also been

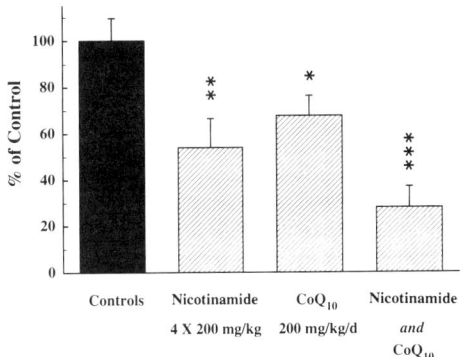

**FIGURE 3.** Effects of treatment with $CoQ_{10}$, nicotinamide or their combination on striatal malonate lesions. The combination produced additive neuroprotective effects. ** $p < 0.01$, *** $p < 0.001$.

reported to show efficacy in the treatment of patients with mitochondrial encephalopathies.[47] We therefore examined whether administration of nicotinamide could protect against malonate-induced striatal lesions. Rats were treated with nicotinamide at four doses of 50, 100, 200, 250 or 500 mg/kg i.p. Nicotinamide produced dose-responsive significant neuroprotective effects in this model with a maximal protection of 60%.

Subsequently we examined whether the combination of nicotinamide with $CoQ_{10}$ might be more efficacious than either compound alone. Pretreatment with oral $CoQ_{10}$ at 200 mg/kg/d produced a significant 33% attenuation of lesion size, while nicotinamide 200 mg/kg × 4 attenuated the lesion size by 43%. The combination of both agents exerted additive effects reducing the lesion size to 72% (FIG.

---

**FIGURE 4.** Schematic representation of the NMDA receptor-mediated cascade of cell death and potential steps of therapeutic intervention. *Upper panel:* Mitochondria provide ATP that fuels a multitude of ion pumps which produce and maintain voltage and ion gradients across neuronal membranes, thereby creating a resting potential of $-80$ mV. The cytoplasmatic $Ca^{2+}$ concentration is maintained several magnitudes lower than outside the cell by means of ATPases that actively move $Ca^{2+}$ out of the cell or into intracellular storage organelles such as the endoplasmatic reticulum (ER). *Lower panel:* Excitotoxicity may occur as a consequence of a defect in energy metabolism. This mechanism is thought to be due to membrane depolarization due to ATP depletion, followed by relief of the voltage-dependent $Mg^{2+}$ block of the NMDA receptor, leading to an ion influx, especially the inward movement of $Na^+$ and $Ca^{2+}$. The intracellular $Ca^{2+}$ concentration increases dramatically leading to an activation of $Ca^{2+}$-dependent enzymes, including the neuronal nitric oxide (NO) synthase which produces NO·. NO· may interact with superoxide radicals ($O_2\cdot$) to form peroxynitrite ($ONOO^-$).[51] The formation of peroxynitrite does not require transition metals, and once formed it can diffuse over several cell diameters where it can oxidize lipids, proteins and DNA. It also can produce nitronium ions which then nitrate tyrosine residues.[52,53] Peroxynitrite can also be protonated to form ONOOH, which may then decompose to OH·.[54,55] Increased mitochondrial $Ca^{2+}$ concentrations also lead to an increase in $O_2\cdot$.[56] The impairment of electron ($e^-$) flux through the electron transport chain produces $O_2\cdot$. Potential therapeutics in this cascade are: (a) Glutamate release inhibitors, *e.g.*, lamotrigine, (2) NMDA antagonists, *e.g.*, MK-801, memantine, (3) $Ca^{2+}$ chelators, (4) substrates of energy repletion, *e.g.*, $CoQ_{10}$ and nicotinamide, (5) selective neuronal NO-synthase inhibitors, and (6) free radical scavengers, *e.g.*, spin traps.

## Normal conditions

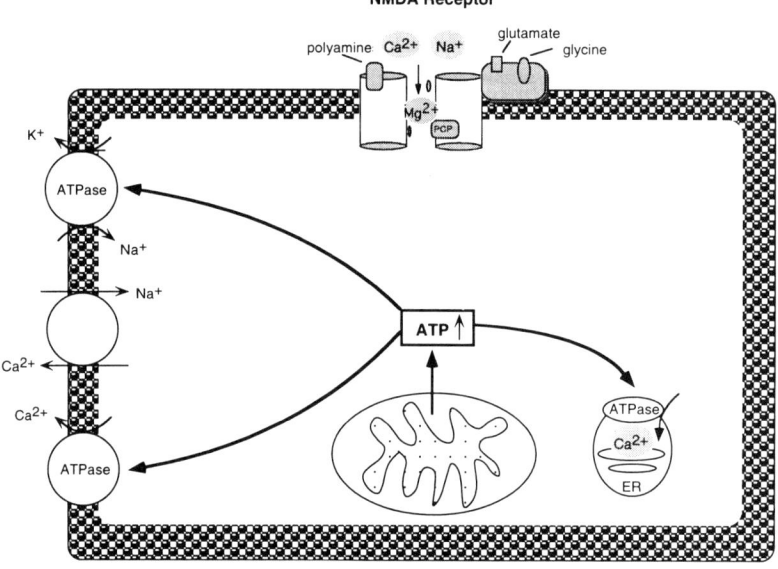

## Energy failure

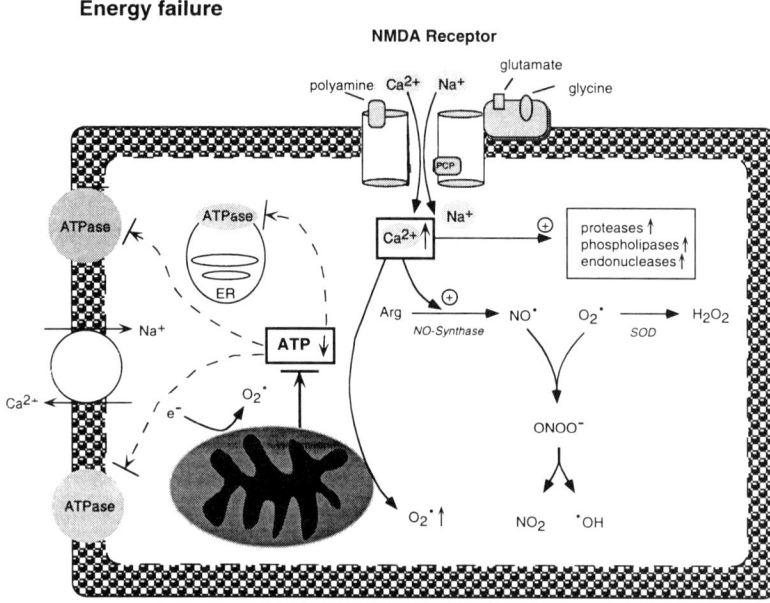

3). The combination was significantly better than nicotinamide alone ($p < 0.05$) or $CoQ_{10}$ alone ($p < 0.01$).

To prove that the neuroprotective effects of $CoQ_{10}$ and nicotinamide are due to energy repletion, we examined the effects of oral $CoQ_{10}$ at a dose of 200 mg/kg for 10 days, nicotinamide 200 mg/kg × 4 i.p., or the combination of both agents on ATP depletions produced by malonate. Malonate alone reduced ATP by 43%. Both $CoQ_{10}$ and nicotinamide treatment prevented ATP depletions as compared with the unlesioned striata of the control animals. Similarly in animals treated with a combination of $CoQ_{10}$ and nicotinamide there was no significant depletion of ATP on the lesioned side, and the ATP content of both the lesioned and unlesioned striata was significantly increased approximately 2-fold.

Although $CoQ_{10}$ is an antioxidant[43] these results showing that it blocks ATP depletions produced by malonate suggests that it may be acting to improve the efficiency of the electron transport chain *in vivo*. Another potential mechanism by which nicotinamide may exert neuroprotective effects is as an inhibitor of poly (adenosine diphosphate (ADP)-ribose) polymerase. In the presence of DNA strand breaks, this chromatin-bound enzyme transfers ADP-ribose from nicotinamide-adenine dinucleotide (NAD) to nuclear proteins and to the ADP-ribose polymer itself, with concomitant release of nicotinamide. This can lead to a depletion of NAD, which can interrupt ATP production and lead to cell death. Both hydrogen peroxide and nitric oxide can produce DNA damage, which associated with cell death and can be prevented by inhibitors of poly (ADP-ribose) polymerase.[48-50]

## CONCLUSIONS

Our results have implications for the pathogenesis of neurodegenerative diseases and offer new strategies for their treatment. There are several potential sites at which therapies may be targeted in neurodegenerative diseases (FIG. 4). If slow excitotoxic cell death is important in neurodegenerative diseases then glutamate release inhibitors, NMDA and non-NMDA antagonists, strategies to improve mitochondrial function, free radical scavengers, neurotrophic factors and $Ca^{2+}$ chelators should be beneficial. It is possible that combinations of therapies, particularly compounds which act at sequential steps in the neurodegenerative process, may have improved efficacy over agents acting at a single step of the cascade. In our paradigms of striatal lesions produced by malonate the combination of S-PBN and MK-801 treatment showed significantly better protection than MK-801 pretreatment alone (FIG. 2). If a combination of therapies is possible in neurodegenerative diseases it might enable one to utilize some compounds at lower dose levels than would otherwise be possible, allowing the avoidance of adverse central nervous system side effects. Once effective treatments are established future prospects will include using both genetic and biochemical markers for identifying patients at risk for neurodegenerative diseases, so that one can initiate therapy prior to the onset of clinical symptoms.

## REFERENCES

1. COYLE, J. T. & P. PUTTFARCKEN. 1993. Oxidative stress, glutamate and neurodegenerative disorders. Science **262**: 689–695.

2. BEAL, M. F. 1992. Role of excitotoxicity in human neurological disease. Curr. Opin. Neurobiol. **2**: 657–662.
3. CHOI, D. W. 1988. Glutamate neurotoxicity and diseases of the nervous system. Neuron **1**: 623–634.
4. ALBIN, R. L. & J. T. GREENAMYRE. 1992. Alternative excitotoxic hypothesis. Neurology **42**: 733–738.
5. BEAL, M. F. 1992. Does impairment of energy metabolism result in excitotoxic neuronal death in neurodegenerative illnesses? Ann. Neurol. **31**: 119–130.
6. BEAL, M. F., B. T. HYMAN & W. KOROSHETZ. 1993. Do defects in mitochondrial energy metabolism underlie the pathology of neurodegenerative disease? TINS **16**: 125–131.
7. SCHULZ, J. B. & M. F. BEAL. 1994. Mitochondrial dysfunction in movement disorders. Curr. Opin. Neurol. **7**: 333–339.
8. BOWLING, A. C., E. M. MUTISYA, L. C. WALKER, D. L. PRICE, L. C. CORK & M. F. BEAL. 1993. Age-dependent impairment of mitochondrial function in primate brain. J. Neurochem. **60**: 1964–1967.
9. DYKENS, J. A., A. STERN & E. TRENKNER. 1987. Mechanisms of kainate toxicity to cerebellar neurons *in vitro* is analogous to reperfusion tissue injury. J. Neurochem. **49**: 1222–1228.
10. LAFON-CAZAL, M., S. PIETRI, M. CULCASI & J. BOCKAERT. 1993. NMDA-dependent superoxide production and neurotoxicity. Nature **364**: 535–537.
11. TIPTON, K. F. & T. P. SINGER. 1993. Advances in our understanding of the mechanisms of the neurotoxicity of MPTP and related compounds. J. Neurochem. **61**: 1191–1206.
12. RAMSAY, R. R., M. J. KRUEGER, S. K. YOUNGSTER, M. R. GLUCK, J. E. CASIDA & T. P. SINGER. 1991. Interaction of 1-methyl-4-phenylpyridinium ion ($MPP^+$) and its analogs with the rotenone/piericidin binding site of NADH dehydrogenase. J. Neurochem. **56**: 1184–1190.
13. CHAN, P., L. E. DELANNEY, I. IRWIN, J. W. LANGSTON & D. DIMONTE. 1991. Rapid ATP loss caused by 1-methyl-4-phenyl-1,2,3,6-tetrahydropyridine in mouse brain. J. Neurochem. **57**: 348–351.
14. STOREY, E., B. T. HYMAN, B. JENKINS, E. BROUILLET, J. M. MILLER, B. R. ROSEN & M. F. BEAL. 1992. 1-Methyl-4-phenylpyridinium produces excitotoxic lesions in rat striatum as a result of impairment of oxidative metabolism. J. Neurochem. **58**: 1975–1978.
15. BROUILLET, E. & M. F. BEAL. 1993. NMDA antagonists partially protect against MPTP induced neurotoxicity in mice. NeuroReport **4**: 387–390.
16. TURSKI, L., K. BRESSLER, K-J. RETTIG, P-A LOESCHMANN & H. WACHTEL. 1991. Protection of substantia nigra from $MPP^+$ neurotoxicity by N-methyl-D-aspartate antagonists. Nature **349**: 414–419.
17. KUPSCH, A., P-A. LOESCHMANN, H. SAUER, G. ARNOLD, P. RENNER, D. PUFAL, M. BURG, H. WACHTEL, G. T. BRUGGENCATE & W. H. OERTEL. 1992. Do NMDA receptor antagonists protect against MPTP-toxicity? Biochemical and immunocytochemical analyses in black mice. Brain Res. **592**: 74–83.
18. SONSALLA, P. K., G. D. ZEEVALK, L. MANZINO, A. GIOVANNI & W. J. NICKLAS. 1992. MK-801 fails to protect against the dopaminergic neuropathology produced by systemic 1-methyl-4-phenyl-1,2,3,6-tetrahydropyridine in mice or intranigral 1-methyl-4-phenylpyridinium in rats. J. Neurochem. **58**: 1979–1982.
19. ZUDDAS, A., G. OBERTO, F. VAGLINI, F. FASCETTI, F. FORNAI & G. U. CORSINI. 1992. MK-801 prevents 1-methyl-4-phenyl-1,2,3,6-tetrahydropyridine-induced parkinsonism in primates. J. Neurochem. **59**: 733–739.
20. LANGE, K. W., P. A. LOSCHMANN, E. SOFIC, M. BURG, R. HOROWSKI, K. T. KALVERAM, H. WACHTEL & P. RIEDERER. 1993. The competitive NMDA antagonist CPP protects substantia nigra neurons from MPTP-induced degeneration in primates. Naunyn-Schmiedebergs Arch. Pharmack. **348**: 586–592.
21. HASEGAWA, E., K. TAKESHIGE, T. OISHI & S. MINAKAMI. 1990. 1-Methyl-4-phenylpyridinium ($MPP^+$) induces NADH-dependent superoxide formation and enhances NADH-dependent lipid peroxidation in bovine heart submitochondrial particles. Biochem. Biophys. Res. Commun. **170**:1049–1055.

22. CHIUEH, C. C., G. KRISHNA, P. TULSI, T. OBATA, K. LANG, S-J HUANG & D. L. MURPHY. 1992. Intracranial microdialysis of salicylic acid to detect hydroxyl radical generation through dopamine autooxidation in the caudate nucleus: effects of MPP$^+$. Free Radic. Biol. Med. **13:** 581–583.
23. ADAMS, JR, J. D., L. K. KLAIDMAN & A. C. LEUNG. 1993. MPP$^+$ and MPDP$^+$ induced oxygen radical formation with mitochondrial enzymes. Free Radic. Biol. Med. **15:** 181–186.
24. CLEETER, M. W. J., J. M. COOPER & A. H. V. SCHAPIRA. 1992. Irreversible inhibition of mitochondrial complex I by 1-methyl-4-phenylpyridinium: evidence for free radical involvement. J. Neurochem. **58:** 786–789.
25. LUDOLPH, A., M. SEELIG, A. LUDOLPH, P. NOVITT, C. N. ALLEN, P. S. SPENCER & M. I. SABRI. 1992. 3-Nitropropionic acid—exogenous animal neurotoxin and possible human striatal toxin. Can. J. Neurol. Sci. **18:** 492–498.
26. BROUILLET, E., B. G. JENKINS, B. T. HYMAN, R. J. FERRANTE, N. W. KOWALL, R. SRIVASTAVA, D. S. ROY, B. R. ROSEN & M. F. BEAL. 1993. Age-dependent vulnerability of the striatum to the mitochondrial toxin 3-nitropropionic acid. J. Neurochem. **60:** 356–9.
27. BEAL, M. F., E. BROUILLET, B. G. JENKINS, R. J. FERRANTE, N. W. KOWALL, J. M. MILLER, E. STOREY, R. SRIVASTAVA, B. R. ROSEN, & B. T. HYMAN. 1993. Neurochemical and histological characterization of striatal excitotoxic lesions produced by the mitochondrial toxin 3-nitropropionic acid. J. Neurosci. **13:** 4181–4192.
28. BEAL, M. F., E. BROUILLET, B. JENKINS, R. HENSHAW, B. ROSEN & B. T. HYMAN. 1993. Age-dependent striatal excitotoxic lesions produced by the endogenous mitochondrial inhibitor malonate. J. Neurochem. **61:** 1147–1150.
29. HENSHAW, R., B. G. JENKINS, J. B. SCHULZ, R. J. FERRANTE, N. W. KOWALL, B. R. ROSEN & M. F. BEAL. 1994. Malonate produces striatal lesions by indirect NMDA receptor activation. Brain Res. **647:** 161–166.
30. ZEEVALK, G. D. & W. J. NICKLAS. 1991. Mechanisms underlying initiation of excitotoxicity associated with metabolic inhibition. Jpn. J. Physiol. **257:** 870–878.
31. DEUTSCH, A. Y., D. L. ROSIN, M. GOLDSTEIN, & R. H. ROTH. 1989. 3-Acetylpyridine-induced degeneration of the nigrostriatal dopamine system: an animal model of olivopontocerebellar atrophy-associated parkinsonism. Exp. Neurol. **105:** 1–9.
32. SCHULZ, J. B., D. R. HENSHAW, B. G. JENKINS, R. J. FERRANTE, N. W. KOWALL, B. R. ROSEN & M. F. BEAL. 1994. 3-Acetylpyridine produces age-dependent excitotoxic lesions in rat striatum. J. Cereb. Blood Flow Metab. in press.
33. KNECHT, K. T. & R. P. MASON. 1993. *In vivo* spin trapping of xenobiotic free radical metabolites. Arch. Biochem. Biophys. **303:** 185–194.
34. CARNEY, J. M., R. P. STARKE, C. N. OLIVER, R. W. LANDUM, M. S. CHENG, J. F. WU & R. A. FLOYD. 1991. Reversal of age-related increase in brain protein oxidation, decrease in enzyme activity, and loss in temporal and spatial memory by chronic administration of the spin-trapping compound *N-tert*-butyl-alpha-phenylnitrone. Proc. Natl. Acad. Sci. USA **88:** 3633–3636.
35. OLIVER, C. N., R. P. STARKE, E. R. STADTMAN, G. J. LIU, J. M. CARNEY & R. A. FLOYD. 1990. Oxidative damage to brain proteins, loss of glutamine synthetase activity, and production of free radicals during ischemia/reperfusion-induced injury to gerbil brain. Proc. Natl. Acad. Sci. USA **87:** 5144–5147.
36. PHILLIS, J. W. & C. CLOUGH-HELFMAN. 1990. Protection from cerebral ischemia injury in gerbils with the spin trap agent *N-tert*-butyl-$\alpha$-phenylnitrone. Neurosci. Lett. **116:** 315–319.
37. YUE, T-L, J-L. GU, P. G. LYSKO, H-Y. CHENG, F. C. BARONE & G. FEUERSTEIN. 1992. Neuroprotective effects of phenyl-t-butyl-nitrone in gerbil global brain ischemia and in cultured rat cerebrellar neurons. Brain Res **574:** 193–197.
38. SCHULZ, J. B., R. HENSHAW & M. F. BEAL. 1994. Involvement of free radicals in excitotoxicity *in vivo*. Neurology **44**(Suppl 2): A178.
39. BEDERSON, J. B., L. H. PITTS, S. M. GERMANO, M. C. NISHIMURA, R. L. DAVIS & H. M. BARTKOWSKI. 1986. Evaluation of 2,3,5-triphenyltetrazolium chloride as a stain

for detection and quantification of experimental cerebral infarction in rats. Stroke **17:** 1304–1308.
40. FLOYD, R. A., J. J. WATSON & P. K. WONG. 1984. Sensitivie assay of hydroxyl radical formation utilizing high pressure liquid chromatography with electrochemical detection of phenol and salicylate hydroxylation products. J. Biochem. Biophys. Methods **10:** 221–235.
41. HALLIWELL, B., H. KAUR & M. INGELMAN-SUNDBERG. 1991. Hydroxylation of salicylate as an assay for hydroxyl radicals: a cautionary note. Free Radic. Biol. Med. **10:** 439–441.
42. LUST, W. D., G. K. FEUSSNER, E. K. BARBEHENN & J. V. PASSONEAU. 1981. The enzymatic measurements of adenine nucleotides and P-creatinine in picomole amounts. Anal. Biochem. **110:** 258–266.
43. FREI, B., M. C. KIM & B. N. AMES. 1990. Ubiquinol-10 is an effective lipid-soluble antioxidant at physiological concentrations. Proc. Natl. Acad. Sci. USA **87:** 4879–4883.
44. NAKAMURA, T., H. SANMA, M. HIMENO & K. KATO. 1989. Transfer of exogenous coenzyme Q to inner membrane of heart mitochondria in rats. *In* Biochemical and clinical aspects of coenzyme $Q_{10}$. Yamamura, Y., K. Folkers & Yu. Ito, Eds. Vol. 2: 3–11. Elsevier/North Holland. Amsterdam.
45. SCHNEIDER, H., J. J. LEMASTER & C. R. HACKEMBROEK. 1982. Lateral diffusion of ubiquinone during electron transfer in phospholipid- and ubiquinone-enriched mitochondrial membrane. J. Biol. Chem. **257:** 10789–10793.
46. OHHARA, H., H. KANAIDE, R. YOSHIMURA, M. OKADA & M. NAKAMURA. 1981. A protective effect of coenzyme $Q_{10}$ on ischemia and reperfusion of the isolated perfused rat heart. J. Mol. & Cell. Cardiol. **13:** 65–74.
47. PENN, A. M., J. W. LEE, P. THUILLIER, M. WAGNER, K. M. MACLURE, M. R. MENARD, L. D. HALL & N. G. KENNAWAY. 1992. MELAS syndrome with mitochondrial tRNA-(Leu)(UUR) mutation: correlation of clinical state, nerve conduction, and muscle 31P magnetic resonance spectroscopy during treatment with nicotinamide and riboflavin. Neurology **42:** 2147–52.
48. ZHANG, J., V. L. DAWSON, T. M. DAWSON & S. H. SNYDER. 1994. Nitric oxide activation of poly(ADP-ribose) synthetase in neurotoxicity. Science **263:** 687–689.
49. SCHRAUFSTATTER, I. U., D. B. HINSHAW, P. A. HYSLOP, R. G. SPRAGG & C. G. COCHRANE. 1986. Oxidant injury of cells. DNA strand-breaks activate polyadenosine diphosphate-ribose polymerase and lead to depletion of nicotinamide adenine dinucleotide. J. Clin. Invest. **77:** 1312–1320.
50. SCHRAUFSTATTER, I. U., P. A. HYSLOP, D. B. HINSHAW, R. G. SPRAGG, L. A. SKLAR & C. G. COCHRANE. 1986. Hydrogen peroxide-induced injury of cells and its prevention by inhibitors of poly(ADP-ribose) polymerase. Proc. Natl. Acad. Sci. USA **83:** 4908–4912.
51. BECKMAN, J. S., T. W. BECKMAN, J. CHEN, P. M. MARSHALL & B. A. FREEMAN. 1990. Apparent hydroxyl radical production by peroxynitrite: implications for endothelial injury from nitric oxide and superoxide. Proc. Natl Acad. Sci. USA **87:** 1621–1624.
52. BECKMAN, J. S., H. ISCHIROPOULOS, L. ZHU, M. VAN DER WOERD, C. SMITH, J. CHEN, J. HARRISON, J. C. MARTIN & M. TSAI. 1992. Kinetics of superoxide dismutase- and iron-catalazed nitration of phenolics by peroxynitrite. Arch. Biochem. Biphys. **298:** 438–445.
53. ISCHIROPOULOS, H., L. ZHU, J. CHEN, M. TSAI, J. C. MARTIN, C. D. SMITH & J. S. BECKMAN. 1992. Peroxynitrite-mediated tyrosine nitration catalyzed by superoxide dismutase. Arch. Biochem. Biophys. **298:** 431–437.
54. CROW, J. P., C. SPRUELL, J. CHEN, C. GUNN, H. ISCHIROPOULOS, M. TSAI, C. D. SMITH, R. RADI, W. H. KOPPENOL & J. S. BECKMAN. 1994. On the pH-dependent yield of hydroxyl radical products from peroxynitrite. Free Radic. Biol Med. **16:** 331–338.
55. VAN DER VLIET, A., C. A. O'NEILL, B. HALLIWELL, C. E. CROSS & H. KAUR. 1994. Aromatic hydroxylation and nitration of phenylalanine and tyrosine by peroxynitrite. Evidence for hydroxyl radical production from peroxynitrite. FEBS Lett. **339:** 89–92.
56. DYKENS, J. A. 1994. Isolated cerebral and cerebellar mitochondria produce free radicals when exposed to elevated $Ca^{2+}$ and $Na^+$: implications for neurodegeneration. J. Neurochem. **63:** 584–591.

# Neuroprotective Effects of Radical Scavengers in an Intact Dorsal Root Ganglion Hypoxia Model

P. R. BÄR

*Department of Neurology*
*University Hospital—AZU*
*Heidelberglaan 100*
*3584 CX Utrecht, The Netherlands*

## INTRODUCTION

The efficacy of potential neuroprotective agents is often tested in cultured cells.[1] Among the advantages of tissue culture are the controlled environment, the accessibility of the target cells and the many ways in which effects can be quantified, both biochemically and morphologically. At the same time, there are some drawbacks too. Cell culture requires dissociation of cells, which means that the cell is no longer in contact with its physiological neighbors. As it is known that in the central nervous system glial and neuronal cells communicate with each other, and that glial cells may play a role in protecting neurons from damage,[2] the absence of certain cell types may hinder correct interpretation of the results. The use of cocultures can be seen as an attempt to reestablish contacts between, *e.g.*, neurons and glial cells, but the physiological 3-dimensional matrix is still far away. Another approach may be the use of more or less intact pieces of tissue, such as slices (cortex, hippocampus) as has long been known in electrophysiology. These structures can be kept 'alive' for hours when appropriate measures are taken. Another example of an organotypic culture system is the dorsal root ganglion (DRG) which can be kept for days or weeks in culture. A technique, called the semisolid medium culture,[3] allows not only for long survival of slices or DRGs, but guarantees they will not disintegrate in culture and that cells will not migrate out of the tissue. Thus, the original structure is kept, and outgrowth of neurites is not obscured by migrating cells.[4] DRGs have been used successfully to study neuroprotection against neurotoxocity of cytostatic drugs such as cisplatin and taxol.[5] In the present study we used DRGs from 12-day-old chick embryos to study the neuroprotective effect of radical scavengers. We used neurite outgrowth to quantify the noxious effect of hypoxia, induced by nitrogen treatment, and we tested the efficacy of two man-made scavengers, one from the 21-aminosteroid group, the other a water-soluble vitamin E analogue.

## MATERIALS AND METHODS

DRGs were dissected from 12-day-old chick embryos and placed with 4 in a 30-mm petri dish. A drop of collagen was applied to each DRG as described.[6]

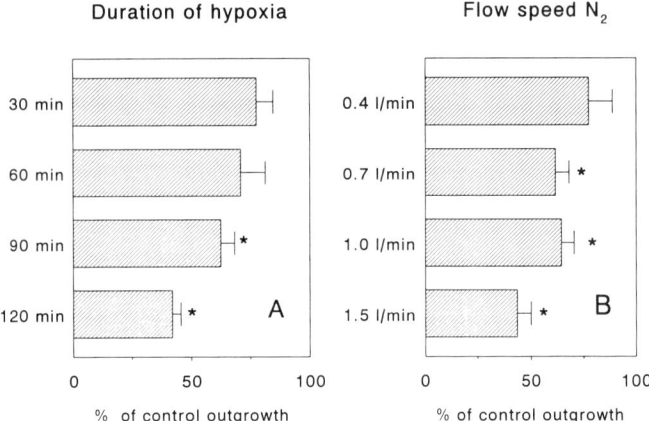

**FIGURE 1.** The influence of the duration of hypoxia (**A**) and the nitrogen gas flow speed (**B**) on the neurite outgrowth of cultured dorsal root ganglia. The outgrowth of parallel cultures not treated with $N_2/CO_2$ is set at 100%. *Asteriks* indicate significant differences with respect to controls ($p < 0.05$).

After 45 min 1.5 ml of MEM (minimal essential medium, 10% fetal calf serum, 1.75 ng/ml $\beta$ nerve growth factor ($\beta$NGF)) was added, and the DRGs were kept at 37°C and 5% $CO_2$.

After 24 h in culture a clear outgrowth could be observed and was quantified using an interactive computerized image analysis system. Next, the DRGs were put in an airtight, thermostated chamber and exposed to hypoxic conditions by blowing a $N_2/CO_2$ (95/5%) mixture via sterile filters through the chamber. Twenty-four hours after this treatment the neurite outgrowth was measured again, so that each DRG acted as its own control. Per experimental condition the data of 2–4 dishes, each containing 4 DRGs, were averaged.

The effect of different hypoxic conditions was tested first by varying duration and gas flow speed. Next, glutathione and nimodipine were tested to assess the role of radicals and calcium influx, respectively, in outgrowth inhibition. Then the two radical scavengers were tested: U74389G (gift from The Upjohn Company, USA) and MDL 73335A (gift from Marion Merril Dow, France). All substances were added immediately before hypoxia.

## RESULTS

The outgrowth assay was validated by measuring DRGs treated with $\beta$NGF (not shown). It appeared that 0, 1, 2, and 4 ng $\beta$NGF produced a linear dose-response curve. The effect of hypoxia is dependent on the duration and the speed of the nitrogen flow (FIG. 1) In following experiments we chose 0.7 l/min during 180 min as standard hypoxic condition. This treatment resulted in an inhibition of outgrowth between 50 and 75%. Nimodipine and glutathione improved neurite

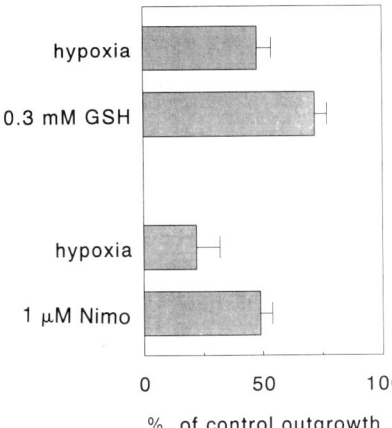

**FIGURE 2.** The protective effect of glutathione (GSH) and nimodipine (Nimo) on the neurite outgrowth of cultures treated with hypoxia for 180 min at a flow speed of 0.71/min. Outgrowth of normal control cultures is set at 100%.

outgrowth at 48 h (FIG. 2). The scavengers were both very effective in protecting the neurons from the damaging effect of hypoxia, up to 80% (FIG. 3).

## DISCUSSION

Neurite outgrowth is a complex activity of fetal or damaged neurons. It requires an intact energy supply, protein synthesis machinery and transport capacity. During anoxia, hypoxia or hypoglycemia, several processes in the cell will be affected to

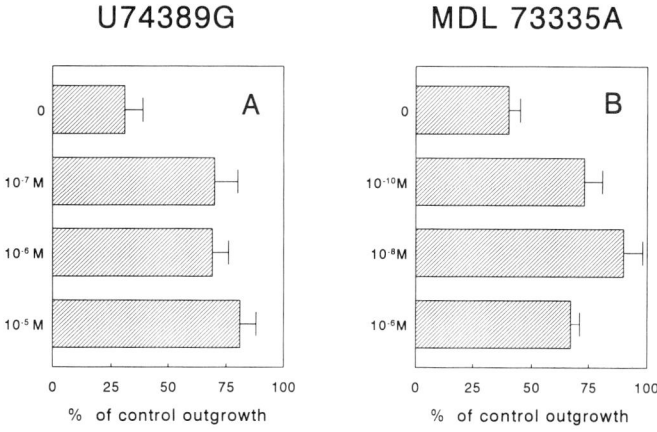

**FIGURE 3.** The neuroprotective effect of two radical scavengers, U74389G, a 21-aminosteroid (**A**) and MDL 73335A, an $\alpha$-tocopherol analogue (**B**). The concentrations used are indicated on the *y-axis;* the *x-axis* gives the percentage outgrowth with respect to untreated control cultures. All treatments were statistically significant ($p < 0.05$).

a more or less severe degree, resulting in energy depletion, excessive neurotransmitter release, dysregulation of the intracellular homeostasis, and overactivation of certain enzymes.[7] Free oxygen radicals are formed in several pathways and are believed to be the cause of severe cellular damage, via lipid peroxidation, but also through their reactions with proteins (enzymes, receptors) and DNA. Thus, full neuroprotection after a hypoxic period, if at all feasible, can only be the result of a multiple approach. Tissue culture has been used to test many possible protective agents, but the data from these studies cannot always be extrapolated to the intact animal or the final target, man. The use of intact structures such as the spinal cord slice[8] or, in this study, the DRG may be one step closer to the *in vivo* situation. We found that neurite outgrowth from DRGs is very sensitive to hypoxia and that several agents are capable of restoring outgrowth. As neurite outgrowth will be affected by many, if not all aspects of intracellular dysregulation, the DRG may well constitute a uniform bioassay to test neuroprotective drugs.

The man-made radical scavengers U74389G and MDL 73335A seem very potent in this assay. The drugs are present in the medium during the hypoxic period, and remain in the culture 24 h after reoxygenation. Radical formation is a relatively late phenomenon, and is believed to have a long-lasting effect and to show a peak when fresh oxygen is supplied. This may partially explain the large effect of scavengers, when compared to, *e.g.*, the effect of nimodipine, which affects the relatively short period of calcium entry via L-channels. The fact that both scavengers have a significant effect indicates that the highly lipophilic 21-aminosteroid[9] and the water-soluble MDL 73335A[10] can penetrate the DRG sufficiently. This is of importance, as it is now known that tirilazad mesylate, which is highly efficient in protecting neurons in tissue culture, *in vivo* probably will not reach neurons, due to its extreme lipophilicity. This is one example where tissue culture experiments, in which no blood-brain barrier is present, do not exactly predict the action of a drug *in vivo*. The high neuroprotective potential of tirilazad mesylate *in vivo* can be explained by its action on the endothelium of the brain capillary bed.[9]

In conclusion, the intact DRG appears to be a sensitive CNS structure that may very well serve as bioassay to test the efficacy of neuroprotective drugs. The anatomical integrity, maintained by culturing in a physiological matrix, is closer to the *in vivo* situation than in dissociated cultures.

## REFERENCES

1. PERUCHE, B., B. AHLEMEYER, H. BRUNGS & J. KRIEGLSTEIN. 1990. Cultured neurons for testing antihypoxic drug effects. J. Pharmacol. Methods **23**: 63–67.
2. VIBULSRETH, S., F. HEFTI, M. D. GINSBERG & R. BUSTO. 1987. Astrocytes protect cultured neurons from degeneration induced by anoxia. Brain Res. **422**: 303–310.
3. MANDYS, V., R. VAN DER NEUT, P. R. BÄR & W. H. GISPEN. 1991. Cultivation of rat foetal spinal cord slices in a semi-solid medium—a new approach for the study of axonal outgrowth and regeneration. J. Neurosci. Methods **38**: 63–69.
4. MANDYS, V., R. TURECEK, W. H. GISPEN & P. R. BÄR. 1994. Organotypic cultures of chick dorsal root ganglia in a semi-solid medium: a model for neurotoxicity testing. Toxicol. In Vitro **8**: 81–90.
5. HOL, E. M., V. MANDYS, W. H. GISPEN & P. R. BÄR. 1994. Protection by an $ACTH_{4-9}$

analogue against the toxic effects of cisplatin and taxol on sensory neurons and glial cells in vitro. J. Neurosci. Res. **39:** 178–185.
6. JOOSTEN, E. A. J., W. H. GISPEN & P. R. BÄR. 1994. Tropism and corticospinal target selection. Neuroscience **59:** 33–41.
7. SIESJÖ, B. K., K. KATSURA, K. PAHLMARK & M-L. SMITH. 1992. The multiple causes of ischemic brain damage: a speculative hypothesis. *In* Pharmacology of Cerebral Ischemia. J. Krieglstein & H. Oberpichler-Schwenk, Eds. 511–525. Wiss. Verl. Ges. Stuttgart.
8. BÄR, P. R., H. RENKEMA, C. M. H. M. VERAART & W. H. GISPEN. 1993. Nimodipine prevents depolarization-induced inhibition of neurite outgrowth from cultured rat spinal cord slices. Cell Calcium **14:** 293–299.
9. HALL, E. D., J. M. MCCALL & E. D. MEANS. 1994. Therapeutic potential of the lazaroids (21-aminosteroids) in acute CNS trauma, ischemia, and subarachnoid hemorrhage. Adv. Pharmacol. **28:** 221–268.
10. BOLKENIUS, F., M. PETTY, M. GRISAR, P. SANDOR & W. DE JONG. 1992. Protection against neurodegeneration by a water soluble analogue of $\alpha$-tocopherol. Neurochem. Int. **21:**(S): B1.

# Discussion

ANONYMOUS: What is the target of 1-methyl-4-phenyl-1,2,3,6-tetrahydropyridine (MPTP) in the whole animal?

S. ALI (*National Center for Toxicological Research, FDA, Jefferson, AR*): As far as the literature is concerned, the nigrostriatal dopamine system is the main target of MPTP-induced neurotoxicity. The effects on the peripheral nervous system are still unclear. Some of our preliminary data suggest that it effects body temperature and produces hypothermia by affecting the peripheral nervous system as well as the cardiovascular system.

M. F. BEAL (*Massachusetts General Hospital, Boston*): In my view, the primary site is the mitochondrial where it acts as a complex I inhibitor. It is accumulated in mitochondria. Direct adenosine triphosphate (ATP) measurements following MPTP in mice show reductions in the striatum, consistent with a mitochondrial effect.

S. JONAS (*New York University*): At what dose and how long did you use ganglioside $GM_1$?

ALI: We used only 10 mg/kg, ip for 5 days (M–F). On Wednesday, we injected $4 \times 10$ mg/kg methamphetamine (METH) to see if the $GM_1$ resulted in any protective effects and we used dopamine (DA) depletion as a neurochemical endpoint. Once we finished the study, we realized that the 10-mg/kg $GM_1$ dose may not be high. Therefore, we are in the process of increasing the dose to see if it has any protective effect against METH- or MPTP-induced neurotoxicity as measured by DA depletion in mice.

A. SCALLET (*National Center for Toxicological Research, FDA, Jefferson, AR*): You emphasized the role of body temperature in the effects of MPTP and amphetamines. It is important to note that two modes of temperature alteration from drugs can take place: 1) re-adjustment of set-point where no defense mechanism takes place or 2) change (reduction) of temperature where thermoregulation defense mechanisms are active (*e.g.*, shivering, brown fat thermogenesis, etc.), since they are trying to restore body temperature to the hypothalamic temperature set-point. Perhaps neurochemical differences between these two states account for some of the varying toxicity of such compounds.

W. SLIKKER (*National Center for Toxicological Research, FDA, Jefferson, AR*): Why is there an apparent age dependence to neurotoxic insult?

ALI: In my view, there are several factors responsible to produce age-dependent neurotoxicity by any neurotoxic insult, such as MPTP, METH, 3-nitropropionic acid (3-NPA) and malonate. These factors could include the generation of free radicals, activities of antioxidant enzymes, such as superoxide dismutase (SOD), catalase, and glutathione synthase, etc., and also the mitochondrial complex-inhibiting ability that may differ between the young and aged animal.

BEAL: Age dependence for MPTP is due to increases in monoamine oxidase $B_1$ and no age dependence is seen with MPTP itself either in our hands or in the studies of Langston and colleagues. Malonate, 3-nitropropionic acid and sodium azide all show marked age dependence. This may be due to a decline in mitochondrial function, which we and others have found in primate brain. There is also an increase in free radical generation by mitochondria with normal aging, which may contribute to the age-dependent neurotoxicity of blockers of mitochondrial electron transport, which act distal to ubiquinone.

S. GOLDIN (*Cambridge NeuroScience*): What are the implications, in terms of side effects and safety, of inhibition of the actions of free radicals which normally play a physiological role?

BEAL: Free radicals play a role in a number of normal physiologic processes including electron transport and killing of bacteria by neutrophils. Nitric oxide is a free radical. The long-term consequences of treatment with free radical scavengers are unknown. They, however, have been administered to animals for months without adverse effects, and antioxidant vitamins have been used in man for years without adverse effects.

D. J. MCCARTHY (*Fisons Pharmaceuticals, Rochester, NY*): Do you think that the malonic acid model is a good predictor of the effectiveness of an agent for treatment of stroke?

BEAL: Malonic acid appears to be an excellent model for predicting potential efficacy of agents for treatment of stroke. It produces a transient partial energy depletion which is similar to the penumbral region of focal ischemic models. It also shows a similar profile in response to neuroprotective agents. The lesions are attenuated by glutamate release blockers, competitive and noncompetitive *N*-methyl-D-aspartate (NMDA) antagonists and free radical scavengers.

G. C. PALMER (*Fisons Pharmaceuticals, Rochester, NY*): Please explain the method to produce 3-nitroproprionic lesions in rats.

BEAL: It is very tricky to get the chronic, less diffuse, low-grade lesion. The dose-response curve is steep; a difference of 1 mg/kg given ip between 12–16 mg/kg can result in dramatically different sized lesions. The age of the animal is also important, since the lesions are markedly age dependent. In view of this, to do therapeutic studies, we have treated animals until controls become symptomatic and at that time have sacrificed treated and untreated animals in pairs. This eliminates problems with control animals becoming symptomatic and developing lesions following varying durations of treatment of 3-nitropropionic acid.

P. R. BÄR (*Utrecht University*): Studies (Italian) with patients with mitochondrial myopathy and high doses of coenzyme $Q_{10}$ produced lower lactate levels, but *no* subjective improvement and *no* increase in muscle $Q_{10}$ levels. Do you have any data on whether $Q_{10}$ reaches your target, *i.e.*, neuronal mitochondria, or does it, due to its high hydrophobicity, remain in the endothelial membrane and have some beneficial effect there (compared to tirilazad meslate, which stays in the vascular membrane too). If so, what could be the neuroprotective mechanism there?

BEAL: There are as yet very few data available concerning coenzyme $Q_{10}$ and its pharmacology in brain. Since it is extremely hydrophobic, one would expect that it may accumulate slowly in brain, similar to observations with vitamin E. This is the reason we choose to treat animals with coenzyme $Q_{10}$ for 9–10 days prior to testing for neuroprotective effects. Single doses have been ineffective. We are presently using an assay to assess the pharmacokinetics of coenzyme $Q_{10}$

in brain but we do not as yet have definitive data. We would expect that it will accumulate slowly in brain parenchyma.

JONAS: You have noted rapid destruction of neurons and glia from 3-nitropropionic acid. Are blood vessels injured early?

BEAL: We have not observed any destruction of blood vessels or any hemorrhage at the site of the lesions, even with high doses.

JONAS: Can you comment on the mechanisms of the clinically stroke-like focal parietal-occipital episodes in mitochondrial encephalomyopathy, lactic acidosis, and stroke (MELAS). Why is there such a bias toward posterior localization? Why do the lesions seen acutely on magnetic resonance imaging (MRI) recede so strikingly? Is the apparent ischemic lesion from obstruction in the arterial tree? If so what are the mechanisms, or is the lesion a biochemical anoxia?

BEAL: The mechanism of ischemic lesions in MELAS is of great interest. It could occur as a consequence of either a microvascular effect or be due to tissue hypoxia at a cellular level, or both. In favor of the former is the observation of marked increases in succinate dehydrogenase-stained mitochondria in endothelial cells in MELAS. The extent of the lesions and their rapid recession, however, favor a contribution of tissue hypoxia. The predilection for parietal-occipital cortex may be due to the relatively high metabolic rate of this cortical region.

# Short-Term Regulation of Neuronal Calcium Channels by Depolarization[a]

JAI LIU,[b] ALETA RUTLEDGE, AND DAVID J. TRIGGLE[c]

*School of Pharmacy*
*State University of New York at Buffalo*
*Buffalo, New York 14260-1200*

## INTRODUCTION

Ion channels are a class of pharmacological receptor which possess drug binding sites for both activator and antagonist ligands. These drug binding sites exhibit discrete structure-activity relationships including stereoselectivity, they are regulated in number and function by a variety of homologous and heterologous influences, and their expression and function are altered in a number of disease states.[1] All of these observations apply to the voltage-gated $Ca^{2+}$ channel which, in fact, represents an homologous family of pharmacological receptors, which is itself a subset of a superfamily of voltage-gated ion channels.[2,3] These subtypes of $Ca^{2+}$ channel may be characterized by their structure, by their electrophysiological characteristics, and by their pharmacologic properties. At least four major types of $Ca^{2+}$ channel have been recognized pharmacologically according to their sensitivity to a variety of clinical and experimental drugs (TABLE 1). The L-type channel has been the best investigated principally because of its importance in determining cardiovascular function and because of the clinical availability of drugs including the prototypical verapamil, nifedipine and diltiazem classes (FIG. 1). The voltage-gated $Ca^{2+}$ channel is a heteromeric association of subunits—alpha$_1$, alpha$_2$-delta, beta and gamma (specific to skeletal muscle)—which are coded for by separate genes. At the present time genes for six alpha$_1$, four beta, one alpha$_2$-delta and one gamma subunit have been cloned.[2,3] Thus, the opportunity exists for a rich variety of voltage-gated $Ca^{2+}$ channel subtypes and functions. Biochemical and expression studies have amply documented that the alpha$_1$ subunit is the major structural and functional component of the $Ca^{2+}$ channel. This subunit carries the permeation and gating functions of the channel and possesses the drug binding sites. However, expression studies have also demonstrated that these same functions of the alpha$_1$ subunit are also substantially modified by the presence of other subunits.[3,6-9] In particular, the beta subunit is of particular importance in modifying functional and pharmacologic activities. Thus, coexpression of beta subunits with the skeletal muscle alpha$_1$ subunit changes activation kinetics and

---

[a] This work was supported by grants from the National Institutes of Health (HL 16003 and NIMH 50281). Additional and generous support from Miles, Inc., West Haven, CT and Fisons Inc., Rochester, NY are gratefully acknowledged.

[b] Present address: National Institute of Diabetes and Digestive and Kidney Diseases, National Institutes of Helath, Laboratory of Bio-Organic Chemistry, Bethesda, MD 20892.

[c] Corresponding author.

TABLE 1. Classification of Voltage-Gated Calcium Channels

| Property | L | T | N | P |
|---|---|---|---|---|
| Conductance, pS | 25 | 8 | 12–20 | 10–12 |
| Activation threshold | high | low | high | moderate |
| Inactivation rate | slow | fast | moderate | rapid |
| Permeation | $Ba^{2+} > Ca^{2+}$ | $Ba^{2+} = Ca^{2+}$ | $Ba^{2+} > Ca^{2+}$ | $Ba^{2+} > Ca^{2+}$ |
| Function | E-coupling cardiovascular system, smooth muscle, endocrine cells and some neurons | cardiac SA node: neuronal spiking repetitive spike activity in neurons and endocrine cells | neuronal only: neurotransmitter release | neuronal only(?): neurotransmitter release |
| Pharmacologic sensitivity: 1,4-dihydropyridines (activators/antagonists), phenylalkylamines, benzothiazepines | sensitive | insensitive | insensitive | insensitive |
| $w$-Conotoxin | sensitive? (some) | insensitive | sensitive | insensitive |
| Octanol, amiloride | insensitive? | sensitive | insensitive | ? |
| Funnel web spider toxin | insensitive | insensitive | insensitive | insensitive |

increases 1,4-dihydropyridine binding site density. Similarly, coexpression of the beta$_1$ and cardiac alpha$_{1C}$ subunits leads to an increase in expressed current and the number of binding sites.[10,11] Similar observations have been made with N-type currents.[12] These and related observations indicate that the physiologic and pharmacologic properties of native $Ca^{2+}$ channels arise from the complete channel complex and that physiologic or pathologic modifications in the assembly of this complex may change channel number and function.

The regulation of the L-type channel under conditions of chronic drug and hormone levels, tissue lesions and clinical and experimental disease states has been well studied.[13] Chronic depolarization has been shown to be a regulatory signal in neuronal and neurosecretory cells downregulating both the number and function of the $Ca^{2+}$ channels.[14–17] Thus, depolarization of PC12 cells or chick retinal neurons for periods of 1–4 days causes a parallel loss of both 1,4-dihydropyridine binding sites and depolarization-induced $Ca^{2+}$ uptake.[15,16] It is of interest that chronic depolarization of cardiac cells in culture failed to show a similar downregulation.[16] Similarly, chronic treatment of PC12 cells with the antagonist nifedipine or the activator Bay K8644 caused up- and downregulation respectively of $Ca^{2+}$ channels as measured by 1,4-dihydropyridine binding, whole cell current, or $^{45}Ca^{2+}$ uptake. Chronic depolarization also regulates drug binding to $Ca^{2+}$ channels by altering the affinities or access of drugs to the several states of the channel. The binding of $Ca^{2+}$ channel antagonists, particularly 1,4-dihydropyridines, is widely established to be voltage-dependent affinity increasing with decreasing membrane potential.[19,20] Thus, voltage regulates $Ca^{2+}$ channel properties in at least two distinct ways.

We recently showed that a rat anterior pituitary neurosecretory cell line, GH$_4$C$_1$, expresses L-type channels and that these channels are regulated acutely

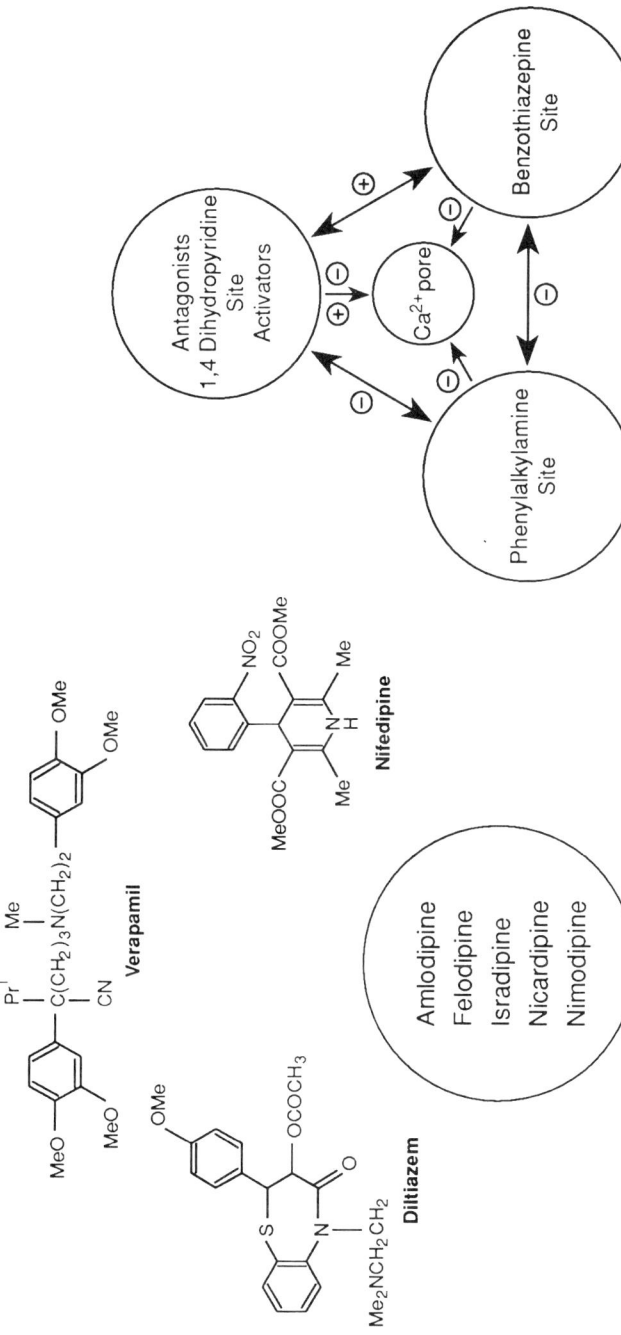

**FIGURE 1.** The organization of drug binding sites at the L-type voltage-gated $Ca^{2+}$ channel. Depicted are the sites for the three principal classes of antagonists represented by verapamil, nifedipine and diltiazem. These sites are linked to the permeation and the gating machinery of the channel and are linked one to the other by complex allosteric relationships. The second-generation 1,4-dihydropyridines, amlodipine, felodipine, nicardipine, nimodipine, interact at the 1,4-dihydropyridine site but exhibit different degrees of cardiovascular selectivity than the first-generation nifedipine.

and chronically by membrane potential.[22] Depolarization causes the anticipated increase in 1,4-dihydropyridine affinity and downregulation of the number and function of the $Ca^{2+}$ channels. Moreover, there appear to be at least two components with different time scales to the down regulation process. A rapid downregulation was observed with periods of depolarization up to two hours. This acute downregulation was membrane-potential dependent and $Ca^{2+}$ dependent and was protected by both $Ca^{2+}$ antagonists and calmodulin antagonists. This downregulation was rapidly reversible and this reversibility was not dependent on protein synthesis, consistent with it not involving major structural reorganization of cell machinery or degradation of channel components.[22] There are obvious parallels apparent between this process and the rapid desensitization seen in G protein-coupled receptors and that which is attributed to a reversible and transient cellular internalization of the receptor in a light membrane vesicle.[23] Our subsequent investigations suggest, however, that the process at the $Ca^{2+}$ channel may be more complex than a simple internalization of the heteromeric channel complex.

## METHODS

### Cell Culture

$GH_4C_1$ cells, a generous gift from Dr. Jane Chisholm, Miles Laboratories, Inc., West Haven, CT, were cultured in Ham's F-10 medium supplemented with 15% horse serum and 2.5% fetal calf serum, as previously described.[22] Cells were used when essentially confluent but still dividing.

### 1,4-Dihydropyridine Binding Assay

$(+)$-[$^3$H]PN 200-110 was used as the 1,4-dihydropyridine ligand in the binding assays in both membranes and intact cells.[22] This ligand was used extensively in previous studies of L-type $Ca^{2+}$ channels, is a single enantiomer, has high affinity, and shows high specific binding. [$^3$H]-$N$-methylscopolamine, a permanently charged ligand, was used to quantitate muscarinic receptors in the $GH_4C_1$ cells. The binding assay in whole $GH_4C_1$ cells under polarized and depolarized conditions (determined by the $K^+$ concentration) and in membrane preparations was described previously.[22] In brief, cells attached to 35- to 60-mm culture dishes were incubated with various concentrations of radioligands in Hank's buffer containing defined concentrations of $K^+$ (by replacement of $Na^+$) at 37°C for 90 min, or varying times for kinetic assays, with or without unlabeled ligand to define specific binding. For membrane binding cells were scraped from the plates and homogenized in Tris buffer followed by centrifugation at 30,000 g for 10 min. The resultant pellet, a microsomal fraction, was resuspended in 50 mM Tris buffer, pH 7.2 and used in conventional radioligand binding experiments.[20–23] Incubation was terminated by filtration through GF/B filters using a Brandel cell harvester.

## $^{45}Ca^{2+}$ Uptake

Uptake studies were carried out at 37°C as described.[20-23] Hank's solution containing 5mM $K^+$ (resting buffer) or various higher concentrations of $K^+$ (stimulating buffer) were used with $^{45}Ca^{2+}$. Incubation was for 20 sec and was terminated by aspiration and replacement with ice-cold Hank's buffer containing $LaCl_3$ (5 mM).

## Poly $A^+$ mRNA Preparation

Poly $A^+$ RNA was extracted from cells after varying periods of depolarization. In brief, cells were rinsed with Hank's solution and lysed in a buffer containing 0.2 mg/ml proteinase K, 0.2 M NaCl, 1.5 mM $MgCl_2$, 2% sodium dodecyl sulfate (SDS) and 0.2 M Tris-HCl, pH 7.5. The lysates were passed through a sterile plastic syringe with a 21 G needle to shear high molecular weight DNA and incubated at 45°C for 1–3 hrs with gentle shaking. Oligo-deoxythymidine (dT) cellulose beads were added to the lysates after the NaCl concentration of the lysates was increased to 0.5 M. The oligo-dT cellulose beads had been swollen in diethylpyrocarbonate (DEPC)-treated $H_2O$, treated with NaOH and equilibrated in binding buffer containing 0.5 M NaCl and 10 mM Tris-HCl at pH 7.5. The binding of poly $A^+$ mRNA to the oligo-cellulose beads was carried out at room temperature for 30–60 min with gentle shaking. Following incubation the binding mixture was centrifuged and the supernatant aspirated. The oligo-dT cellulose beads with mRNA attached were washed free of proteins, DNA, poly A RNA and other contaminants. The beads were resuspended in a small volume of binding buffer and transferred into a spin column inside an Eppendorf tube. The beads were then washed with buffer until the $OD_{260}$ of the flow was <0.05. Poly $A^+$ mRNA was then eluted with DEPC-treated $H_2O$. RNA was quantitated with spectrophotometry at 260 nm. The ratio of 260/280 nm absorbance was between 1.8 and 2.0. The purified RNA was then precipitated with 20 ug tRNA, 0.1 volume of 3 M sodium acetate and 2.5 volumes of ethanol at $-70°C$.

## Northern Analysis

Aliquots (10 ug) of poly $A^+$ RNA were size-fractionated by electrophoresis on an 0.8% agarose/6% formaldehyde gel after denaturing and transferred to nitrocellulose membranes by capillary approach.[24] After ultraviolet cross-linking the membranes were prehybridized at 45°C for 4 hr in solution containing 5 × saline sodium citrate (SSC) (1 × SSC = 0.15 M NaCl + 15 mM sodium citrate), 0.2% SDS, 25 mM sodium phosphate buffer (pH 6.5), 250 ug/ml denatured salmon sperm DNA and 5 × Denhardt's solution. The membranes were then hybridized with specific probes in the same solution at 50°C overnight. At the end of the hybridization the membranes were washed three times with 2 × SSC/0.1% SDS at 37°C for 15 min and then twice with 0.1 × SSC/0.1% SDS at 60°C for 30 min. The membranes were exposed at $-80°C$ on X-ray films (X-Omat, AR, Eastman Kodak Co.) with intensifying screens (DuPont Co.). The relative amounts of specific mRNA species were determined by densitometry. The specific probes employed were cDNA encoding the alpha$_1$ subunit of rat brain D subtype of the voltage-gated $Ca^{2+}$ channel and cDNA encoding 18S ribosomal protein. The cDNAs were cleaved from plasmids with restriction enzymes and labeled by random priming with [$^{32}$P]alpha-deoxycytidine triphosphate (dCTP). The specific activities of the probes were above $10^8$ cpm/ug DNA.

## Western Analysis

Membrane proteins as prepared for the binding assay from GH$_4$C$_1$ cells were fractionated by SDS-polyacrylamide gel electrophoresis (PAGE) after denaturation at 95°C for 5 min in loading buffer containing 1% SDS, 25% glycerol, 1% mercaptoethanol and 15 mN Tris at pH 6.8. The proteins were first run on a stacking gel of 2% acrylamide/bisacrylamide (30:0.5) mixture, 0.1% SDS, 0.5 mg/ml ammonium persulphate and 0.1 M Tris-HCl at pH 6.8. The electrophoresis was continued on a separation gel which was made of varied concentrations of acrylamide/bisacrylamide (30:0.14) mixture depending on the size of target proteins, 0.1% SDS, 0.1% TEMED, 0.5 mg/ml ammonium persulphate and 0.5 M Tris-HCl at pH 6.8. For studies on the beta-subunit of the $Ca^{2+}$ channel 10% gels were used; for studies on the alpha$_2$ subunit 6% gels were used. The running buffer consisted of 0.1% SDS and 0.2 M Tris-glycine at pH 8.6. Proteins were transferred onto nylon membranes with standard Western blotting techniques. The membranes were incubated for >2 hr in blocking buffer (5% nonfat milk, 0.2% Tween-20 dissolved in phosphate-buffered saline (PBS) at pH 7.4. Antibodies in blocking buffer were then added to the blots at appropriate concentrations and incubated for 5–12 hr. After incubation the unbound antibodies were washed away and the membranes were then incubated with horseradish peroxidase-labeled second antibodies in blocking buffer for 2 hr. Finally, the blots were washed three times with PBS containing 0.2% Tween-20 and the specific proteins were detected by enhanced chemiluminescence (ECL) procedures. The sizes of detected proteins were determined based on prestained molecular weight markers including myosin (205 kD), beta-galactosidase (116.5 kD), phosphorylase B (106 kD), ovalbumin (49.5 kD), carbonic anhydrase (32.5 kD) and lysosyme (18.5 kD).

## MATERIALS

### Radioligands

[$^3$H]PN 200-110 (isopropyl-4-(2,1,3-benzoxadiazol-4-yl)-1,4-dihydro-5-methoxycarbonyl-2,6-dimethyl-3-pyridinecarboxylate, sp. act. 87.0 Ci/mmol) was purchased from Dupont-New England Nuclear, Boston, MA. [$^3$H]N-methylscopolamine, sp. act. 72.0 Ci/mmole was purchased from Amersham, Arlington Heights, IL.

TABLE 2. Binding of [$^3$H]PN 200-110 to Intact Cells in Polarizing and Depolarizing Conditions[a]

| Condition | $K^+$ (mM) | $K_D$ (nM) | $B_{max}$ (fmoles/mg$^{-1}$) | $k_{on}$ ($\times 10^8$ M$^{-1}$ min$^{-1}$) | $k_{off}$ ($\times 10^{-2}$ min$^{-1}$) |
|---|---|---|---|---|---|
| Polarizing | 5 | 2.15 ± 0.42 | 214 ± 48 | 0.175 ± 0.04 | 3.28 ± 0.23 |
| Depolarizing | 50 | 0.11 ± 0.02 | 24 ± 6 | 3.08 ± 0.4 | 3.34 ± 0.31 |

[a] From Liu et al.[22] Reprinted by permission from *Molecular Pharmacology*.

### Cell Culture Medium

F-10 medium, horse serum, fetal bovine serum, Roswell Park Memorial Institute (RPMI) 1640 vitamins (100 × concentrated), RPMI 1640 amino acids (50 × concentrated), and antibiotics were obtained from GIBCO, Grand Island, NY. Hank's solution was made fresh every month. It contains NaCl 125 mM, KCl 5 mM, $MgCl_2$ 1.25 mM, $CaCl_2$ 1.35 mM, dextrose 10 mM, $NaH_2PO_4$ 10 mM, and HEPES 10 mM at pH 7.4: with the addition of RPMI 1640 vitamins and amino acids this medium was used as the polarizing solution. Depolarizing medium was made by increasing the KCl concentration with concomitant reduction of NaCl.

### Antibodies

Secondary antibodies for immunoblotting, which are linked to horse radish peroxidase, and ECL Western blotting detecting reagents were purchased from Amersham, Arlington Heights, IL.

## RESULTS AND DISCUSSION

Our previous data showed that $GH_4C_1$ cells depolarized for ninety minutes showed an increased affinity fro PN 200-110 binding that was characterized by an increase in the association (on) rate constant and a decrease in the maximum binding density (TABLE 2.) The decrease in 1,4-dihydropyridine binding site density was time dependent and reversible (FIG. 2) and was accompanied by a loss of depolarization-induced $^{45}Ca^{2+}$ uptake (FIG. 3). This change in the number and function of voltage-gated channels is not accompanied by any change in the expression of mRNA (FIG. 4). Under the same conditions the density of surface muscarinic receptors measured by N-methylscopolamine is increased from 18 to 37 fmole/mg protein without change in ligand affinity (FIG. 5). This increase in surface muscarinic receptor density is blocked by staurosporine (50 nM) present during the depolarization, consistent with a role for protein kinase C in this upregulation process. In contrast, the downregulation of the $Ca^{2+}$ channels is a $Ca^{2+}$-calmodulin-dependent process.[22] The relationship between muscarinic receptor upregulation and $Ca^{2+}$ channel downregulation under depolarizing conditions is not estab-

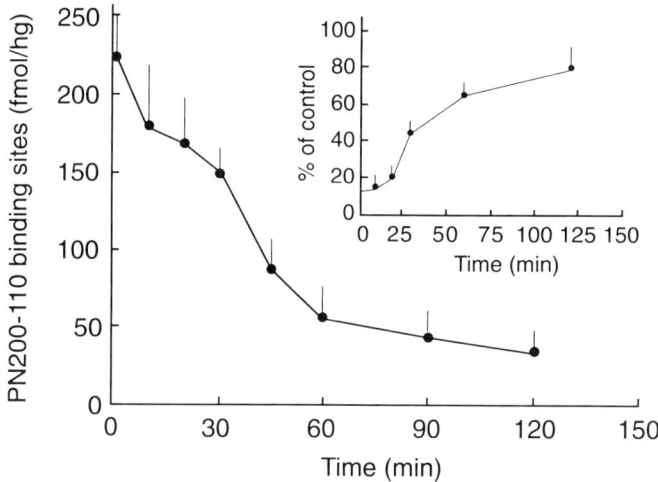

**FIGURE 2.** The time course of the loss of [$^3$H]PN 200-110 binding sites from GH$_4$C$_1$ cells following depolarization for 2 hours with 50 mM K$^+$. The *inset* shows the recovery of binding sites from a 2-hour depolarization period. *Bars* indicate the standard error of the mean; n = 5. (From Liu et al.[22] Reprinted by permission from *Molecular Pharmacology*.)

lished. However, these components are linked functionally through G proteins, and these may mediate the coordinate regulation observed.

Our previous hypothesis concerning the rapid downregulation of L-type channel number and function in neuronal and neurosecretory cells was that there was internalization of the channel complex into the cell in a membrane vesicle inaccessible to ligand binding in the intact cell protocol and devoid of cellular function.[22,25] This is a model directly analogous to that demonstrated for G protein-coupled receptors including the beta-adrenergic receptor. Almost certainly, this hypothesis is oversimplified. Immunoblot analysis of membranes from GH$_4$C$_1$ cells during polarized and depolarized conditions revealed, using a monoclonal antibody against alpha$_2$ subunits, that there was no significant change after depolarization relative to control for 2 or 12 hours (FIG. 6). Similarly, a polyclonal antibody directed against the beta subunit, a 58 kD protein, revealed downregulation by approximately 40% and 60% after 1 and 2 hours depolarization respectively in 50 mM K$^+$. A similar depolarization with the Na$^+$ channel activator veratridine (10 uM) also revealed a similar downregulation (FIG. 7). This downregulation of the beta subunit is Ca$^{2+}$ dependent and is blocked by the Ca$^{2+}$ antagonist D 600 (FIG. 8). The decrease in the amount of membrane-associated beta subunit during depolarization was partially restored by reincubating the cells in a polarizing medium (FIG. 9). These observations on the regulation of the beta subunit parallel the original observations on the regulation of 1,4-dihydropyridine binding and Ca$^{2+}$ uptake.[22]

These data suggest that the L-type voltage-gated Ca$^{2+}$ channel of the neurose-

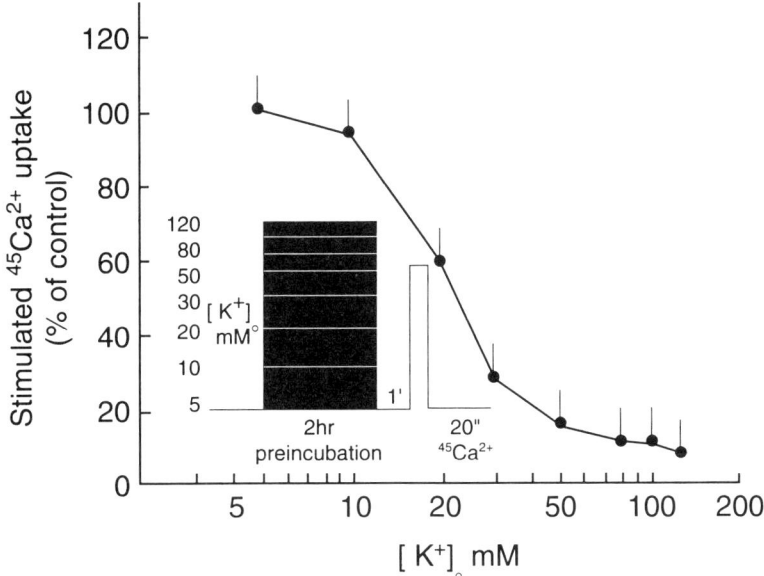

FIGURE 3. The decrease in stimulated $^{45}Ca^{2+}$ uptake in $GH_4C_1$ cells caused by predepolarization with the indicated concentrations of $K^+$. The cells were preincubated at the indicated concentrations for 1 hour, shifted to polarizing conditions (5 mM $K^+$) for one minute, and $^{45}Ca^{2+}$ uptake was then measured over a 20-sec period in response to a standard 50 mM $K^+$ challenge. *Bars* indicate standard error of the mean; n = 4. (From Liu *et al.*[22] Reprinted by permission from *Molecular Pharmacology*.)

cretory cell $GH_4C_1$ is downregulated during depolarization by a reversible process that involves dissociation or partial dissociation of the functionally active heteromeric complex. Three possible schemes are depicted in FIGURE 10. Our data do not permit distinction between the schemes of FIGURE 10B and 10C. However, the scheme depicted in FIGURE 10A, the internalization of the entire heteromeric complex, is eliminated by the antibody studies. The scheme of FIGURE 10C involving the dissociation of the beta-subunit will accommodate the observations made and is also consistent with expression studies showing the important role of the beta subunit in upregulating the permeation and binding characteristics of the coexpressed $alpha_1$ subunit. Recent work by Campbell and his colleagues has revealed that the beta subunit binds to the cytoplasmic linker between domains I and II of the $alpha_1$ subunit.[26] This binding site may represent a locus for voltage- and $Ca^{2+}$-dependent dissociation and association.

The regulation of voltage-gated $Ca^{2+}$ channels by depolarization may have both pathologic and physiologic significance. Abnormal and persistent elevations of intracellular $Ca^{2+}$ are known to cause cell damage and death.[27] During neuronal ischemia the extracellular $K^+$ concentrations may reach very high levels and the resultant depolarization generate $Ca^{2+}$ overload.[28] The downregulation of neuronal channels may represent a cell protection mechanism. $Ca^{2+}$ channel regula-

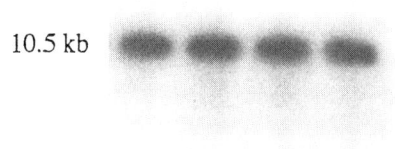

10.5 kb

**FIGURE 4.** The effect of membrane depolarization by 50 mM $K^+$ for periods of 1, 2 or 12 hours on the content of mRNA encoding the $alpha_1$ subunit of the L-type $Ca^{2+}$ channel in $GH_4C_1$ cells. The experiment was repeated twice with identical results.

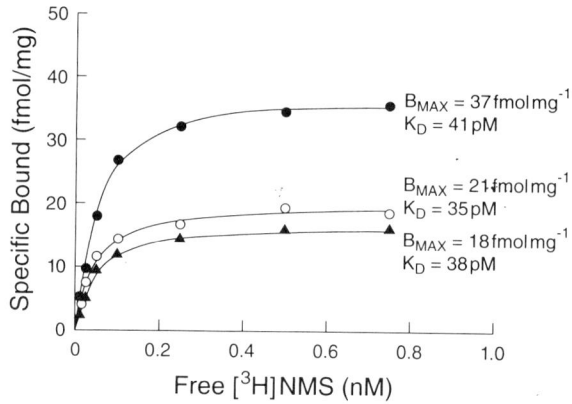

**FIGURE 5.** The regulation of muscarinic receptors by depolarization and its inhibition by staurosporine. N-methylscopolamine ([$^3$H]NMS) binding was performed in intact $GH_4C_1$ cells in polarizing medium (5 mM $K^+$, ▲) or depolarizing medium (50 mM $K^+$) with (○) or without (●) 50 nM staurosporine. The binding data were obtained by Scatchard analysis of the saturation curves. The data shown are the mean of two essentially identical experiments.

tion by membrane potential may also contribute to physiologic control mechanisms. Thus, the loss of electrical activity may promote neuronal death,[29] and depolarization is necessary for the growth of some neuronal cells in culture including cerebellar granule neurons.[30] Additionally, depolarization can rescue cells

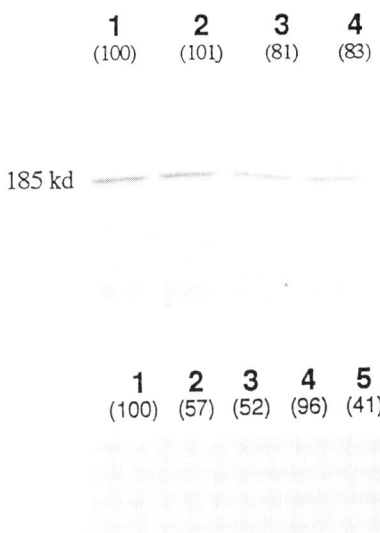

**FIGURE 6.** The regulation by depolarization of the amount of the alpha$_2$ subunit of the Ca$^{2+}$ channel in GH$_4$C$_1$ cells. Cells were incubated for 2 hours in 5 mM K$^+$ *(lane 1)* or 50 mM K$^+$ *(lane 2)* or for 12 hours in 5 mM K$^+$ *(lane 3)* or 50 mM K$^+$ *(lane 4)*. Membrane proteins were loaded at 50 ug and 40 ug for 2 and 12 hour incubation respectively and subject to SDS-PAGE and immunoblotting analysis. The *numbers in parentheses* indicate the relative densities. The experiment was repeated three times with very similar results.

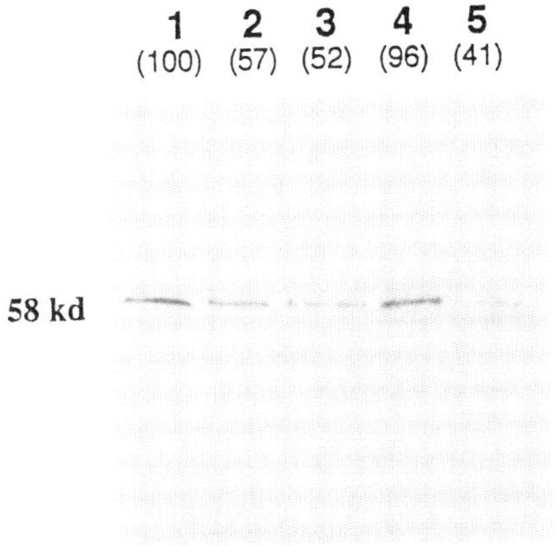

**FIGURE 7.** The regulation by depolarization of the amount of the beta subunit of the Ca$^{2+}$ channel in GH$_4$C$_1$ cells. Cells were incubated in 5 mM K$^+$ *(lanes 1 and 4)*, 50 mM K$^+$ for 1 hour *(lane 2)* or 2 hours *(lane 3)* or 50 mM K$^+$ with 10 uM veratridine *(lane 5)*. The *numbers in parentheses* indicate the relative densities. The experiment was repeated twice with very similar results.

dying from trophic factor deprivation through a Ca$^{2+}$-dependent mechanism.[31] However, given the critical roles that N- and P- and other types of Ca$^{2+}$ channels play in neuronal function, it will be of importance to determine whether their properties and numbers are similarly regulated by membrane potential.

## SUMMARY

The 1,4-dihydropyridine-sensitive voltage-gated Ca$^{2+}$ channel is widely distributed in excitable cells. The channel and its several associated drug binding sites are known to be up- and downregulated by a variety of homologous and heterologous influences including membrane depolarization. The neurosecretory GH$_4$C$_1$ cell line possesses L-type channels. Depolarization of these cells by elevated K$^+$ increases the binding affinity of 1,4-dihydropyridines and decreases the number of 1,4-dihydropyridine binding sites and functional channels. There is a coordinate

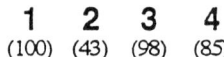

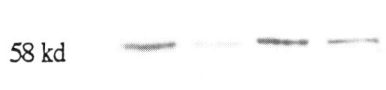

**FIGURE 8.** The $Ca^{2+}$ dependence of the regulation of the beta subunit of the $Ca^{2+}$ channel in $GH_4C_1$ cells. $GH_4C_1$ cells were incubated for 2 hours in 5 mM $K^+$ *(lane 1)*, 50 mM $K^+$ *(lane 2)*, 50 mM $K^+$ in the presence of 1 uM D600 *(lane 3)* or 50 mM $K^+$ without extracellular $Ca^{2+}$. The *numbers in parentheses* indicate the relative densities. The experiment was repeated twice with essentially similar results.

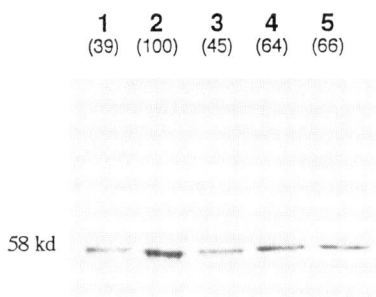

**FIGURE 9.** The recovery of membrane-associated beta subunits of the $Ca^{2+}$ channel in $GH_4C_1$ cells from depolarization-induced downregulation. The cells were incubated in 5 mM $K^+$ *(lane 2)* or 50 mM $K^+$ *(lane 1)* and then returned to polarizing medium for 30 min, 1 hour or 2 hours *(lanes 3–5)*. The *numbers in parentheses* indicate the relative densities. The experiment was repeated twice with very similar results.

upregulation of the number of muscarinic receptors. This membrane potential- and $Ca^{2+}$-calmodulin-dependent process of channel downregulation may involve internalization of the channel heteromeric complex or, more plausibly, a dissociation of the complex and a concomitant loss of both binding and permeation functions.

## ACKNOWLEDGMENTS

We thank Dr. Kevin P. Campbell of the University of Iowa for a polyclonal antibody against the beta subunit, Dr. Terry Snutch, University of Vancouver, British Columbia for rat brain D type cDNA and Dr. S. Froehner, Dartmouth Medical School, Dartmouth, NH, for an antibody against the skeletal muscle $alpha_2$ subunit.

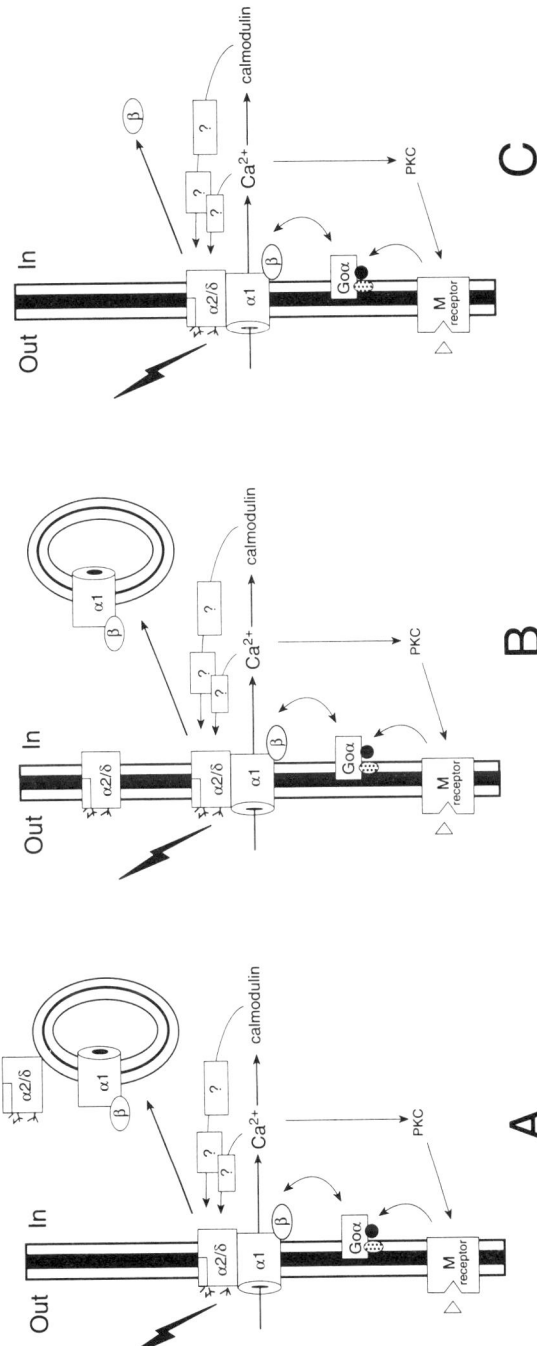

**FIGURE 10.** Schematic representation of the regulation of the $Ca^{2+}$ channel of $GH_4C_1$ cells by depolarization. **(A)** The entire heteromeric complex is internalized in a vesicle fraction. **(B)** The alpha$_1$-beta portion of the complex is internalized. **(C)** The beta subunit is dissociated from its association with the alpha$_1$ subunit. Also depicted is the coordinate upregulation of the muscarinic receptor and, from data not presented here (J. Liu and D. J. Triggle, unpublished observations), evidence that the alpha subunit of the G protein $G_0$ is upregulated by depolarization of $GH_4C_1$ cells but with a longer (24-hour) time-course.

## REFERENCES

1. RAMPE, D. & D. J. TRIGGLE. 1994. Ion channels as targets for drug design. Drug Dev. Res. **33:** 189–372.
2. TSIEN, R. W., P. T. ELLINOR & W. A. HORNE. 1991. Molecular diversity of voltage-dependent $Ca^{2+}$ channels. Trends Pharmacol. Sci. **12:** 349–354.
3. PEREZ-REYES, E. & T. SCHNEIDER. 1994. Calcium channels: structure, function and classification. Drug Dev. Res. **33:** 295–318.
4. ADAMS, B. A., T. TANABE, A. MIKAMI, S. NUMA & K. G. BEEAM. 1990. Intramembrane charge movement restored in dysgenic skeletal muscle by injection of dihydropyridine cDNAs. Nature **346:** 569–572.
5. CATTERALL, W. A. & J. STRIESSNIG. 1992. Receptor sites for $Ca^{2+}$ channel antagonists. Trends Pharmacol. Sci. **13:** 255–262.
6. HULLIN, R., M. BIEL, V. FLOCKERZI & F. HOFMANN. 1993. Tissue-specific expression of calcium channels. Trends Cardiovasc. Med. **3:** 48–53.
7. LACERDA, A. E., H. S. KIM, P. RUTH, E. PEREZ-REYES, V. FLOCKERZI, F. HOFMANN, L. BIRNBAUMER & A. M. BROWN. 1991. Normalization of current kinetics by interaction between the $alpha_1$ and beta subunits of the skeletal muscle dihydropyridine-sensitive $Ca^{2+}$ channel. Nature **352:** 527–530.
8. WELLING, A., E. BOSSE, A. CAVALIE, R. BOTTLENDER, A. LUDWIG, W. NASTAINCZYK, V. FLOCKERZI & F. HOFMANN. 1993. Stable co-expression of calcium channel $alpha_1$, beta and $alpha_2$/delta subunits in a somatic cell line. J. Physiol. **471:** 749–765.
9. HOFMANN, F., M. BIEL & V. FLOCKERZI. 1994. Molecular basis for $Ca^{2+}$ channel diversity. Annu. Rev. Neurosci. **17:** 399–418.
10. PEREZ-REYES, E., A. CASTELLANO, H. S. KIM, P. BERTRAND, E. BAGGSTROM, A. E. LACERDA, X-Y. WEI & L. BIRNBAUMER. 1992. Cloning and expression of a cardiac brain beta-subunit of the L-type calcium channel. J. Biol. Chem. **267:** 1792–1797.
11. WEI, X-Y, E. PEREZ-REYES, A. E. LACERDA, G. SCHUSTER, A. M. BROWN & L. BIRNBAUMER. 1993. Heterologous regulation of the cardiac $alpha_1$ subunit by skeletal muscle beta and gamma subunits. Implications for the structure of cardiac L-type $Ca^{2+}$ channels. J. Biol Chem. **266:** 21943–21947.
12. STEA, A., S. J. DUBEL, M. PRAGNELL, J. P. LEONARD, K. P. CAMPBELL & T. P. SNUTCH. 1993. A beta-subunit normalizes the electrophysiological properties of a cloned N-type $Ca^{2+}$ channel $alpha_1$ subunit. Neuropharmacology **32:** 1102–1116.
13. FERRANTE, J. & D. J. TRIGGLE. 1990. Drug- and disease-induced regulation of voltage-dependent calcium channels. Pharmacol. Rev. **42:** 29–44.
14. DELORME, A. E. & R. MCGEE. 1986. Regulation of voltage-dependent $Ca^{2+}$ channels of neuronal cells by chronic changes in membrane potential. Brain Res. **397:** 189–192.
15. DELORME, A. E., C. S. RABE & R. MCGEE. 1988. Regulation of the number of functional voltage-sensitive $Ca^{2+}$ channels in PC-12 cells by chronic changes in membrane potential. J. Pharmacol Exp. Ther. **244:** 838–843.
16. FERRANTE, J., D. J. TRIGGLE & A. RUTLEDGE. 1991. The effects of chronic depolarization on L-type 1,4-dihydropyridine-sensitive, voltage-dependent $Ca^{2+}$ channels in chick neural retina and rat cardiac cells. Can. J. Physiol. Pharmacol. **69:** 914–920.
17. FRANKLIN, J. L., D. J. FICKBOLM & A. L. WILLARD. 1992. Long-term regulation of neuronal calcium current by prolonged changes of membrane potential. J. Neurosci. **12:** 1726–1735.
18. SKATTEBOL, A., D. J. TRIGGLE & A. M. BROWN. 1989. Homologous regulation of voltage-dependent $Ca^{2+}$ channels by 1,4-dihydropyridines. Biochem. Biophys. Res. Commun. **160:** 929–936.
19. HONDEGHEM, L. M. & B. G. KATZUNG. 1984. Antiarrhythmic agents: the modulated receptor mechanism of action of sodium and calcium blocking drugs. Annu. Rev. Pharmacol. Toxicol. **24:** 387–423.
20. WEI, X-Y., A. RUTLEDGE & D. J. TRIGGLE. 1989. Voltage-dependent binding of 1,4-

dihydropyridine $Ca^{2+}$ channel antagonists and activators in cultured rat neonatal rat ventricular myocytes. Mol. Pharmacol. **35:** 541–552.
21. COHEN, C. J. & R. T. MCCARTHY. 1987. Nimodipine block of calcium channels in rat anterior pituitary cells. J. Physiol. (London) **387:** 196–225.
22. LIU, J., R. BANGALORE, A. RUTLEDGE & D. J. TRIGGLE. 1994. Modulation of L-type $Ca^{2+}$ channels in clonal rat pituitary cells by membrane depolarization. Mol. Pharmacol. **45:** 1198–1206.
23. PERKINS, J. P., W. P. HAVSDORFF & R. J. LEFKOWITZ. 1991. Mechanisms of ligand-induced desensitization of beta-adrenergic receptors. *In* Beta-Adrenergic Receptors. J. P. Perkins, Ed. 125–140. Humana Press. Clifton, NJ.
24. MANIATIS, T., E. F. FRITSCH & J. SAMBROOK. 1982. Molecular Cloning. Cold Spring Harbor Press. Cold Spring Harbor, NY.
25. BANGALORE, R., A. RUTLEDGE & D. J. TRIGGLE. 1993. Neuronal calcium channels. Regulated receptors. Drugs Dev. **2:** 103–110.
26. PRAGNELL, M., M. DE WAARD, Y. MORI, T. TANABE, T. P. SNUTCH & K. P. CAMPBELL. 1994. Calcium channel beta subunit binds to a conserved motif in the I-II cytoplasmic linker of the $alpha_1$ subunit. Nature **368:** 67–70.
27. CHEUNG, J. Y., J. V. BONVENTRE, C. D. MALIS & A. LEAF. 1986. Calcium and ischemic injury. N. Engl. J. Med. **314:** 1670–1676.
28. SIESJO, B. 1990. Calcium in the brain under physiological and pathological conditions. Eur. Neurol. **30**(Suppl. 2): 3–9.
29. LIPTON, S. A. 1986. Blockade of electrical activity promotes the death of mammalian retinal ganglion cells in culture. Proc. Natl. Acad. Sci. USA **83:** 9774–9778.
30. GALLO, V., A. KINGSBURY, R. BALAZS & O. S. JORGENSEN. 1987. The role of depolarization in the survival and differentiation of cerebellar granule cells in culture. J. Neurosci. **7:** 2203–2213.
31. KOIKE, T., D. P. MARTIN & E. M. JOHNSON. 1989. Role of $Ca^{2+}$ channels in the ability of membrane depolarization to prevent neuronal death induced by trophic-factor denervation: evidence that levels of internal $Ca^{2+}$ determine growth factor dependence of sympathetic ganglion cells. Proc. Natl. Acad. Sci. USA **86:** 6421–6425.

# Potential Interactions between Nimodipine and Adrenal Hormones

ROBERT L. ISAACSON AND JULIE A. VARNER

*Department of Psychology*
*Binghamton University*
*Binghamton, New York 13902-6000*

A quiet revolution has been occurring in the field of adrenal steroids over the past ten years. It began with the documentation of two types of glucocorticoid receptors with greatly different affinities for corticosterone in the rat brain. For example, the classical adrenal cortical hormone receptors of the hippocampus[1] were found to have such great affinity for corticosterone that almost all of them would be bound to whatever small amounts might be in the general circulation. As a consequence, very little response would be possible with large increases in hormonal levels, such as found during the circadian cycle or under stress, but there is evidence that early estimates of type I receptor occupancy may have been too high.[2] With the discovery of low-affinity receptors that are only partially occupied under nonstress conditions,[3,4] a mechanism for a wider range of corticosterone-induced responses was found. Originally the two forms of corticosterone receptors were called types I and II (or 1 and 2) but the current terminology describes the high-affinity receptor as the mineralocorticoid receptor and the low-affinity receptor as the glucocorticoid receptor. The designations of receptor types is largely based on inferences from the binding of selected agonists and specific antagonists to the receptors.[5] A summary of some of the characteristics of the two receptor classes is given in TABLE 1. A review of the use of these relatively new distinctions among receptors is available.[6]

de Kloet has stressed the importance of the balance between mineralocorticoid and glucocorticoid receptor activation for the understanding of functional effects. The interactions between the two types of receptors are complex and, at times, antagonistic. For example, giving a mineralocorticoid prior to a glucocorticoid may block the usual effects of the latter in adrenalectomized rats.[7] However, certain of the effects mediated by glucocorticoids may depend on some degree of occupancy of the mineralocorticoid receptors. It has been suggested that the absence of mineralocorticoid receptor activation *or* the continued excessive occupancy of glucocorticoid receptors may lead to disruptions of neural circuitry and cell death.[8] The interactions between the two receptor types may help explain why *both* adrenalectomy and excessive administrations of glucocorticoids may lead to cellular disturbances and apparent cell loss in the hippocampus.[9,10]

Calcium plays an important role as a mediator of the neuronal responses to the activation of the two types of receptors. "Sustained" calcium conductance is increased when the glucocorticoid receptor occupancy rates are high, and this leads, in turn, to enhanced hyperpolarizing afterpotentials after $Na^+$ spikes as well as to prolongation of the $Ca^{2+}$ response. High mineralocorticoid receptor

TABLE 1. Summary of Selected Characteristics of Type I and Type II Adrenal Cortex Hormone Receptors

| |
|---|
| Type I. Mineralocorticoid<br>  High affinity: ALDO, CORT<br>  Low affinity: dexamethasone<br>  Location: hippocampal & septal area<br>    Neuroprotective?<br>Type II. Glucocorticoid<br>  High affinity: RU 28362, dexamethasone<br>  Low affinity: ALDO, CORT<br>  Antagonist: RU 38486<br>  Location: widely distributed<br>    Degeneration? |

occupancy rates are associated with *reduced* hyperpolarizing afterpotentials.[8] The changes in the calcium conductances are mediated by channels that appear to resemble those of the voltage-dependent L channels known to be antagonized by the dihydropyridines. In fact Mazzanti, Thibault, and Landfield found that nimodipine reduced the calcium-dependent hyperpolarizing afterpotentials in hippocampal slices from both young and aged rats.[11] Thus, there is a suggestion of a biochemical link of the steroid-induced changes to nimodipine.

The sites of greatest binding of the corticosterone to the mineralocorticoid receptor are in the hippocampus. This is also the site of greatest nimodipine binding.[12] Thus, the septal-hippocampal area, as well as the median eminence, shares characteristics of high corticosterone binding, high nimodipine binding, and high levels of nerve growth factor receptors. Another similarity in the effects of corticosterone and nimodipine is that both increase the metabolic activity of the hippocampus—the latter agent producing a more global enhancement of activity,[13] the former one localized to the septal-hippocampal axis.[14]

We believed there was likely to be an interaction between nimodipine and an animal's response to stress, because of the drug's potentiation of the effects of hypnotic drugs, first documented in the case of barbiturates by Hoffmeister, Benz, Heise, Krause, and Neuser.[15] These authors showed that the time of onset of barbiturate effects was shortened and sleep duration extended. In our laboratory this effect has been seen while exposing mice to ethyl ether atmospheres (unpublished observations). These informal observations were extended to the potentiation of motor incoordination and hypothermia induced by ethanol in the Binghamton heterozygous mouse.[16] We went on to demonstrate that these effects could not be explained on the basis of the rate of metabolism or elimination of ethanol[17] and to show that nimodipine could potentiate the hypothermia produced by diazepam but *not* the motor incoordination produced by this benzodiazepine.[18] In our informal studies of the potentiation of ether-induced sleep by nimodipine and in the study of Isaacson *et al.*,[16] the drug was given by intraperitoneal injection, and control injections were made using the same vehicle as that in which the drug was dissolved. No uninjected control group was used—only the vehicle-injected control group.

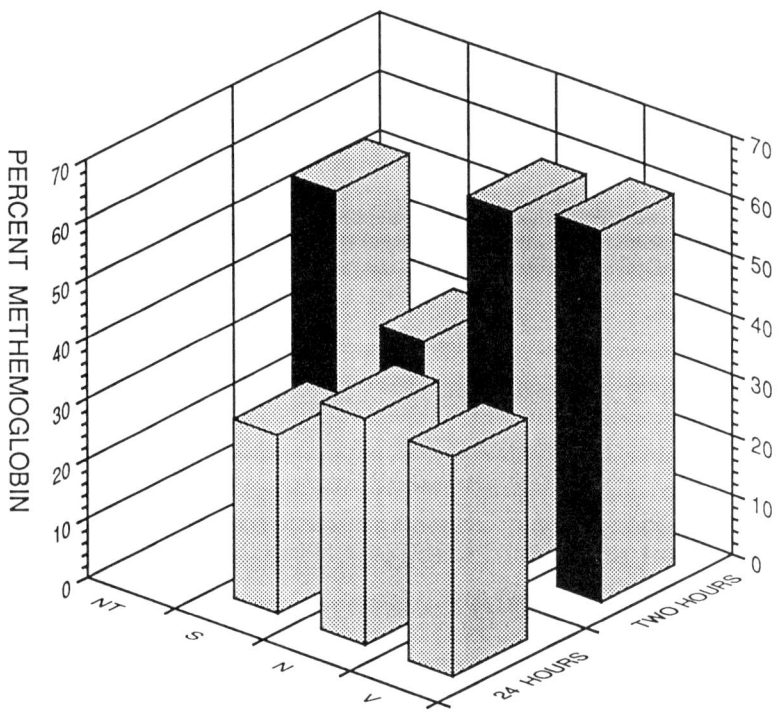

**FIGURE 1.** The percent methemoglobin in the blood of rats 2 or 24 hours after nimodipine (N), verapamil (V), or vehicle administration (S) and 25 minutes after sodium nitrite injection. NT = no treatment group. (Adapted from Fahey and Isaacson.[19])

Shortly after our studies of the relationship between ethanol and nimodipine, Fahey and Isaacson undertook to determine the effect of nimodipine on the production of methemoglobinemia induced by the administration of sodium nitrite.[19] We investigated the effects of pretreatment of the animals with nimodipine or with verapamil or with the saline vehicle used in that experiment. Thankfully, we also included a group that received no injection prior to the administration of the nitrite. The effect of these pretreatments is shown in FIGURE 1. Blood samples were always taken 25 min after the nitrite administration. The "pretreatments" were given either 2 hr or 24 hr before the nitrite. The only group different from the others was the group that received a saline injection 2 hr before the nitrite. The untreated group and the two groups given the L channel antagonists were similar in percent of methemoglobin in the blood. At the 24-hr delay between the pretreatment injections and the nitrate, all of the groups had less methemoglobinemia than did the untreated group. This suggests that the effects of the calcium channel antagonists were diminished by 24 hours after administration, but the effects of the stress involved with the injections were not. What was apparent was that some aspect of the stress response related to handling and injection reduced the amount of methemglobin produced by the nitrite. We suspected that an enhanced release

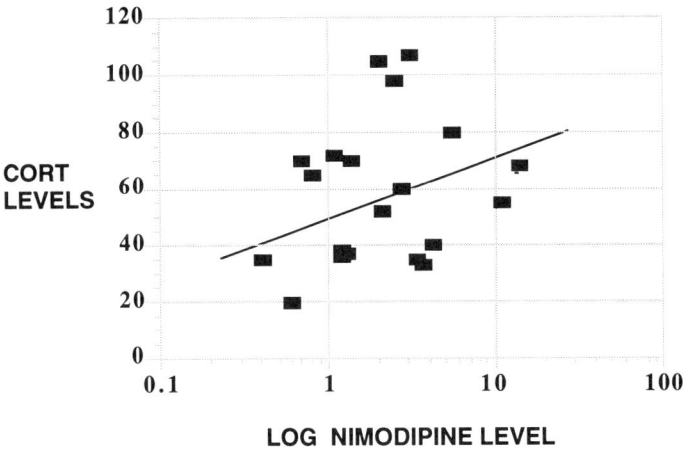

**FIGURE 2.** Corticosterone levels of rats maintained on a diet containing 1000 ppm nimodipine for about two weeks before blood was taken for hormone and drug assays. CORT = corticosterone and drug levels in ng/ml. Unpublished observations.

of corticosterone might be involved with this reaction, but this is not certain. It did lead us to try to examine the interactions of corticosterone and nimodipine in greater detail. We have been doing this in several ways since these early 1990 results. Here we present some data from these studies conducted over the last 5 years (see Acknowledgments).

In some of our early experiments rats were maintained on a diet containing 1000 ppm nimodipine in standard lab chow for at least 10 days prior to the sampling of blood via cardiac puncture after etherization. Half the animals were subjected to an ether stress one hour before the blood samples were taken. The other half were not; these will be called the "No Stress" group. FIGURE 2 shows the relationship between nimodipine and corticosterone levels taken at the middle of the light cycle. A weak positive relationship was found. A somewhat stronger relationship was found when corticosterone levels were compared with metabolite 2 levels (assays of plasma nimodipine kindly prepared by Dr. George Krol, Institute for Dementia Research, Miles, Inc., West Haven, CT). This is shown in FIGURE 3. When the effect of ether stress was studied, no relationships were found between either the nimodipine or its metabolite and corticosterone levels. Given the weak relationships between nimodipine and circulating corticosterone under the baseline condition, the wisest conclusion would be that nimodipine has little if any effect on corticosterone levels, *per se*. This would represent a situation like that with thyrotropin-releasing hormone (TRH) in the hypothalamus, *i.e.*, it is not influenced by dihydropyridine antagonists.

The ability of the injection procedure to affect levels of methemoglobin formed 24 hours later when the animals were given the sodium nitrite is of substantial interest. Just how long the carryover effects of the handling and injection stress last is a worthwhile experimental question as is asking whether or not corticoste-

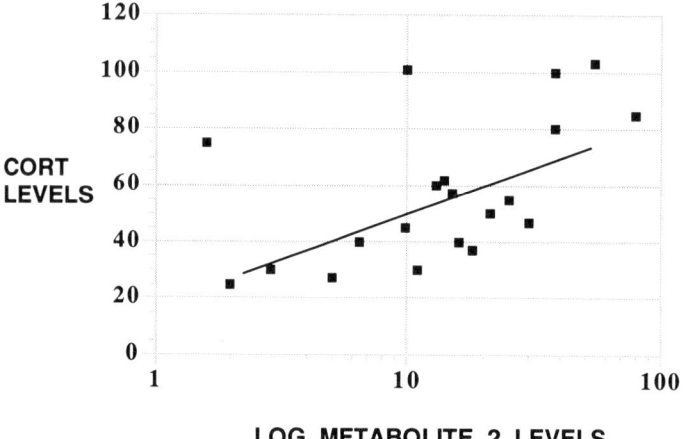

**FIGURE 3.** Corticosterone (CORT) levels and nimodipine metabolite 2 levels for animals shown in FIGURE 2. Corticosterone and drug levels in ng/ml. Unpublished observations.

rone levels would parallel these long-lasting effects. Such carryover stress effects of injections and handling, as well as the disruption and resetting of the circadian rhythms by consistent environmental stimulation, e.g., the introduction of wet mash food into the rats' cages at regular times of the day, are factors that subtly affect experiments with hormonal systems of a cyclic nature. We found this out through bitter experience in some of our initial studies trying to determine the relationship between nimodipine and corticosterone levels. The ease with which circadian pituitary-adrenal rhythms can be disturbed by even minor changes in the laboratory routines has been well documented.[20]

In a recently completed experiment[21] we found more evidence supporting the ability of nimodipine to alter corticosterone levels after mild but not strong stressors. In this experiment controlled release pellets (100 $\mu$g/day) of nimodipine or placebo pellets were implanted subcutaneously between the shoulders of the rats while they were under a general anesthesia. Other rats received no surgical intervention whatsoever. The corticosterone response of the animals in all three groups to the exposure to ether fumes was identical as illustrated in FIGURE 4. However, baseline measures of corticosterone differed among the groups. The (surgically) untreated group and the nimodipine group had virtually identical levels whereas the placebo pellet groups' level was significantly elevated. This suggested that the implantation of the inert pellet might have represented a continuing source of irritation and stress, thus inducing the higher level of corticosterone. To investigate this possibility, another experiment was undertaken. In it, four groups of rats were studied. These were an untreated group, a nimodipine pellet group, a placebo pellet group, and a surgical control group. This latter group received the anesthetic and the small cut in the skin between the shoulders necessary for the insertion of the pellets. We anticipated that *only* the placebo pellet group would show the elevated baseline corticosterone levels when blood was collected 21 days later.

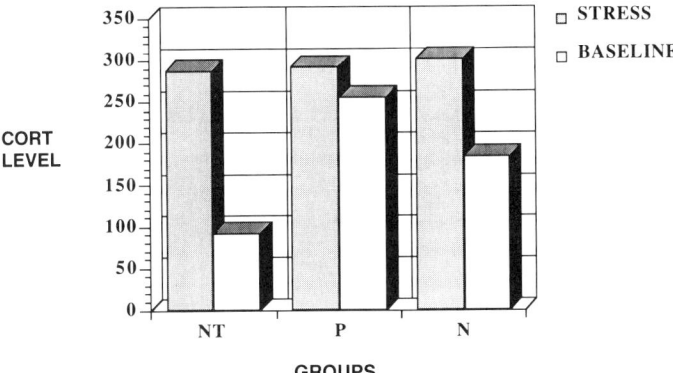

**FIGURE 4.** Corticosterone (CORT) levels of groups of rats implanted s.c. with slow-release nimodipine (N), placebo pellets (P), or not handled or subjected to other intervention (NT) under baseline conditions or after ether stress. (Data from Becker et al.[21]).

Our wizardly forecast was wrong. As can be seen in the FIGURE 5, the group with the highest levels of corticosterone was the surgical intervention group. The placebo pellet group had an elevated corticosterone level, but, although not easily seen in the figure, the variance of levels within this group was extremely high. It was 7 times larger than the variance of any other group—basically a bimodal distribution. About half the rats had very high levels, the other half having levels about the same as the untreated or nimodipine pellet groups. To return to the major surprise, however, the results indicated that we were wrong about the pellet being the cause of the prolonged elevation of the corticosterone levels. It was not the pellet that was the culprit—it was the anesthesia and the minor surgery. The

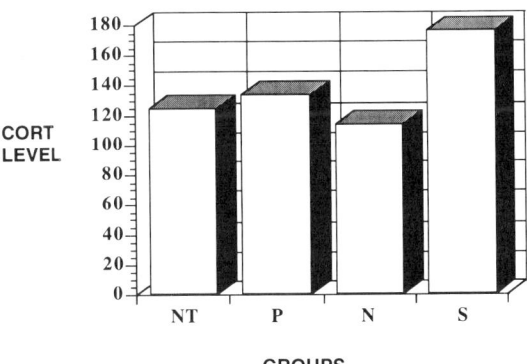

**FIGURE 5.** Corticosterone (CORT) levels of groups of rats implanted s.c. with slow-release pellets of nimodipine (N) or placebo (P) pellets, rats subjected to control surgical procedures and anesthesia (S), or rats receiving no treatment or intervention (NT). (From Isaacson, Varner, Becker, and Dokas, in preparation.)

next question should be, "Is it the surgery or the anesthesia (ketamine and xylazine) or both that produces the prolonged high levels of this adrenal hormone?"

What take-home messages are there in these data? One of the most important is the absolute necessity for the use of untreated, undisturbed control groups in any study. Almost anything that is done to, or occurs in the environment of, the rat will affect the pituitary-adrenal axis. As a consequence, comparisons of drug- or hormone-treated animals relative to placebo-treated controls alone may misrepresent the real consequences of the treatment. Above we discussed the seemingly synergistic effects of ethanol and nimodipine. Given what we know now and the limitations in the studies done but a few years ago, it is possible that what was observed was not an additive or synergistic effect of nimodipine and ethanol but rather the nimodipine blockade of the stress-induced arousal caused by the placebo injections. Stress can counteract the motoric debilitations produced by alcohol and, as a consequence, if nimodipine reduces this stress then the animals would be more impaired but not due to a functional interaction of the two drugs. What must be done in the face of this new information is to repeat the studies done in our laboratory and elsewhere showing cooperativeness between nimodipine and sedatives using untreated control groups. The drug "interaction" may really be an artifact of the stress response in the vehicle-treated controls.

In terms of neuroplasticity the rule of thumb remains that nimodipine generally enhances plasticity and neurite growth while corticosterone impedes these processes. The negative effects of corticosterone on the reinnervation processes have been well documented.[22,23] It is likely that some of the detrimental effects are due to impaired expression of actin and tubulin.[24] To the extent that nimodipine can reduce the expression of the stress response and reduce corticosterone levels subsequent to chronic or mild stress stimuli, neuroplasticity will be enhanced. At the present time it is not clear whether it is the chronic aspect of a stressor or its mildness that allows nimodipine to be effective. There is some evidence that the degree of stimulation may be the important factor based on work using neurons in cell cultures. For example, nimodipine will significantly attentuate the increase in intracellular calcium of cultured chick neurons induced by the addition of 250 $\mu$M pregnenolone sulfate to the media but does not affect the increase when the level of pregnenolone sulfate is raised to 500 $\mu$M.[25] It may be that the response to mild stresses can be attenuated by nimodipine but, as seen in our data, the response to the strenuous stress of ether exposure is unchanged.

Regardless, nimodipine is undoubtedly influencing the levels of circulating corticosterone under most conditions except those of extreme stress. In so doing it is altering the balance between mineralocorticoid and glucocorticoid receptor occupancy that would occur in the absence of the drug. Thus, it alters the genomic, posttranslational, and membrane actions of the adrenal hormones. As a consequence, changes in mood and behavioral dispositions would be anticipated. Such have been reported. Recently, nimodipine was shown to alter the reward value of morphine.[26] It has also been shown to reduce "learned helplessness" induced by inescapable footshock[27] and to facilitate the effects of antidepressants in experimental tests of depression.[28,29] These effects are not surprising given the results of the present study and, indeed, may be mediated in part by the drug-induced change in the hormonal response to stress. It is also likely that the balance between adrenal cortical hormone receptor occupancies may provide insight into a possible relationship between "mood" and rate of recovery from brain damage. Perhaps both mood and enhanced neuronal plasticity reflect a favorable balance of type I and II corticoid receptor occupancies and that under mild or low-level chronic stress, nimodipine may help produce this favorable balance.

## ACKNOWLEDGMENTS

The following people have been associated with these projects over the years: Linda Dokas, Department of Biochemistry, Medical School of Ohio, Toledo; Jeanne M. Fahey, Anne M. Danks, Donna Maier, Adam Mandel, Julie Varner, Lora Becker, and John Parsons while they were at Binghamton University.

## REFERENCES

1. McEwen, B. S., J. M. Weiss & L. S. Schwartz. 1969. Uptake of corticosterone by rat brain and its concentration by certain limbic structures. Brain Res. **16:** 227–241.
2. Spencer, R. L., E. A. Young, P.H. Choo & B. S. McEwen. 1990. Adrenal steroid type I and type II receptor binding: estimate of *in vivo* receptor number, occupancy, and activation with varying level of steroid. Brain Res. **514:** 37–48.
3. Reul, J. M. H. M. Y E. R. de Kloet. 1985. Two receptor systems for corticosterone in the rat brain: microdistribution and differential occupation. Endocrinology **117:** 2505–2511.
4. McEwen, B. S., E. R. de Kloet & W. Rostene. 1986. Adrenal steroid receptors and actions in the central nervous system. Physiol. Rev. **66:** 1121–1150.
5. Coirini, H., A. M. Magarinos, A. F. De Nicola, T. C. Rainbow & B. S. McEwen. 1985. Further studies of brain aldosterone binding sites employing new mineralocorticoid and glucocorticoid receptor markers *in vitro*. Brain Res. **361:** 212–216.
6. de Kloet, E. R. 1991. Brain corticosteroid receptor balance and homeostatic control. Front. Neuroendocrinol. **12:** 95–164.
7. Veldhuis, H. D. & E. R. de Kloet. 1983. Antagonistic effects of aldosterone on corticosterone-mediated changes in exploratory behavior of adrenalectomized rats. Horm. Behav. **17:** 225–232.
8. Karst, H., W. J. Wadman & M. Joëls. 1994. Corticosteroid receptor-dependent modulation of calcium currents in rat hippocampal CA1 neurons. Brain Res. **649:** 234–242.
9. Sapolsky, R. M., L. C. Krey & B. S. McEwen. 1985. Prolonged glucocorticoid exposure reduces hippocampal neuron number: implication for aging. J. Neurosci. **5:** 1222–1227.
10. Sloviter, R. S., G. Valiquette, G. M. Abrams, E. C. Ronk, A. I. Sollas, L. A. Paul & S. L. Neubort. 1989. Selective loss of hippocampal granule cells in the mature rat brain after adrenalectomy. Science **243:** 535–538.
11. Mazzanti, M. L., O. Thibault & P. W. Landfield. 1991. Dihydropyridine modulation of normal hippocampal physiology and young and aged rats. Neurosci. Res. Commun. **9:** 117–126.
12. Glossmann, H., A. Goll, M. Rombusch & D. R. Ferry. 1985. Molecular pharmacology of $Ca^{2+}$ channels: receptor binding studies. *In* Nimodipine—Pharmacological and Clinical Properties. E. Betz, K. Deck & F. Hoffmeister, Eds. 56–73. F. K. Schattauer Verlag. Stuttgart.
13. d'Avella, D., R. Cicciarello, F. La Torre, P. Princi, R. P. Greenberg, S. d'Aquino & A. P. Caputi. 1984. The effect of the calcium antagonist nimodipine upon local cerebral glucose utilization in the rat brain. Life Sci. **34:** 2583–2588.
14. Doyle, P., C. Guillaume-Gentil, F. Rohner-Jeanrenuad & B. Jeanrenaud. 1994.

Effects of corticosterone administration on local cerebral glucose utilization of rats. Brain Res. **645:** 225–230.
15. HOFFMEISTER, F., U. BENZ, A. HEISE, H. P. KRAUSE & V. NEUSER. 1982. Behavioral effects of nimodipine in animals. Arzneim. Forsch. Drug Res. **32:** 3–47.
16. ISAACSON, R. L., J. C. MOLINA, L. J. DRASKI & J. E. JOHNSTON. 1985. Nimodipine's interactions with other drugs. I. Ethanol. Life Sci. **36:** 2195–2199.
17. GILLIAM, D. M., R. L. ISAACSON, R. G. BURRIGHT, J. E. JOHNSTON, J. M. FAHEY & D. VARGAS. 1988. Nimodipine's effect on alcohol disposition in mice. Alcohol **5:** 259–261.
18. DRASKI, L. J., J. E. JOHNSTON & R. L. ISAACSON. 1985. Nimodipine's interaction with other drugs. II. Diazepam. Life Sci. **35:** 2123–2128.
19. FAHEY, J. M. & R. L. ISAACSON. 1990. Pretreatment effects on nitrite-induced methemoglobinemia: saline and calcium channel antagonists. Pharmacol. Biochem. Behav. **37:** 457–459.
20. LEVINE, S. & G. D. COOVER. 1976. Environmental control of suppression of the pituitary-adrenal system. Physiol Behav. **17:** 35–37.
21. BECKER, L. A., J. A. VARNER, L. DOKAS & R. L. ISAACSON. 1994. Nimodipine treatment effect on classic ether stress and plus maze performance. Soc. Neurosci. **20:** 71.
22. DEKOSKY, S., S. W. SCHEFF & C. W. COTMAN. 1984. Elevated corticosterone levels: a possible cause of reduced axon sprouting in aged animals. Neuroendocrinology **38:** 33–38.
23. SCHEFF, S. W. & S. DEKOSKY. 1983. Steroid suppression of axonal sprouting in the hippocampus of the dentate gyrus of rat: dose response relationship. Exp. Neurol. **82:** 183–191.
24. POIRER, J., D. DEA, A. BACCICHET & S. GAUTHIER. 1992. Modulation of $\gamma$-actin and $\alpha_1$-tubulin expression by corticosterone during neuronal plasticity in the hippocampus. Mol. Brain Res. **15:** 263–268.
25. FAHEY, J. M., D. G. LINDQUIST, G. A. PRITCHARD & L. G. MILLER. 1994. Pregnenolone sulfate potentiation of NMDA-mediated increases in intracellular calcium in cultured chick cortical neurons. Brain Res. In press.
26. KUZMIN, A. V., N. A. PATKINA & E. E. ZVARTAU. 1994. Analgesic and reinforcing effects of morphine in mice. Influence of Bay K-8644 and nimodipine. Brain Res. **652:** 1–8.
27. MARTIN, P., S. LAURENT, J. MASSOL, M. CHILDS & A. J. PUECH. 1989. Effects of dihydropyridine drugs on reversal by imipramine of helpless behavior in rats. Eur. J. Pharmacol. **162:** 185–188.
28. CZYRAK, A., E. MOGILNICKA & J. MAJ. 1989. Dihydropyridine calcium channel antagonists as antidepressant drugs in mice and rats. Neuropharmacology **28:** 299–233.
29. CZYRAK, M., E. MOGILNICKA, J. SIWANOWICZ & J. MAJ. 1989. Some behavioral effects of subchronic administration of calcium channel antagonists. Naunyn Schmiedebergs Arch. Pharmacol. **339**(Suppl.): R48.

# The Effects of Nimodipine on the EEG of Substance Abusers

RONALD I. HERNING,[a] XIAOYAN GUO, AND W. ROBERT LANGE

*Molecular Neuropsychiatry Section*
*Neuroscience and Medical Affairs Branches*
*National Institutes of Health*
*National Institute on Drug Abuse*
*Intramural Research Program*
*Addiction Research Center*
*Baltimore, Maryland 21224*

## INTRODUCTION

Cocaine abusers have an increased risk of neurological and cerebrovascular complications such as strokes,[1] seizures,[2] transient ischemic attacks,[3] and headaches.[4] Blood flow deficits[5-9] and electroencephalogram (EEG) abnormalities[10-13] associated with cocaine abuse may reflect this increased risk for these medical complications. An increased EEG beta has been observed in cocaine-dependent individuals, and was correlated with the self-reported amount of cocaine used in the week before evaluation.[13] The increase in fast EEG activity may be a manifestation of the subtle perfusion deficits in cocaine abusers, since vertebral-basilar artery insufficiency has been associated with increases in EEG beta.[14] The reductions in blood flow may lead to neuron loss similar to that observed in aging, since neuron loss which accompanies aging is related to increases in EEG beta abundance.[15] Bursts of beta activity have been reported in awake elderly individuals.[16]

Nimodipine, a dihydropyridine calcium channel blocker, may be useful in reversing the perfusion deficits and EEG changes observed in cocaine abusers. Nimodipine is known to increase cerebral blood flow by dilatation of cortical arterioles[17,18] and to reduce vasospasm.[19] The EEG of geriatric patients was normalized after chronic treatment with nimodipine.[20] The present study tests the efficacy of single or acute multiple daily doses of nimodipine in reducing EEG beta and increasing EEG alpha of substance abusers.

## METHODS

### Subjects

Fourteen male substance abusers were studied in a double-blind, placebo controlled study. All subjects used alcohol and marijuana as well as cocaine and/or

[a] Address for correspondence: Ronald I. Herning, Ph.D., Molecular Neuropsychiatry Section, NIH/NIDA/IRP/ARC, P.O. Box 5180, Baltimore, MD 21224.

TABLE 1. Subject Characteristics and Drug History

| Measure | Mean | SD |
|---|---|---|
| Age (years) | 31.0 | 3.2 |
| SCL-90: General Severity Index | 45.4 | 10.8 |
| Addiction Severity Index | | |
| severity rating: 0 (no problem) to 9 (life-threatening situation) | | |
| Medical | 0.00 | 0.00 |
| Employment/Support | 0.86 | 2.00 |
| Family/Social Relationships | 0.29 | 1.07 |
| Psychological | 0.21 | 0.80 |
| Legal | 0.79 | 1.12 |

heroin, but no subject had any current active medical or psychiatric disorder (except substance abuse or dependence) as determined by medical history, Addiction Severity Index[21] (ASI), physical examination, and clinical laboratory testing. None had a history of seizures or head injury with loss of consciousness. The drug history was also determined from the ASI. All subjects were seronegative for human immunodeficiency virus. Participants lived on closed residential research unit in which abstinence was monitored by testing randomly obtained urine samples. The subjects' demographic characteristics and drug histories are presented in TABLES 1 and 2, respectively. This study was approval by the Johns Hopkins Bayview Medical Center Institutional Review Board for Human Research.

*Experiment Design*

For safety reasons, a pseudo-random series of ascending doses of oral nimodipine (Nimotop, Miles Inc.) was given. Placebo doses were inserted randomly and doses were repeated to maintain the double-blind. Single 30- and 60-mg doses of nimodipine and placebo were given during the first phase. During the second

TABLE 2. Addiction Severity Index: Drug History

| Drug | Recent Use: Number of Days Used in the Last 30 Days | | | Lifetime Use: Number of Months | | |
|---|---|---|---|---|---|---|
| | N | Mean | SD | N | Mean | SD |
| Cocaine | 10 | 8.4 | 7.6 | 11 | 68.7 | 27.9 |
| Alcohol | 14 | 6.6 | 4.2 | 14 | 166.5 | 55.9 |
| Heroin | 5 | 6.2 | 3.9 | 6 | 94.0 | 109.3 |
| Marijuana | 8 | 7.0 | 9.5 | 11 | 154.1 | 56.6 |
| Amphetamines | | | | 5 | 26.8 | 25.5 |
| Barbiturates | 1 | 3.0 | | 3 | 92.0 | 69.2 |
| Benzodiazapines | 1 | 4.0 | | 2 | 30.0 | 25.4 |
| Hallucinogens | | | | 5 | 48.0 | 38.9 |
| PCP | | | | 2 | 66.0 | 76.4 |
| Inhalants | | | | 2 | 43.0 | 57.3 |

phase, three doses were administered each test day at 0000, 0600 and 1000, with at least 48 hours between test days. The sequence was 0/30/30 mg, 30/30/30 mg, 30/30/60 mg and 60/30/60 mg with 0/0/0 mg inserted randomly in the dosing sequence.

## EEG Recording Procedures

This report focuses on the multichannel EEG collected during recording sessions with the eyes closed and eyes open. The recordings were obtained one and two hours after the test dose. The EEG was recorded from the following International 10/20 scalp sites: $F_3$, $C_3$, $P_3$, $O_1$, $F_4$, $C_4$, $P_4$, and $O_2$. The EEG recording was monopolar with an ipsolateral reference site at $A_1$ or $A_2$. Silver/silver chloride electrodes were used at all locations. The EEG was amplified by a Neurodata Acquisition System, Model 12 (Grass Instruments, Quincy, MA) and filtered with HZI Research Center (Tarrytown, NY) signal conditioning unit using a 1.0- to 50.0-Hz half amplitude bandpass. The output from the amplifier was collected with a Dell, 333D, personal computer (Austin, TX) with a Data Translation, Model DT2808 (Marlboro, MA) analog to digital convertor. Monitoring of EEG artifact was performed both during on-line collection and during off-line processing.

During the EEG recording, the subjects rested in a reclining chair in a sound-attenuated electronically shielded chamber. A minimum of three minutes of EEG was recorded during the three conditions. During these three-minute recordings, the percent of EEG activity was determined for delta (1.3–3.5 Hz), theta (3.6–7.5 Hz), alpha (7.6–13.5 Hz), and beta (13.6–50.0 Hz) EEG bands using the clinical or zero crossing method with the Brain Function Monitoring™ (HZI Research Center) software.

## Statistical Analysis

Separate analyses were performed for the single and multiple dosing phases of the study. A separate analysis of variance (ANOVA) was performed for each condition (eyes closed, eyes open) and for each EEG band (delta, theta, alpha, beta). These ANOVAs had three within subject factors: dose, time (one and two hours post drug) and electrode ($F_3$, $C_3$, $P_3$, $O_1$, $F_4$, $C_4$, $P_4$, $O_2$). The levels of dose factor for the single dose phase were placebo and 30 and 60 mg of nimodipine and for the multiple dose phase were 0/0/0 mg, 0/30/30 mg, 30/30/30 mg, 30/30/60 mg and 60/30/60 mg of nimodipine.

## RESULTS

### EEG Delta and Theta

Nimodipine did not significantly alter the percent of EEG delta and theta in the eyes closed or open conditions for the single or multiple dose phases of this study.

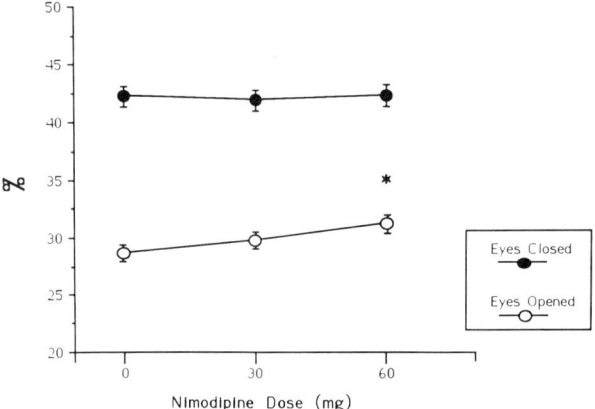

**FIGURE 1.** The means for EEG alpha during the single dose phase are plotted for the eyes closed and eyes open conditions. The one- and two-hour session are averaged together. The *asterisk* indicates a significant ($p < 0.05$) increase in EEG alpha after the 60-mg dose as compared to the placebo dose in the eyes open condition.

### *EEG Alpha*

In the eyes closed condition during the single dose phase, an increase in alpha (dose × time × electrode interaction: $F(14,182) = 2.12, p < 0.05$) was observed at $O_2$ electrode at one but not at two hours after the 30-mg dose of nimodipine. Increases in alpha were not observed at other electrodes or at any electrode with 60-mg dose. During the single dosing phase in the eyes open condition, the results for alpha were clearer. Nimodipine increased EEG alpha in a dose-dependent manner (dose main effect: $F(2,26) = 4.43, p < 0.05$). The means averaged over both times and all electrodes are shown for EEG alpha in FIGURE 1.

In the multiple dose phase EEG alpha was also increased. In the eyes closed condition, the dose × time interaction was significant ($F(4,40) = 2.93, p < 0.05$). Nimodipine increased alpha at the 30/30/30-mg dose relative to the placebo at one and decreased alpha at the same dose at two hours. In the eyes open condition, nimodipine significantly increased alpha (dose main effect: $F(4,40) = 2.98, p < 0.05$). The increase was observed at lower dose combinations only at the one hour and at both test times at the highest dose (see FIG. 2).

### *EEG Beta*

In the eyes closed condition during the single dose phase, decreases in beta (dose × time × electrode interaction: $F(14,182) = 2.53, p < 0.01$) were observed at $P_4$ at one hour for the 30-mg dose and at $P_3$ at one hour at the 60-mg dose, but not at two hours after either nimodipine dose. In the eyes open condition, nimodipine tended to decrease beta (dose main effect: $F(2,26) = 2.39, p < 0.12$). The

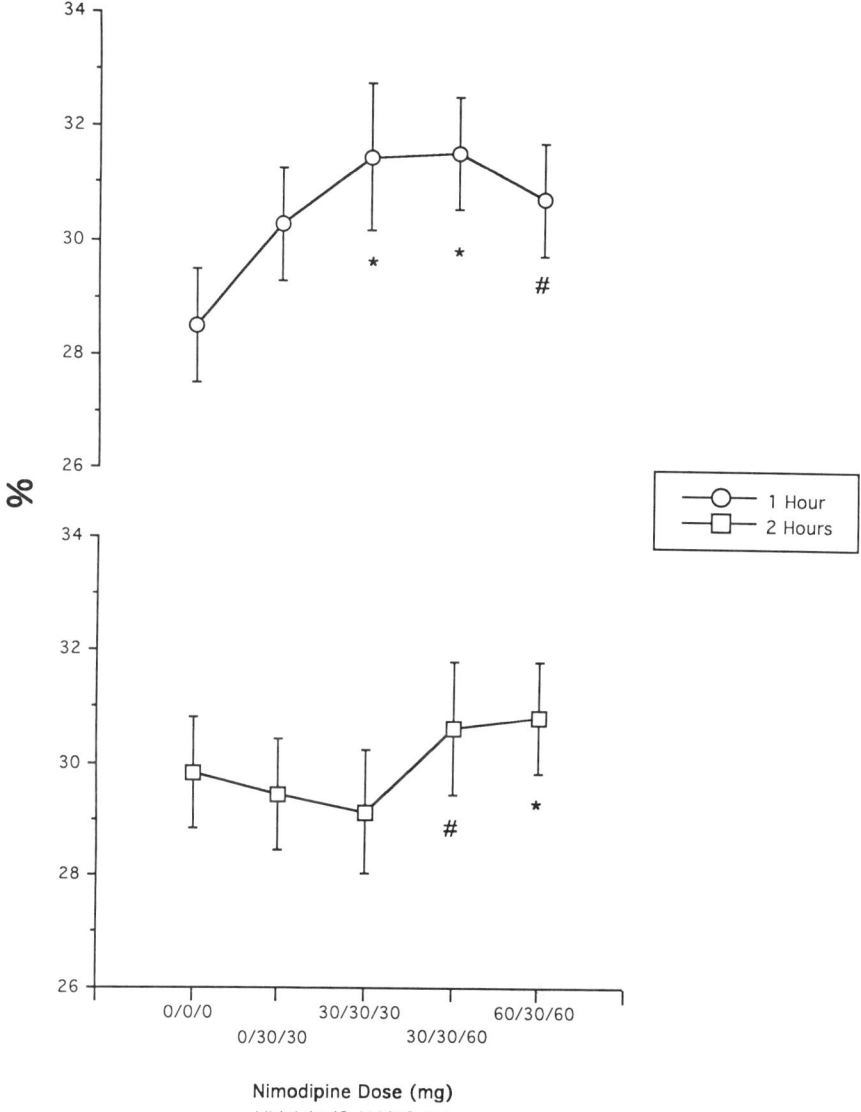

**FIGURE 2.** The means for EEG alpha during the multiple dose phase are shown for the eyes open condition at one hour *(top)*. The *asterisk* indicates a significant ($p < 0.05$) increase in EEG alpha at the indicated dose as compared to the placebo dose. The *pound sign* indicates a trend ($p < 0.10$). The means for the two-hour session are plotted at the *bottom*. (N = 11.)

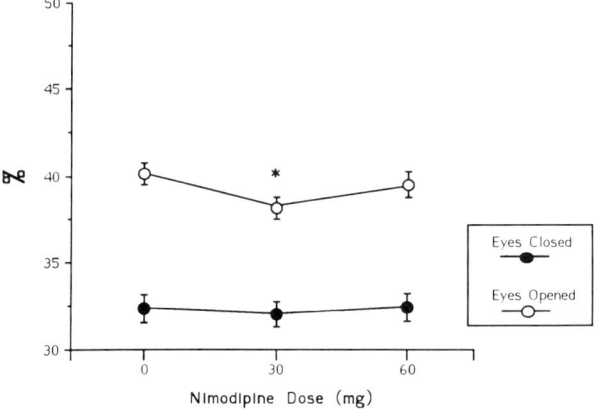

**FIGURE 3.** The means for EEG beta during the single dose phase are plotted for the eyes closed and eyes open conditions. The *asterisk* indicates a significant ($p < 0.05$) decrease in EEG beta after the 30-mg dose as compared to the placebo dose in the eyes open condition.

means averaged over both times and all electrodes are shown for beta in FIGURE 3.

In the multiple dosing phase, there was no clear effect of nimodipine in the eyes closed condition (dose main effect: $F(4,40) = 0.17$, ns) or the eyes open condition (dose main effect: $F(4,40) = 1.42$, ns). Since nimodipine had different effects at one versus two hours on the EEG alpha in the eye open condition, separate ANOVAs were performed for the one- and two-hour test sessions. Nimodipine decreased beta at one hour (dose main effect: $F(4,40) = 2.40, p < 0.06$), but not at two hours (dose main effect: $F(4,40) = 0.36$, ns). The means averaged over electrodes are plotted in FIGURE 4.

## DISCUSSION

Nimodipine increased EEG alpha and decreased EEG beta in substance abusers. The EEG changes were larger in the eyes open condition. EEG alpha increases were greater and more robust than the decreases in EEG beta. The increase in EEG alpha was dose dependent with the 60-mg dose producing the largest increase in the single dose phase and the 60/30/60-mg dose producing an increase at both the one- and two-hour test sessions in the multiple dose phase of the study.

It is unclear why the decreases in EEG beta were small. Our determination of beta abundance was based on a single wide beta band, *i.e.*, 13.6–50.0 Hz. Some investigators divide this band into two or three subbands. Nimodipine may have shifted the abundance of beta from one frequency range to another in this total frequency range. If nimodipine produced such an alteration, there would be no net change in the amount of EEG beta. The data can and will be reanalyzed to

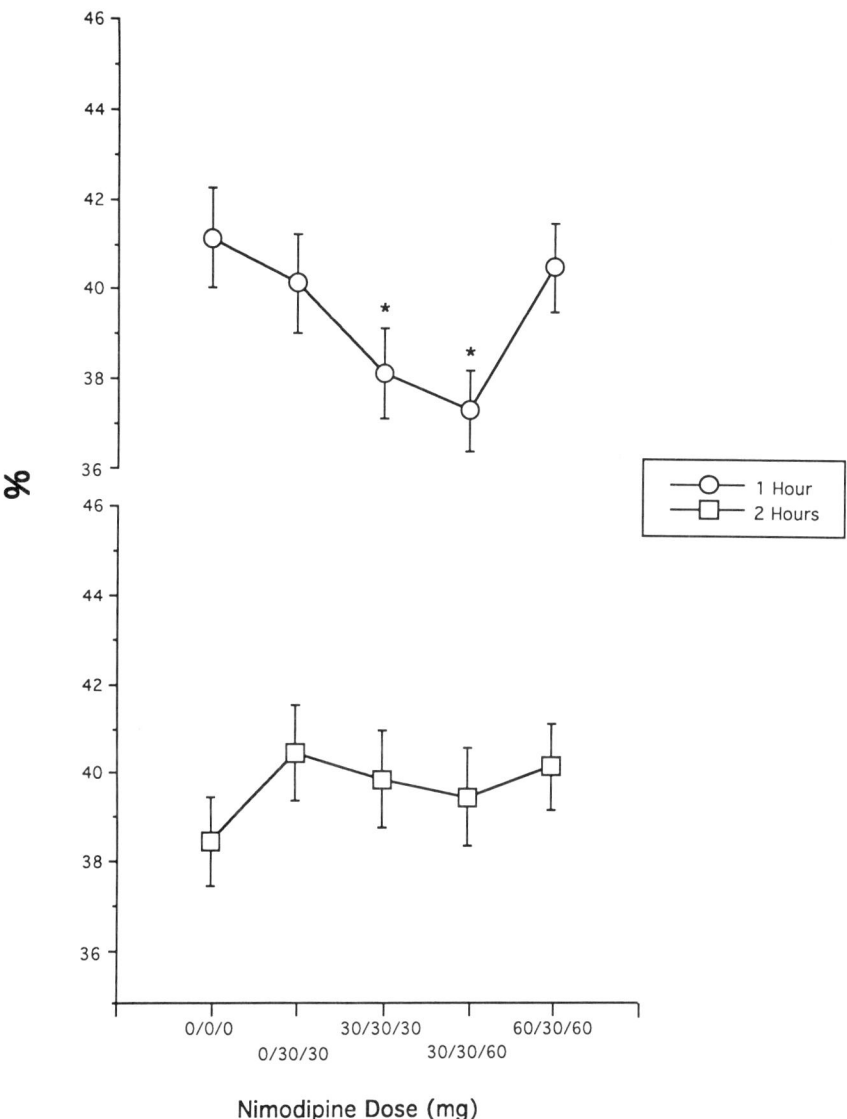

**FIGURE 4.** The means for EEG beta during the multiple dose phase are plotted for the eyes open condition at one hour *(top)*. The *asterisk* indicates a significant ($p < 0.05$) decrease in EEG alpha at the indicated dose as compared to the placebo dose. The means for the two-hour session are displayed at the *bottom*. (N = 11.)

resolve this issue, since it is important to understanding the nature of the EEG changes observed with nimodipine.

Nimodipine may be useful in the treatment of cocaine dependence. The changes were small, but in the appropriate direction to normalize the EEG in cocaine abusers who have a reduced abundance of alpha and an increased abundance of beta.[13] Chronic nimodipine dosing may produce larger changes in the EEG than we observed with single doses. In particular, chronic dosing may have more clearly decreased EEG beta activity. The EEG of geriatric patients was normalized after chronic treatment with nimodipine.[20] Chronic nimodipine dosing in cocaine-dependent individuals is now needed to confirm its efficacy in normalizing the EEG of cocaine-dependent patients in an inpatient setting.

Nimodipine appears to have anticraving effects which would also provide strong rationale for its use in the treatment of cocaine dependence. It reduced self-administration of morphine in mice[22] and reduced craving in cocaine-dependent patients.[23] The relationship between the EEG alterations in cocaine-dependent patients and cocaine craving is not known. However, the reduction of craving may be enhanced by normalizing brain function.

It is important to note that the present study was also designed to determine whether single doses of nimodipine were safe to administer to substance abusers. No untoward reductions in blood pressure were noted in this study. While decreases in blood pressure with chronic nimodipine dosing appear unlikely, it is possible they may occur. Likewise, this study did not address the issues concerning its safety during interactions with cocaine.

## SUMMARY

Cocaine abusers have increased EEG beta and areas of reduced cortical blood flow. Since, nimodipine has neuroprotective effects and increases blood flow, we investigated the efficacy of single and multiple doses of the nimodipine in normalizing the EEG of substance abusers. Fourteen subjects received single (0, 30, 60 mg) and eleven received multiple daily (up to 150 mg in 12 hours) doses of nimodipine to determine whether this drug would increase EEG alpha and decrease beta in substance abusers. The EEG was recorded from eight scalp locations ($F_3$, $C_3$, $P_3$, $O_1$, $F_4$, $C_4$, $P_4$ and $O_2$) for three minutes during eyes closed, and eyes open conditions. Single and multiple doses of nimodipine produced significant increases in EEG alpha and decreases in EEG beta in the eyes open condition. Thus, nimodipine may have potential therapeutic implications in the treatment of cocaine dependence. Chronic nimodipine dosing in cocaine-dependent individuals is now needed to confirm its efficacy in the treatment of cocaine dependence.

### REFERENCES

1. SLOAN, M. A. & T. A. MATTIONI. 1992. Concurrent myocardial and cerebral infarctions after intranasal use. Stroke **23**:427–430.
2. HOLLAND, R. W., J. A. MARX, M. P. EARNEST & S. RANNIGER. 1992. Grand mal

seizures temporally related to cocaine use: clinical and diagnostic features. Ann. Emerg. Med. **21:**772–776.
3. SPIVEY, W. H. & B. EUERLE. 1990. Neurologic complications of cocaine abuse. Ann. Emerg. Med. **19:**1422–1428.
4. DHOPESH, V., I. MAANY & C. HERRING. 1990. The relationship of cocaine to headache in polysubstance abusers. Headache **31:**17–19.
5. VOLKOW, D. N., N. MULLANI, K. L. GOULD, S. ADLER & K. KRAJEWSKI. 1988. Cerebral blood flow in chronic cocaine users: a study with positron emission tomography. Br. J. Psychiatry **151:**641–648.
6. WEBER, D. A., P. KLEINER, N. D. VOLKOW, D. SACKER & M. IVANNVIC. 1990. SPECT regional cerebral blood flow (rCBF) studies in crack users and control subjects. J. Nucl. Med. **31:**876–877.
7. MENA, I., B. MILLER, K. GARRENT, L. LEEDOM, I. KHALKHALI & A. DJENDEREDJIAN. 1990. Neurospect in cocaine abuse. Eur. J. Nucl. Med. **16:**5137–5143.
8. TUMEH, S. S., J. S. NAGEL, R. J. ENGLISH, M. MOORE, & B. L. HOLMAN. 1990. Cerebral abnormalities in cocaine abusers: demonstration by SPECT perfusion brain scintigraphy. Radiology **176:**821–824.
9. HOLMAN, B. L., P. A. CARVALHO, J. MENDELSON, S. K. TEOK, R. NARDIN, J. HALLGRING, N. HEBBEN & K. A. JOHNSON. 1991. Brain perfusion is abnormal in cocaine-dependent polydrug users: a study using technetium-99m-NMPAO and AS-PECT. J. Nucl. Med. **32:**1206–1210.
10. ALPER, K. R., R. J. CHABOT, A. H. KIM, L. S. PRICHEP & E. R. JOHN. 1991. Quantitative EEG correlates of crack cocaine dependence. Psychiatry Res. Neuroimaging **35:**95–105.
11. BAUER, L. O. 1993. Electroencephalographic evidence for residual CNS hyperexcitability during cocaine abstinence. Am J. Addict. **2:**287–298.
12. BAUER, L. O. 1994. Photic driving of EEG alpha in recovering cocaine-dependent and alcohol-dependent patients. Am. J. Addict. **3:**49–57.
13. HERNING, R. I., X. GUO, L. L. WEINHOLD, W. R. LANGE & D. A. GORELICK. 1994. Neurophysiological signs of cocaine dependence: excessive EEG beta activity. Biol. Psychiatry. In press.
14. NIEDERMEYER, E. 1963. The electroencephalogram and vertebral-basilar artery insufficiency. Neurology **13:**412–422.
15. SHEARER, D. E., R. Y. EMMERSON & R. E. DUSTMAN. 1989. EEG relationships to neural aging in elderly: overview and bibliography. Am J. EEG Technol. **29:**43–63.
16. IYAMA, A, T. INOUYE, S. UKAI & K. SHINOSAKI. 1992. Spindle activity in the waking EEG of older adults. Clin. Electroencephalogr. **23:**137–141.
17. GODFRAIND, T., N. MOREI & C. DESSY. 1990. Calcium antagonists and vasoconstrictor effects on intracerebral microarterioles. Stroke **21:**IV-59–IV-63.
18. OLIVER, D. N., I. C. DORMEHL, I. F. REDELINGHUYS, N. HUGO & G. BEVERLEY. 1993. Drug effects on cerebral blow flow in the baboon model-acetazolamide and nimodipine. Nukleamedizin **32:**292–298.
19. FLECKENSTIEN-GRUIN, G. & A. FLECKENSTEIN. 1990. Prevention of cerebrovascular spasms with nimodipine. Stroke **21:**IV-64–IV-71.
20. ULRICH, G. & R. D. STIEGLITZ. 1988. Effect of nimodipine upon electroencephalographic vigilance in elderly persons with minor impairment of brain functions. Arzneim.-Forsch. **30:**392–396.
21. MCLELLAN, A. T., J. CACCIATO, J. GRIFFITH, P. MCCAHN & C. P. O'BRIEN. 1985. Guide to the Addiction Severity Index: background, administration and field testing results. Washington, DC, U.S. Printing Office, Treatment Research Report DHHS Publication Number ADM 85-1419.
22. KURZMIN, A. V. & N. P. PATKINA. 1994. Analgesic and reinforcing effects of morphine in mice: influence of Bay K-8644 and nimodipine. Brain Res. **652:**1–8.
23. DEUTSCH, S. I., R. B. ROSSE, T. N. ALIM & C. D. JENTGEN. 1993. Nimodipine during early cocaine abstinence. Biol. Psychiatry **33:**153A–154A.

# Nimodipine Improves Information Processing in Substance Abusers

RONALD I. HERNING,[a] XIAOYAN GUO, AND W. ROBERT LANGE

*Molecular Neuropsychiatry Section*
*Neuroscience and Medical Affairs Branches*
*National Institutes of Health*
*National Institute on Drug Abuse*
*Intramural Research Program*
*Addiction Research Center*
*Baltimore, Maryland 21224*

## INTRODUCTION

A decline in the amplitude of the P3 component of the event-related potential (ERP), which is obtained from the scalp electroencephalogram (EEG) during cognitive tasks, with repeated testing has been observed in substance abusers.[1] P3 reflects resources allocated to the evaluation of task-relevant stimuli and the updating of recent memory.[2,3] Reductions in P3 amplitude or increases in P3 latency are observed during fatigue or boredom in normal subjects and are reversed by stimulants.[4-8] Cocaine blocked the reduction in P3 amplitude produced by repeated testing in substance abusers.[1] Since nimodipine improved cognitive performance in young, old, and brain-damaged animals[9-15] and cognitive status in dementia,[16,17] it may also reverse this cognitive deficit in substance abusers. Thus, we examined whether nimodipine can improve information processing in substance abusers by monitoring the P3 in two information processing tasks.

## METHODS

### Subjects

Twelve male substance abusers were studied. They used alcohol, marijuana, cocaine and/or heroin, but no subject had a current medical or psychiatric disorder (except substance abuse or dependence) as determined by medical history interview, Addiction Severity Index (ASI),[18] physical examination, and clinical laboratory testing. The drug history was also determined by the ASI. They were seronegative for human immunodeficiency virus. The subjects lived on a closed residential research unit in which abstinence was monitored by randomly obtained urine samples. The subjects' demographic characteristics and drug histories are pre-

---

[a] Address for Correspondence: Ronald I. Herning, Ph.D., Molecular Neuropsychiatry Section, NIH/NIDA/IRP/ARC, P.O. Box 5180, Baltimore, MD 21224

sented in TABLES 1 and 2, respectively, of the previous paper.[19] The study was approved by the Johns Hopkins Bayview Medical Center Institutional Review Board for Human Research.

## Experimental Design

On each test day the subjects received either placebo, 30 or 60 mg of nimodipine (Nimotop, Miles Inc.) in a random double-blind experimental design. All subjects had previously received the placebo and two doses of nimodipine as a part of the previous study.[19] This study was performed on separate days and was independent of the EEG recording in the previous study. The subjects were tested on the auditory rare event monitoring task (AREM) and the paired letter continuous performance task (CPT) before as well as one and two hours after the oral administration of the test drug.

During the AREM task the subject was required to count the number of rare tones in a sequence of rare and frequent tones. At the end of the sequence the subject reported his count to the researcher. The tones were presented at the rate of one every two seconds by the Neurological Workload Test Battery (NWTP) (Systems Research Laboratories, Dayton, OH). The task lasted four minutes. Twenty percent of the tones were of the rare type. Rare tone frequency was 1000 Hz and the frequent tone frequency was 2000 Hz. Both tones were 100 ms long and were 70 decibels standard pressure level. The tones were presented to the subject through a headset (TDH-39). During testing the subject was seated in a reclining chair in a soundproof, electrically shielded chamber.

For the CRT task, event-related responses were elicited visually using letters presented on a TV monitor by the NWTB system. The subject monitored a series of letters displayed on the screen, one at a time, and was required to press a push button with his preferred hand when any letter repeated itself. This task lasted about five minutes. The letters subtended 10° of visual angle, remained on the screen for 600 ms and were presented at a rate of one every two seconds. The mean luminance of the screen was 40 cd/m$^2$. The TV monitor was 30 cm from the subject's eyes.

## EEG Recording Procedure

The EEG was recorded from seven scalp locations ($F_z$, $C_z$, $P_z$, $F_3$, $F_4$, $P_3$ and $P_4$) using the International 10/20 System. The scalp locations were referred to the left ear tip. Eye movement (EOG) was recorded from above the left eye referred to the temporal side of that eye and from above the left eye referred to the left ear. Beckman Ag/AgCl electrodes were used at all sites and the electrode impedance was below 5K Ohms. The EEG was amplified with a Neurodata Acquisition System, Model 12 (Grass Instruments, Quincy, MA). The half amplitude bandpass of each amplifier was from 0.1 to 30 Hz. The amplifiers were calibrated with a 5-Hz, 50-μvolt square wave (Grass Calibrator, Model SWC1B). The output of the amplifiers was recorded on a Dell, System 325, personal computer (Austin, TX)

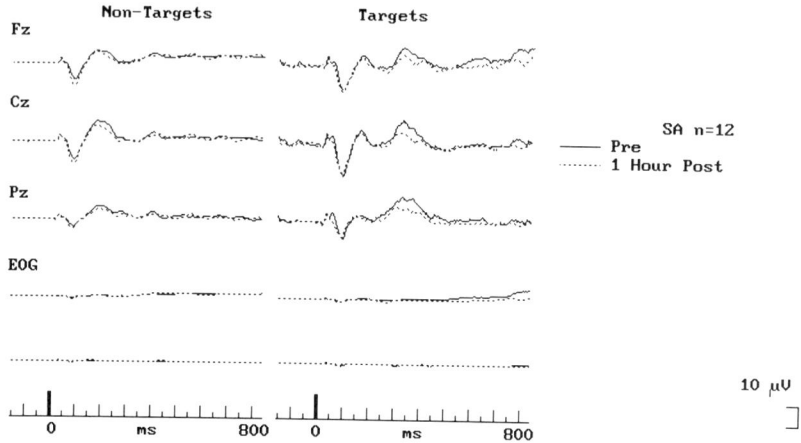

**FIGURE 1.** The average ERPs for the substance abusers (SA) are displayed for the AREM task at the placebo day. The pre-placebo session is compared to a session about an hour later. The centerline electrodes $F_z$ (frontal), $C_z$ (central) and $P_z$ (parietal) are plotted with two eye movement (EOG) channels for the target and non-target tones. Positive is up.

with a Data Translation, Model DT2821-F-SE (Marlboro, MA) analog to digital convertor. Each channel was sampled at 5.0-msec intervals using software developed by NIDA for this purpose. The sampling interval began 150 ms before stimulus onset and ended 850 ms after onset. An average ERP was calculated separately for the target and nontarget stimuli.

### ERP Measurement

Principal components analysis (PCA) was used to objectively extract multiple independent components from the ERP.[20] The resultant factor scores were further analyzed by analysis of variance (ANOVA) techniques. Seven hundred and fifty-six rare ERP waveforms (12 subjects × 3 test days × 3 test times × 7 electrodes) were used in the PCA. The ERPs which were originally digitized at 5-ms intervals were reduced to 60 variables for the AREM task and 80 for CPT by sampling every 10.0 ms to allow for PCA using the CRUNCH statistical package (Oakland, CA) since this package allowed for a maximum of 80 variables. The PCA with a Varimax rotation was performed on the covariance matrix and factor scores were calculated.

## RESULTS

The average ERP waveforms for the AREM task are displayed in FIGURE 1 for the placebo day. The P3 component can be seen at about 300 ms after stimulus onset for the target tones. It is reduced by about 50% at about one hour after the

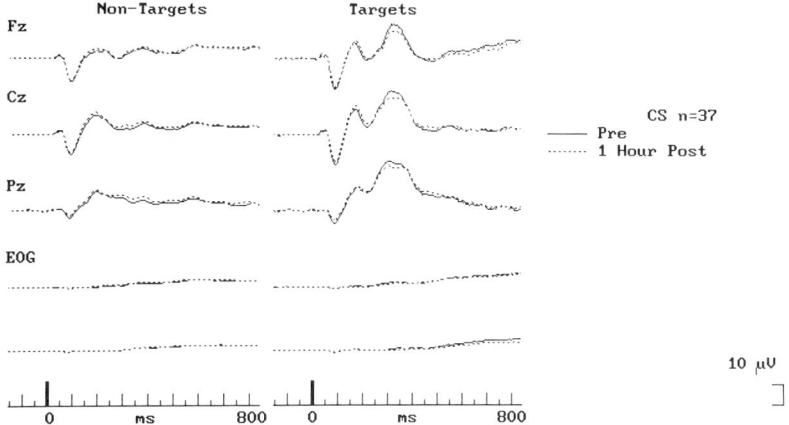

**FIGURE 2.** The average ERPs for the control subjects (CS) are displayed for the AREM task. The pre or first session is compared to a session about an hour later. The centerline electrodes $F_z$ (frontal), $C_z$ (central) and $P_z$ (parietal) are plotted with two eye movement (EOG) channels for the target and non-target tones. Positive is up.

first session. In a sample of 37 control subjects (no history of drug abuse and negative urine toxicology for abused drugs) tested twice on the same task, only a small reduction in P3 was observed (see FIG. 2). In comparing both figures plotted with the same scale, the substance abusers also have a much smaller P3 component than the control subjects.

## PCA Analysis

The PCA on the ERPs from the AREM task extracted six factors which accounted for 81.8% of the variance: SW (47.9%), N1 (12.7%), P3A (7.7%), P2B (5.3%), P3B (4.5%) and P2A (3.6%). Change scores (post drug minus prefactor score) were calculated and a dose (placebo, 30 mg, 60 mg) by time (1 hour, 2 hours) by electrode ANOVA was performed on these values. The dose factor was significant for P3A ($F(2,22) = 3.40$, $p < 0.05$). P3A was reduced after placebo and 60 mg of nimodipine, but not after the 30-mg dose of nimodipine. The pattern of results was similar at all electrode locations, but was largest at $P_z$. The means for $P_z$ are plotted in FIGURE 3. No significant dose effects were observed for P3B.

The PCA on the ERPs from the visual paired letter CPT extracted six factors which accounted for 91.3% of the variance: SW (60.7%), P3 (13.1%), P1 (7.2%), P2A (4.6%), N1 (3.2%) and P2B (2.6%). Change scores (post drug minus prefactor score) were calculated and a dose (placebo, 30 mg, 60 mg) by time (1 hour, 2 hours) by electrode ANOVA was performed on these values. A significant dose by electrode interaction was observed ($F(12,132) = 2.62$, $p < 0.004$). When P3 was further investigated by separate analyses for each electrode, the dose by time interaction was significant for the $P_3$ ($F(2,22) = 13.35$, $p < 0.005$) and $P_4$ ($F(2,22)$

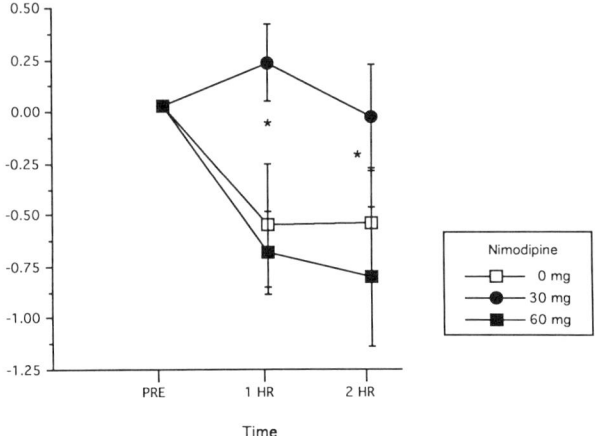

**FIGURE 3.** The P3A change scores for the $P_z$ are shown for the AREM task. *Negative values* indicate a reduction and *positive values* indicate an increase in P3A relative to the pre-drug session. The *asterisks* indicate a significant difference between the placebo and 30-mg dose of nimodipine.

$= 5.13$, $p < 0.01$) electrode sites. P3 at these electrode sites were reduced after placebo and 60 mg, but not after the 30-mg nimodipine dose (see FIG. 4).

## DISCUSSION

Nimodipine blocked the decline in P3 amplitude observed with repeated testing in substance abusers. The decrease with repeated testing was observed in the auditory rare event monitoring task and the visual continuous performance task and was blocked in both tasks with 30 mg of nimodipine. The changes with nimodipine were largest at parietal electrode sites. The block of the P3 reduction with nimodipine was observed with the 30-mg, but not the 60-mg dose of nimodipine.

In a previous study, P3 was also reduced with repeated testing on the placebo day and cocaine blocked the decline.[1] The reduction in P3 on the placebo day was significantly correlated with self-reported tiredness at 60 minutes. Substance abusers appear to fatigue more rapidly during cognitive tasks. This deficit in cognitive processing may be a premobid characteristic of those at risk for substance abuse. A similar decline in P3 amplitude with repeated testing was observed in extroverts.[21] The P3 is reduced in children with attention deficit hyperactivity disorder (ADHD).[22] Methylphenidate (Ritan, Ciba) blocks the reduction in P3 in these ADHD children.[23,24] P3 is also reduced in adolescents who use drugs, but not in aggressive adolescents who do not use drugs.[25] Both ADHD and aggressive children are to be at risk for substance abuse, but the former have a reduced P3 and the latter do not. Further prospective research in children at risk for drug abuse is needed to determine whether this reduction in P3 existed before the individuals began using drugs.

The P3 reflects neural processing involved in stimulus evaluation[2] and in updat-

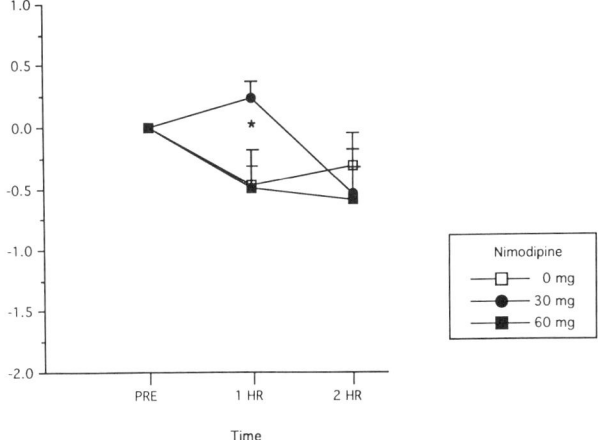

**FIGURE 4.** The P3 change scores for the $P_3$ are shown for the CPT task. *Negative values* indicate a reduction and *positive values* indicate an increase in P3 relative to the pre-drug session. The *asterisk* indicates a significant difference between the placebo and 30-mg dose of nimodipine.

ing recent memory.[3] Lesions at the temporal-parietal cortical junction reduce the auditory and somatosensory P3.[26] The P3 deficit we observed may be due to temporal-parietal cortical perfusion deficits reported in this population.[27–29] Thus, the improvement in information processing with nimodipine may be due to nimodipine's ability to increase in cortical blood flow.[30,31] In most but not all studies investigating the cognitive effects of nimodipine, the drug was administered chronically.[9–17] We observed the effect with a single 30-mg dose. Thus, the improvement in our study was not due to changes in dendritic branching and synaptic density.

Although the results are promising, it is unclear why no improvement was observed with the 60-mg dose of nimodipine in either of the cognitive tasks or at any of the electrode sites. The results with the 60-mg dose resembled that of the placebo dose rather than the 30-mg dose. The dose-response curve may not be linear and testing with 15, 30, and 45 mg of nimodipine would help resolve this issue. More seriously drug-impaired subjects may require the 60-mg dose to improve this cognitive process. The real issue, however, is whether or not chronic nimodipine dosing would improve information processing and whether improved cognitive functioning would improve treatment outcome for the cocaine-dependent patients.

In conclusion, acute doses of nimodipine improved information processing in substance abusers. Further research is needed to determine whether chronic administration of nimodipine may alleviate the cognitive deficits observed in substance abusers during abstinence and prevent treatment relapse.

## SUMMARY

We examined whether nimodipine can improve information processing in healthy drug abusers using cognitive event-related potential (ERP) methodology.

Placebo and 30- and 60-mg doses of nimodipine were administered on separate days in a random double-blind design to twelve male subjects, who used cocaine and/or opiates as well as alcohol and marijuana. The subjects performed the auditory rare event monitoring (AREM) task and the paired letter version of the visual continuous performance task (CPT) before oral drug administration as well as one and two hours after drug ingestion. The EEG was recorded from 7 scalp locations. The P3 component of the ERPs to the target stimulus was reduced with repeated testing on the placebo day. The 30-mg dose of nimodipine blocked the decrease in P3, which reflects stimulus evaluation in both tasks. Chronic administration of nimodipine may alleviate the cognitive deficits observed in substance abusers during abstinence and prevent treatment relapse.

## REFERENCES

1. HERNING, R. H., B. G. GLOVER & X. GUO. 1994. The effects of cocaine on the P3B in cocaine abusers. Neuropsychobiology. In press.
2. DONCHIN, E. & M. G. H. COLES. 1988. Is the P300 component a manifestation of context updating? Behav. Brain Sci. **38:** 387–401.
3. JOHNSON, R. 1993. On neural generators of the P300 component of the event-related potential. Psychophysiology **30:** 90–97.
4. COONS, H. W., L. J. PELOQUIN, R. KLORMAN, R. M. RYAN, L. O. BAUER, R. A. PERLMUTTER & L. F. SALZMAN. 1981. Effects of methylphenidate on young adults' event-related potentials. Electroencephalogr. Clin. Neurophysiol. **51:** 373–387.
5. STRAUSS, J., J. L. LEWIS, R. KLORMAN, L. J. PELOQUIN, R. A. PERLMUTTER & L. F. SALZMAN. 1984. Effects of methylphenidate on young adult's performance and event-related potentials in a vigilance and a paired-associates learning test. Psychophysiology **21:** 601–612.
6. PELOQUIN, L. J. & R. KLORMAN. 1986. Effects of methylphenidate on normal children's mood, event-related potentials and performance in memory scanning and vigilance. J. Abnorm. Psychol. **95:** 88–98.
7. BRUMAGHIM, J. T., R. KLORMAN, J. STRAUSS, J. D. LEVINE & M. G. GOLDSTEIN. 1987. What aspects of information processing are affected by methylphenidate? Findings on performance and P3b from two studies. Psychophysiology **24:** 361–373.
8. FITZPATRICK, P., R. KLORMAN, J. T. BRUMAGHIM & R. W. KEEFOVER. Effects of methylphenidate on stimulus evaluation and response processes: evidence from performance and event-related potentials. Psychophysiology **25:** 292–307.
9. LEVY, A., R. M. KONG, M. J. STILLMAN, B. SHUKITT-HALE, T. KADAR, T. M. RAUCH & H. R. LIEBERMAN. 1991. Nimodipine improves spatial working memory and elevates hippocampal acetylcholine in young rats. Pharmacol. Biochem. Behav. **39:** 781–786.
10. NELSON, C., S. FINGER & D. SIMONS. 1993. Effects of nimodipine on two neurologic measures sensitive to sensorimotor cortex damage. Exp. Neurol. **119:** 302–308.
11. DISTERHOFT, J. F., J. R. MOYER, L. T. THOMPSON & M. KOWALSKA. 1993. Functional aspects of calcium-channel modulation. Clin. Neuropharmacol. **16**(Suppl 1): S12–S16.
12. DE JONGE, M. C. & J. TRABER. 1993. Nimodipine: cognition, aging, and degeneration. Clin. Neuropharmacol. **16**(Suppl 1): S25–S30.
13. INGRAM, D. K., J. A. JOSEPH, E. L. SPANGLER, D. ROBERTS, J. HENGEMIHLE & R. J. FANELLI. 1993. Chronic nimodipine treatment in aged rats: analysis of motor and cognitive effect and muscarinic-induced striatal dopamine release. Neurobiol. Aging **15:** 55–61.
14. KOWALSKA, M. & J. F. DISTERHOFT. 1994. Relationship of nimodipine dose and serum concentration to learning enhancement in aging rabbits. Exp. Neurol. **127:** 159–166.
15. MERVIS, R. F., N. KUNTZ, D. BURTON, R. DVORAK, R. TANDON, M. S. WOOD & P.

R. Soloman. 1995. Structural-functional correlates of neuroprotection in the aging rabbit by a calcium channel blocker: nimodipine reverses neurocortical dendritic atropy and improves memory retention. This volume.
16. Tollefson, G. D. 1990. Short-term effects of the calcium channel blocker nimodipine (Bay-e-9736) in the management of primary degenerative dementia. Biol. Psychiatry **27:** 1133–1142.
17. Parnetti, L., U. Senin, M. Carosi & H. Baasch. 1993. Mental deterioration in old aging: result of two multicenter, clinical trial with nimodipine. Clin. Ther. **15:** 394–406.
18. McCellan, AT. T., J. Cacciata, J. Griffith, P. McCahn & C. P. O'Brien. 1985. Guide to the addiction severity index: background, administration and field testing results. Washington, DC, U.S. Printing Office, Treatment Research Report DHHS Publication Number ADM 85-1419.
19. Herning, R. I., X. Guo & W. R. Lange. 1995. The effect of nimodipine on the EEG of substance abusers. This volume.
20. Squires, K. C., E. Donchin, R. I. Herning & W. McGarty. 1977. On the influence of task relevance and probability on ERP components. Electroencephalogr. Clin. Neurophysiol. **42:** 1–14.
21. Ditraglia, G. M. & J. Polich. 1991. P300 and introverted/extraverted personality types. Psychophysiology **28:** 177–184.
22. Satterfield, J. H., A. M. Schell, T. W. Nicholas, B. T. Satterfield & T. E. Freese. 1990. Ontogeny of selective attention effects on event-related potentials in attention-deficit hyperactivity disorder and normal boys. Biol. Psychiatry **28:** 879–903.
23. Klorman, R., L. F. Salzman, L. O. Bauer, H. W. Coons, A. D. Borgstedt & W. I. Halpern. 1983. Effects of two doses of methylphenidate on cross-situational and borderline hyperactive children's evoked potentials. Electroencephalogr. Clin. Neurophysiol. **56:** 169–185.
24. Overtoom, K., M. N. Vertatem & H. Van Engeland. 1993. Methylphenidate influences both early and late ERP waves of ADHD-children in a continuous performance task. Psychophysiology **30:** S49.
25. Herning, R. I., J. E. Hickey, W. B. Pickworth & J. H. Jaffe. 1989. Auditory event-related potentials in adolescents at risk for drug abuse. Biol. Psychiatry **25:** 598–609.
26. Yamaguchi, S. & R. T. Knight. 1992. Effects of temporal-parietal lesions on somatosensory P3 to lower limb stimulation. Electroencephalogr. Clin. Neurophysiol. **84:** 139–148.
27. Volkow, D. N., N. Mullani, K. L. Gould, S. Adler & K. Krajewski. 1988. Cerebral blood flow in chronic cocaine users: a study with positron emission tomography. Br. J. Psychiatry **151:** 641–648.
28. Weber, D. A., P. Klieger, N. D. Volkow, D. Sacker, M. Ivannvic. 1990. SPECT regional cerebral blood flow (rCBF) studies in crack users and control subjects. J. Nucl. Med. **31:** 876–877.
29. Holman, B. L., P. A. Carvalho, J. Mendelson, S. K. Teoh, R. Nardin, K. Hallgring, N. Hebben & K. A. Johnson. 1991. Brain perfusion is abnormal in cocaine-dependent polydrug users: a study using technetium-99m-NMPAO and AS-PECT. J. Nucl. Med. **32:** 1206–1210.
30. Godfraind, T., N. Morei & C. Dessy. 1990. Calcium antagonists and vasoconstrictor effects on intracerebral microarterioles. Stroke **21:** IV-59–IV-63.
31. Oliver, D. N., I. C. Dormehl, I. F. Redelinghuys, N. Hugo & G. Beverley. 1993. Drug effects on cerebral blow flow in the baboon model-acetazolamide and nimodipine. Nukleamedizin **32:** 292–298.

# Discussion

S. ALI (*National Center for Toxicological Research, FDA, Jefferson, AR*): Have you performed these studies with other drugs of abuse such as methylenedioxymethamphetamine (MDMA), phencyclidine hydrochloride (PCP), or methamphetamine (METH)?

R. HERNING (*National Institute on Drug Abuse, NIH, Bethesda, MD*): We have not studied these drugs with electroencephalogram (EEG) or event-related potential (ERP) measures in humans.

ALI: What is the neurochemical mechanism(s) of nimodipine, and is it a neuroprotective agent against cocaine addiction?

HERNING: Based on our data and SPECT blood flow studies in cocaine-dependent subjects, it appears these individuals have reduced cortical blood flow. Nimodipine is known to increase blood flow, thus, the simplest mechanism to explain the results. Increases in EEG alpha power were correlated with increases in blood flow in studies when both were measured in the same individuals. It is possible that nimodipine operates directly on neurons in the cortex, but we have no direct measure of such action in humans.

P. BOKSA (*Douglas Hospital Research Center, Verdun Quebec*): How can you eliminate the possibility that the decreases in performance in event-related tasks on the part of substance abusers are due to motivation deficits and not due to cognitive deficits, *i.e.*, that substance abusers just do not care about doing the task, are antisocial and do not care if they live up to your expectations, etc.?

HERNING: This is an important question. In the performance data, in a continuous performance task (CPT) in cocaine-dependent individuals, the percent correct was about 99% for controls and about 95% in abstinent cocaine-dependent patients. Task performance was quite acceptable, but brain potential were altered. In an early study of aggressive and antisocial teens, the P3 amplitude was not different from carefully matched control subjects. However, on the tasks given to cocaine-dependent individuals, the P3 is reduced compared to controls. The tasks are not extremely difficult or long. Although we have not studied motivation influence on task performance and ERPs in substance abusers, our subjects performed the task quite well, antisocial teens had no reduction in P3 and the tasks are relatively easy! The evidence suggests motivation may not be important on these tasks, but may be important on more difficult tasks.

S. GOLDIN (*Cambridge NeuroScience*): Does sustained depolarization also increase the affinity for L-type Ca channels for other classes of Ca antagonists, *e.g.*, phenylalkylamines (verapamil) and benzthiazapines (diltiazem)?

D. TRIGGLE (*State University of New York, Buffalo*): Yes. As representatives of the three major structural classes of clinically available $Ca^{2+}$ channel antagonists, verapamil and diltiazem also show use-dependent blocking properties. These use-dependent properties appear as both voltage dependence and frequency dependence. Thus, all 1,6-dihydropyridines show structural-dependent, voltage-dependent binding, and affinity increasing with decreasing membrane potential. Verapamil and diltiazem show frequency dependence. Thus, indicating their antiarrhythmic properties.

**DISCUSSION** 161

ANONYMOUS: Are you, or have you, tested for $N$-type channel downregulation during $K^+$ depolarization in PC-12 cells treated with neural growth factors?

TRIGGLE: No; but we are looking at downregulation of non-L-type $Ca^{2+}$ channels in several neuronal and neurosecretory cells.

A. J. MERCER (*Wellcome Research Laboratories, Beckenham, UK*): What is the effect of nimodipine at the doses you gave on the performance of healthy controls?

HERNING: We have not given nimodipine to healthy controls. At this point we have collected normative ERP data on the task used to detect alterations in cocaine-dependent individuals, since normal values do not exist for brain potentials elicited in these tasks. However, one can speculate. If a normal control was fatigued by repeated testing or by sleep deprivation, these doses of nimodipine would protect against these conditions which would alter information processing. If there were not deficits in information processing, then there would be no enhancement of performance. This speculation is based on what we know about the effects of stimulants on the ERP component. Stimulants only reverse deficits in ERP components!

W. SLIKKER (*National Center for Toxicological Research, FDA, Jefferson, AR*): Considering the known influence of glucocorticoids on both neuronal structure and animal behavior, have you considered that the effects of nimodipine may be partially mediated by glucocorticoids as postulated by Dr. Isaacson?

Dr. Isaacson's data is most interesting. It is possible that our P300B (P3B) results are mediated through the glucocorticoids. The source of the P3B in humans is thought to be in the hippocampus or closely related limbic structures. We show an improvement in P3B with nimodipine. Besides EEG and ERPs, a variety of hormones were collected in our sample of cocaine-dependent subjects. We have not as yet correlated the EEG and ERP changes with the level of these hormones.

R. F. MERVIS (*NeuroMetrix Research, Inc., Columbus, OH*): The hypothesis is interesting. Landfield and others have shown that increased levels of glucocorticoids lead to cell death in the brain, particularly in the hippocampus. Nimodipine treatment would tend to restore calcium homeostasis and would attenuate potential cellular damage stemming from high levels of glucocorticoids. However, at this time, no specific studies have been carried out to define that correlations between these parameters. This would seem to be a fruitful area for future research.

A. SCALLET (*National Center for Toxicological Research, FDA, Jefferson, AR*): You mentioned that you Golgi-stained formalin-fixed sections of brain as opposed to blocks. Is there a published method for this?

MERVIS: Formalin-fixed rabbit brains were shipped to my laboratory. Coronal blocks of parietal cortex (approximately 4 mm thick) were removed and Golgi-stained "en bloc" using a rapid Golgi variant. I did not mean to imply that thin sections of brain were stained.

SCALLET: Is the circuit thought to underlie the eye-blink conditioning related to the parietal cortex layer 5 pyramids? Why do you think you got a correlation between the behavioral and Golgi response to nimodipine in aging? Would Purkinje or Granule cerebellar cells correlate better?

MERVIS: Actually, eye-blink conditioning is believed to be mediated primarily through hippocampal circuits (and, perhaps, via the cerebellum). The cortex may not be a major player in this conditioning paradigm. However, we chose to evaluate cortical pyramids because: 1) it was a region which stained particularly well; and 2) we reasoned that nimodipine's effects on neuronal morphology would not be localized, *i.e.*, if it influenced cortical pyramids it would also most likely affect the hippocampus (and other regions) as well. So essentially, looking at the cortex was a first step in a much larger scheme. Clearly, we next intend to evaluate neurons in the hippocampus and, perhaps, later Purkinje cells in the cerebellum. In any event, the enlarged dendritic domains in the rabbits' cortices probably implied that had these animals been behaviorally tested in another (cortically-mediated) learning paradigm, their memory may well have been improved (relative to age-matched controls).

# Adenosine: a Prototherapeutic Concept in Neurodegeneration

DAG K. J. E. von LUBITZ,[a,c] MARGARET F. CARTER,[a] MARK BEENHAKKER,[a] RICK C-S. LIN,[b] AND KENNETH A. JACOBSON[a]

[a]*Laboratory of Bioorganic Chemistry*
*Molecular Recognition Section*
*National Institute of Diabetes and Digestive and Kidney Diseases/NIH*
*Bethesda, Maryland 20892*
*and*
[b]*Department of Physiology and Biophysics*
*Hahnemann University*
*Philadelphia, Pennsylvania 19102*

## ADENOSINE AND BRAIN: THE VIEWS AND THE VISTAS

Ten years ago, Newby introduced a new description of adenosine: "the retaliatory metabolite."[1] The theoretical notion that adenosine may protect against tissue injury[2] evolved rapidly into a practical demonstration of powerful neuroprotective effects of endogenous adenosine and its analogues.[3-5] Subsequent improvement in understanding both the effects of adenosine receptor stimulation and the pathological processes that accompany numerous neurological disorders ultimately led to proposals that adenosine-based therapies may be effective not only in stroke and seizures, but also in Alzheimer's, Huntington's and Parkinson's diseases, and a number of psychiatric pathologies.[5,6]

## ADENOSINE AND BRAIN: THE FUNCTIONS

### Endogenous Brain Adenosine and Pathologic Stress

Technical difficulties complicate the exact measurement of extracellular brain adenosine concentration.[4] Currently, the level of free adenosine level in the interstitial brain space of unanesthetized, freely moving animals is estimated at 50–300 nM.[4] More importantly, however, several laboratories have consistently reported that the amount of extracellular adenosine increases dramatically following cerebral metabolic stress caused by seizures, hypoxia, or ischemia.[4]

In focal ischemia (and probably global as well), the reduction of cerebral blood flow (CBF) correlates with the concomitant elevation of both adenosine and gluta-

---

[c]DvL is a Special Fellow of the Cystic Fibrosis Foundation, Washington, DC, and of Gilead Sciences, Foster City, CA.

mate.[7] However, while increased release of adenosine occurs at CBF values of 25 ml/100 g/min, further reduction of CBF (20 ml/100 g/min) is necessary to elevate concentration of the extracellular glutamate. Quite recently, Hoehn and White[8,9] showed that release of excitatory amino acids elicited by electrical field stimulation also results in the release of adenosine—an effect mediated in part by both $N$-methyl-D-aspartate (NMDA) and $\alpha$-amino-3-hydroxy-5-methylisoxazole-4-proprionic acid (AMPA) receptors. It appears, therefore, that glutamate-mediated hyperexcitation of neurons (such as seen in cerebral ischemia) may provide an additional, and somewhat unexpected, stimulus for further increase in adenosine release. These observations indicate that, in view of the powerful inhibitory effect of adenosine on the release of several excitatory neurotransmitters (see below), it is quite likely that increase in the concentration of interstitial adenosine, which both precedes and accompanies massive intraischemic release of glutamate,[10-13] constitutes part of a mechanism whose operation provides a transient, endogenous protection of the brain against injury.[5]

### Cerebral Receptors of Adenosine

Endogenous adenosine acts at three principal G-protein-associated receptor subtypes: $A_1$, $A_2$ and $A_3$.[14,15] Both the molecular structure and the nature of the effector coupling are known for all three subtypes.[16,17] Cerebral $A_1$ receptors are linked to several second messenger systems, and one of their characteristic responses to stimulation is inhibition of adenylate cyclase.[14] Activation of $A_2$ receptors stimulates adenylate cyclase,[14] whereas activation of $A_3$ receptors inhibits it, and also stimulates phosphoinositide metabolism.[18] Although their specific distribution varies,[19] all three adenosine receptor subtypes are found in the brain.[15,20] $A_1$ receptors are predominantly found in the hippocampus, IV–VI laminas of the cortex, striatum, amygdala, and superior colliculus, and appear to be codistributed with NMDA receptors.[21,22]

$A_2$ receptors, of which two subclasses ($A_{2a}$ and $A_{2b}$) exist, abound on smooth muscle and endothelial cells of cerebral blood vessels, where they mediate vascular effects of adenosine.[23] High-affinity $A_{2a}$ receptors are particularly well represented in the striatum and other dopamine-rich regions of the brain,[19] where they are colocalized with dopamine $D_2$ receptors, and exert profound modulatory effect on dopaminergic transmission.[24] Adenosine receptors on glial cells belong, most likely, to the low-affinity $A_{2b}$ subclass.[4] Cerebral distribution of $A_1$ and $A_2$ receptors follows an intriguing pattern, *i.e.*, $A_2$ appear to be less abundant within regions where the density of $A_1$ sites is elevated, and vice versa. Differences in the anatomical distribution of $A_1$ and $A_2$ receptors may have striking behavioral consequences.[25] $A_3$ receptors are found throughout the brain but their density is much lower than that of either $A_1$ or $A_2$.[20] The cell type on which they are located is unknown.

### Physiological Effects of Adenosine Receptor Stimulation

The principal function of adenosine in the brain is that of an inhibitory neuromodulator.[26,27] The inhibitory effects of adenosine are mediated mainly via both pre- and postsynaptic $A_1$ receptors.

Activation of presynaptic $A_1$ sites inhibits neuronal calcium uptake[28–30] and results in reduced release of several neurotransmitters, *e.g.*, acetylcholine, noradrenaline, dopamine, serotonin, and glutamate.[31–34]

Stimulation of both pre- and postsynaptic $A_1$ receptors causes activation of potassium[35–37] and chloride[38] conductances. The resultant elevation of the membrane potential and the depression of the membrane resistance[35,39] decrease neuronal excitability and firing rate.[35,40,41]

Apart from the involvement of adenosine $A_2$ receptors in regulation of CBF[23] adenosine $A_2$ receptors are responsible for accumulation of cyclic adenosine monophosphate (cAMP) in the brain.[4] The details of $A_2$ receptor involvement in neuronal physiology are still poorly understood, although existing evidence indicates that excitatory $A_2$ receptors are present in the hippocampus[42] and may be involved in potentiation of calcium-dependent neurotransmitter release[43,44] and in modulation of electrically evoked release of gamma-aminobutyric acid (GABA) in globus pallidus.[45] It is also known that in the striatum, $A_2$ receptors mediate control of gene expression in enkephalinergic neurons,[46] and that $A_2$ activation attenuates activity of the colocalized dopamine $D_2$ receptors through reduction of their affinity for $D_2$ agonists.[25,47,48] Finally, participation of $A_2$ receptors in generation of astrocytic edema has been also suggested.[49]

## ADENOSINE AND NEUROPROTECTION: THE THEORETICALS

The first experimental confirmation of neuroprotective properties of adenosine analogues in cerebral ischemia has been provided by Evans *et al.*[52] and von Lubitz *et al.*[53,54] A variety of *in vitro* and *in vivo* models of hypoxic/ischemic models of neuronal injury have been used in most of the subsequent studies of neuroprotection afforded by adenosine, its analogues, and inhibitors of its uptake.[4] Moreover, the effect of these approaches has been also investigated in seizures[55] and in either clinical[56] or *in vitro* hypoglycemia.[57] Since pathophysiology of cerebral ischemia has been extensively reviewed,[58–60] for the purpose of the present review suffice to say that the arrest of brain blood supply results in a rapid depolarization of neuronal membranes,[61] massive release of excitatory neurotransmitters[11] and excitation of postsynaptic glutamate receptors (NMDA and non-NMDA[59]), followed by influx of calcium and its release from intracellular stores.[62] The latter process triggers a series of cascading events[60] that ultimately lead to neuronal demise.

From the preceding brief discussion of the effects of adenosine receptor stimulation it is apparent that adenosine analogues may be applicable in interrupting several ischemia-associated events, *e.g.*, membrane (hypoxic) depolarization, neurotransmitter release, hyperexcitation of NMDA receptors, and calcium influx.

### *Endogenous Adenosine and Hypoxic Depolarization*

Rapid depolarization of neuronal membrane is one of the initial events evoked by either impaired or entirely interrupted supply of the cerebral blood flow.[63]

Moreover, duration of hypoxic depolarization may be the determining factor that dictates the subsequent fate of neurons, *i.e.*, their survival or death.[64]

Hypoxic depolarization is associated with enhanced influx of calcium through voltage-gated calcium channels,[59] and concomitant increase in neurotransmitter release. Since intraischemic liberation of endogenous adenosine precedes that of glutamate,[7] and since intraischemically released adenosine both significantly delays the onset of hypoxic depolarization[65] and reduces glutamate release,[66] it appears that adenosine-mediated protective processes take place already at the very beginning of the insult.

### *Adenosine $A_1$ Receptors and Excitatory Neurotransmitter Release*

Significant reduction of intraischemic release of glutamate by the $A_1$ receptor agonist $N^6$-cyclopentyladenosine (CPA) and the $A_1/A_2$ agonist $N$-ethylcarboxamidoadenosine (NECA) has been demonstrated in the 4-vessel occlusion rat model of ischemia.[66] Reduction of glutamate release by the $A_1$ agonist $N^6$-cyclohexyladenosine (CHA) has been also reported in focal ischemia in the rat[3] and in forebrain ischemia in the gerbil (Marangos and von Lubitz, unpublished). However, while glycine levels were significantly attenuated by CHA in a study of global ischemia in rabbits,[67] the reduction of glutamate showed only a dose-dependent but statistically insignificant trend. Nonetheless, even if in the latter study glutamate release was affected only to a limited extent, the protective effect of adenosine agonist is still likely.

Glycine is necessary for activation of the ion-gated channel of the NMDA receptor which regulates calcium influx.[68] Moreover, several studies have showed that glycine antagonists and partial agonists have a neuroprotective effect.[69,70] Therefore, it is conceivable that, despite a variable effect on the liberation of glutamate, CHA-mediated reduction in glycine release may diminish the functional efficiency of the NMDA receptor-associated ion-gated channel, and thereby decrease the subsequent calcium overload.

### *Endogenous Adenosine and Glutamate Uptake Sites*

Postischemic release of glutamate is comparatively brief and abates within approximately 30 min.[11] However, postischemic depression of CBF seen after severe ischemia (hypoperfusion stage) may result in secondary hypoxia.[71] Hence, a supplementary elevation in the extracellular glutamate concentration is also quite possible and may, unless astrocytic transport mechanisms remain intact, lead to exacerbation of the excitotoxic processes initiated by the primary event. Interestingly, Anderson *et al.*[72] have showed that even a brief (5-min) ischemia results in a prolonged upregulation of high-affinity excitatory amino acid (EAA) transport sites. At the same time, Schmidt *et al.*[73] have showed that a brief 10-min exposure to adenosine produces a significant increase in the density of high-affinity glutamate and aspartate uptake sites in rat hippocampal slices. Therefore, it is possible that intraischemic elevation of brain adenosine[74] may, apart from its effect on neurotransmitter release, also result in a sustained upregulation of EAA transporters. Consequently, due to its control of both release and uptake of EAAs, endogenous adenosine may play an important role in prevention of excitotoxic damage following very brief ischemic periods, the absence of which has been noted by several authors.[75,76]

### Postsynaptic Effects of Adenosine and Neurodegeneration

The intensity of excitatory synaptic input depends on the amount of NMDA-mediated influx of $Ca^{2+}$ [77] which, in turn, increases membrane depolarization and acts as a synaptic amplifier. Since the evoked influx of calcium is tightly controlled by postsynaptic $A_1$ receptors even at low extracellular $Ca^{2+}$ concentrations,[29,30,78] such control tends to attenuate calcium-mediated synaptic amplification.[4] Consequently, adenosine and its postsynaptic $A_1$ receptors regulate critical input frequencies required to operate postsynaptic NMDA receptors, as was recently demonstrated by Schubert and his colleagues.[30,79]

The additional, albeit indirect, benefit of reduced NMDA receptor-mediated depolarization elicited by interaction of adenosine with its $A_1$ receptors is the effect on voltage-sensitive $K^+$ currents.[35] Depolarization appears to block these currents and enhances neuronal excitability and firing rate.[80] Hence, vigorous activation of $A_1$ receptors by elevated concentrations of extracellular adenosine may counteract NMDA receptor-mediated depolarization, and drive the membrane potential toward voltage ranges at which depolarization-dependent block of potassium conductance is either less likely or does not occur.[4]

Apart from its enhancing effect on potassium conductance,[36,37,81] adenosine stimulates voltage-dependent $Cl^-$ conductance as well.[38,82] It has been suggested that the opening of this conductance may diminish accumulation of intraneuronal $Cl^-$ during repetitive firing[4] which, unless prevented, will eventually impair GABAergic inhibition.[83] Elevation in extracellular adenosine during periods of enhanced neuronal activity[41] may, therefore, assist in maintaining GABA-mediated inhibition, and constitute another functional aspect of the protective adenosine/adenosine receptor complex.

### Adenosine $A_2$ Receptors and Neurodegeneration

The concept of $A_2$ receptor involvement in neurodegeneration has not been pursued with the same vigor as that of $A_1$ receptors. There is, however, indirect, evidence that $A_2$ receptors may play a pivotal role in neuronal death observed in the striatum, and possibly also in the substantia nigra. Contrary to general belief, it is the dorsolateral aspect of striatum rather than the hippocampal CA4 sector[75] that appears to be endowed with the highest sensitivity to ischemic insult.[84,85] Light microscopic evidence of neuronal impairment in the striatum is clearly discernible already 1 h after a very light ischemic episode, while acute ischemic damage in the hippocampal CA4 appears 6–12 h after the event.[84] Rapid, intraischemic release of dopamine and glutamate,[85,86] persistent elevation of cAMP,[87] and eventual loss of dopamine $D_2$ receptors[86] precede morphologic damage of striatal neurons.

Globus et al.[85] have showed that, while increased concentration of intrastriatal dopamine alone has no adverse effect, elevated concentration of both dopamine and glutamate is associated with striatal vulnerability to ischemia. Since dopamine $D_2$ receptors attenuate the effect of glutamatergic stimulation,[88] it is possible that accelerated postischemic loss of $D_2$ receptors, rather than elevated concentration of both neurotransmitters per se may constitute one of the critical factors resulting in the apparent potentiation of glutamate-evoked damage. The most characteristic aspect of this damage is its containment to the medium-sized spiny neurons containing enkephalin and substance P,[84] i.e., neurons receiving glutamatergic input from both substantia nigra and neocortex.[88] Moreover, the same medium-sized GABAergic enkephalin-containing neurons are also characterized by the highest density of adenosine $A_2$ receptors.[24]

Based on the existing evidence, and on the fact that stimulation of adenosine $A_2$ receptor decreases the affinity of $D_2$ receptors to agonist stimulation,[48] it is possible to construct a chain of conjectural events that may ultimately lead to the selective neuronal loss in the striatum. Most likely, the initial intraischemic surge of adenosine agitates high-affinity $A_{2a}$ receptors located on enkephalin-containing GABAergic neurons. At the same time, the colocalized $D_2$ receptors which attenuate glutamatergic excitation supplied by cortical and nigro-striatal fibers[88] will be stimulated by dopamine, whose concentration also increases. However, the activated $A_2$ receptors decrease affinity of the colocalized $D_2$ sites to dopamine,[24] thereby diminishing the efficiency of their counterexcitatory effect. Ultimately, combination of $A_2$-$D_2$ interactions and postischemic loss of $D_2$ receptors[86] will result in a progressive shift toward unopposed glutamatergic hyperexcitation whose intensity will, eventually, attain the level sufficient to induce excitotoxic damage of enkephalin-containing GABAergic neurons.

Contrary to $A_1$ receptors, the time course of ischemia-induced adenosine $A_2$ receptor disappearance is unknown. However, cerebral ischemia causes elevation in striatal cAMP that persists for at least 4 h after the reperfusion.[87] Since stimulation of $A_2$ receptors leads to production of cAMP,[4,14] its prolonged postischemic presence may indicate that the functional $A_2$ receptors are preserved for several hours following the insult. Moreover, it was shown recently that $A_2$ receptor stimulation enhances ischemia-evoked release of glutamate and aspartate.[44] Thus, although the mechanism involved in this process is unknown, the sustained operation of $A_2$ receptors may amplify the damage to enkephalin-containing GABAergic neurons even further.

Allowing that this speculative sequence of events is correct, its repercussions on "downstream" damage caused by ischemia may be significant. Both global and prolonged forebrain ischemia cause damage in the substantia nigra as well as in the striatum and the hippocampus.[89,90] Hence, possible involvement of $A_2$ receptors in development of the rapid damage to the inhibitory enkephalin-containing neurons in the striatum may contribute to the subsequent loss of inhibitory input to the substantia nigra, and amplify the adverse effects of ischemia-associated hyperstimulation also in that region.

The pattern of striatal neuron loss in cerebral ischemia is very similar to that observed in Huntington's chorea[84] and, although the postischemic fate of $A_2$ receptors is presently unknown, a significant decrease in their density was recently observed in striatal tissue of patients with Huntington's disease.[91] Since striatal adenosine $A_2$ receptors appear to play an important role in pathophysiology of basal ganglia associated with Huntington's and Parkinson's diseases,[25,46,92] drugs acting at these receptors may prove very useful in the treatment of these disorders. Involvement of $A_2$ receptors in neurodegenerative processes of different etiology is the subject of current, intensive studies at our laboratory.

Striatum apart, stimulation of adenosine $A_2$ receptors may result in an improved postischemic survival of neurons in other regions through, *e.g.*, improvement of postischemic CBF[93] or prevention of postischemic inflammatory processes.[94] Normalization of postischemic CBF may be obtained through $A_2$ receptor-mediated vasodilation[5,23,95] and through antithrombotic effects.[96,97] Moreover, since stimulation of $A_2$ receptors prevents activation of neutrophils, it may, through concomitant reduction in free radical release, diminish the damage to the endothelial lining of cerebral blood vessels.[98] Finally, stimulation of leukocyte $A_2$ receptors decreases their adherence to capillary walls, and appears to be involved in preventing postischemic "plugging" of cerebral capillaries.[99]

## ADENOSINE AND NEUROPROTECTION: THE PRACTICALS

### *Effects of Acute Administration*

The results of experimental studies of the neuroprotective effects of adenosine, its analogues, and agents affecting its turnover are the subject of several recent reviews.[3-5,100,101] Most of those studies concentrate on investigations of either forebrain or global cerebral ischemia, and use survival and/or neuropathology as the measures of outcome.

Due to their well-known physiological properties and their relevance in treatment of cerebral ischemia, $A_1$ receptors are the chief subject of the existing experimental work.[3,4] Significant neuroprotection has been reported in virtually all studies of focal (but see Roussel *et al*, 1991), global, and forebrain ischemia in which $A_1$ receptor agonists have been administered either shortly before or after the insult, whose duration ranged from 5 to 30 min.[3,4] However, since the maximum interval between pretreatment and ischemia was 15 min, and maximum postischemic delay did not exceed 30 min, the dimension of the therapeutic window within which acutely administered adenosine agonists are effective is uncertain. It is known, however, that rapid downregulation of $A_1$ receptors follows even a mild anoxic or ischemic episode,[103,104] and that 14–24 h after ischemia, $A_1$ receptors become dysfunctional.[4] Thus, since the strength of adenosine modulation depends on the density of $A_1$ receptors,[105] the therapeutic window for administration of $A_1$ analogues is probably not an extensive one.[4]

The veracity of neuroprotective effects of $A_1$ receptor agonists has been confirmed by studies in which $A_1$ antagonists have been used.[4] Uniformly, administration of antagonists has resulted in severe exacerbation of mortality,[106] and in amplified neuronal destruction.[4]

Contrary to the effects of $A_1$ receptor agonists, the results following acute administration of agents active at $A_2$ receptors is virtually unknown. Recently, however, Gao and Phillis[107] showed that pretreatment with a weakly selective $A_2$ antagonist CGS 15943 resulted in protection of the hippocampus against ischemic damage. Our own results (von Lubitz et al., in preparation) indicate that $A_2$ antagonists administered prior to 10-min ischemia protect not only hippocampus but striatum as well.

Presently, only one report describes the effect of acute $A_3$ receptor stimulation on the outcome of forebrain ischemia.[50] The study shows that preischemic administration of a small dose (100 μg/kg) of a selective $A_3$ agonist, $N^6 - $ (3-iodobenzyl)-adenosine-5′-methylcarboxamide (IB-MECA), results in an extensive hippocampal damage and a very high mortality (90%) within the initial 24 h after ischemia.

Despite their neuroprotective efficacy, the acute treatment with adenosine $A_1$ agonists is accompanied by two major side effects, i.e., hypothermia and hypotension. Since hypothermia results in a significant reduction of postischemic neuronal damage,[107] it is possible that $A_1$ agonists mediate their neuron-sparing effect chiefly through the depression of brain temperature. However, both in vitro studies[108] and studies in which brain temperature has been carefully maintained[106] indicate that the protective effect is preserved also in the normothermic environment. Moreover, it must be remembered that, in the context of therapies aimed at stroke and brain ischemia, the comparatively mild hypothermic impact of $A_1$ receptor agonists may constitute a benefit rather than a hindrance.

Failure of cerebral perfusion pressure after ischemia is among the most critical factors that influence clinical recovery,[109,110] and hypotension and cardiodepression accompanying administration of $A_1$ agonists constitute potentially serious side effects of $A_1$ receptor-based therapies. Cardiovascular side effects of $A_1$ receptor agonists may be countered by coadministration of peripheral adenosine antagonists. However, von Lubitz and Marangos[111] have showed that, although concomitant postischemic administration of the $A_1$ receptor agonist CHA and the peripheral adenosine antagonist 8-P-sulphophenyladenosine (8-SPT) in gerbils resulted in a full normalization of CHA-evoked hypotension, the combined CHA/8-SPT treatment does not improve either survival or neurological impairment scores beyond those attained with CHA alone.

### Effects of Chronic Administration

Among all disorders for which adenosine-based therapies have been envisaged, only stroke offers a target for their acute administration while most, if not all, other central nervous system (CNS) diseases require chronic, frequently even lifelong, exposure. However, very little is known about the chronic effects of agents acting at adenosine receptors in the context of neuronal pathologies. The pioneering study of Rudolphi et al.[112] showed that chronic treatment with caffeine—a nonspecific $A_1/A_2$ antagonist—resulted in protection against ischemic damage in gerbils (i.e., the exactly opposite effect to that obtained with acute administration of another nonspecific antagonist, theophylline).[76] Von Lubitz et al.[106,112,113,115] have investigated the consequences of chronic administration of drugs acting at adenosine receptors further, and have used the highly potent $A_1$ agonist CPA or antagonist 8-cyclopentyl-1,3-dipropylxanthine (CPX). The work of the latter authors has confirmed the results of Rudolphi and his colleagues,[76,112] and has also showed that while acute treatment with a selective $A_1$ receptor agonist is highly protective, chronic treatment with the same drug has a profoundly aggravating effect in several measures of postischemic recovery, *i.e.,* survival, neurological status, and preservation of ischemia-vulnerable brain regions. Treatment with $A_1$ receptor antagonists, on the other hand, produced a diametrically opposite effect, *i.e.,* acute administration enhanced, and chronic administration protected against the damage.[106] The same authors also showed that while acute treatment with adenosine $A_3$ receptor agonist enhanced ischemia-associated damage, chronic treatment was highly ameliorative.[50] Preliminary studies with agents acting at $A_2$ receptors indicate the same pattern of regimen-dependent reversal. Interestingly, regimen-dependency of the therapeutic outcome of adenosine-based treatment has been also described in NMDA-evoked seizures[50,113,116] and in the water maze model of learning and memory.[114]

## ADENOSINE AND NEUROPROTECTION: THE PUZZLES AND THE PARADOXICALS

Despite numerous and convincing demonstrations of neuroprotective effects of endogenous adenosine, and despite highly alluring results of experimental treatment of cerebral ischemia with agents acting at all three adenosine receptor subtypes, a number of unsolved puzzles exists. We have already mentioned the fact that, although critical from the therapeutic point of view, time limits for efficient administration of acute adenosine therapies in stroke and cerebral ischemia are unknown. Glial response to the activation of their $A_1$ and $A_2$ receptors is also very poorly known, although there are indications that both glycogenolysis[117] and astrocytic edema[118] may ensue.

Degradation of endogenous adenosine contributes to the generation of highly destructive free radicals.[119] Since administration of free radical scavengers virtually eliminated production of superoxide species during and after cerebral ischemia,[119] therapies based upon elevation of endogenous adenosine may be less effective than those employing stimulation of adenosine receptors with appropriate analogues. Unquestionably, the problem requires a detailed and urgent examination. Finally, there is virtually no information on the interplay of individual adenosine receptor subtypes, although there are indications that such interplay may be critical for neuronal function and survival.[50]

The paradoxical effects of adenosine receptor-based therapies require further studies as well. The regimen-dependent nature of the outcome has been already mentioned. Prolonged stimulation by agonists or blockade by antagonists both *in vitro* and *in vivo* produces, respectively, either down- or upregulation of adenosine receptor density.[18,49,120] However, in some studies, no changes of either receptor density or ligand binding properties ($K_d$) were observed during prolonged exposure to selective $A_1$ agonists and antagonists, and to a nonselective $A_1/A_2$ antagonist theophylline *in vivo*.[106,115,116] On the other hand, Fastbom and Fredholm have showed that prolonged exposure to theophylline upregulates adenosine receptors, and Shi et al.[122] have reported that chronic treatment with caffeine (a nonspecific $A_1/A_2$ antagonist) both upregulates $A_1$ receptors and results in very dramatic density shifts of some receptor types (e.g., GABA, dopamine, noradrenaline), while having no effect on others (e.g., NMDA). Finally, chronic caffeine-mediated upregulation of $A_1$ sites and its functional consequences were the most likely source of protection against ischemia reported by Rudolphi et al.[112]

Although the protective effect of chronically administered $A_1$ antagonists is easily explained when accompanied by receptor upregulation, the nature of the mechanisms behind ameliorative actions of a chronic antagonist regimen observed in absence of increased density of $A_1$ receptors remains entirely obscure. Changes in G-protein-mediated receptor-effector coupling have been proposed as a putative answer to the regimen-dependent shifts seen after chronic exposure to both nonselective and selective agonists and antagonists.[106,115,116] Significant alterations in $G_{S\alpha}$ and $G_{I\alpha}$ proteins that were unaccompanied by a corresponding change in their mRNAs have been seen in rat adipocytes following chronic treatment with $A_1$ receptor antagonist.[123] However, whether similar phenomena take place in the brain remains to be demonstrated.

The effect of acute stimulation of $A_1$ and $A_3$ receptors offers another paradox. While both receptors are negatively coupled to adenylate cyclase (i.e., reduce its levels), acute preischemic activation of $A_1$ causes extensive neuroprotection. Acute activation of $A_3$ receptors, on the other hand, has an equally extensive but damaging result in cerebral ischemia,[50] although it is protective against NMDA-evoked seizures.[51] Moreover, chronic administration of $A_3$ receptor agonist protects equally well against cerebral ischemia and against chemically and electrically evoked seizures.[50,51]

Clearly, there are a number of questions that require additional, extensive studies. On the other hand, even if several aspects of adenosine action on a living cell, be it a neuron, a cardiac myocyte, or a nephron are unknown, Newby's "retaliatory metabolite" has already found its practical application in cardiology. Thus, under the name "Adenocard™," adenosine is now clinically used in treatment of supraventricular tachycardias, and it is not a premature hope that soon the concept of adenosine-based therapies will also find its application in treatment of the disorders of the brain.

## REFERENCES

1. NEWBY, A. C. 1984. Adenosine and the concept of "retaliatory metabolites." TIPS **9:** 42–48.
2. PHILLIS, J. W. & P. H. WU. 1981. The role of adenosine and its nucleotides in central synaptic transmission. Progr. Neurobiol. **16:** 187–239.
3. MILLER, L. P. & C. HSU. 1992. Therapeutic potential for adenosine receptor activation in ischemic brain injury. J. Neurotrauma **9**(Suppl. 2): S563–577.
4. RUDOLPHI, K. A., P. SCHUBERT, F. E. PARKINSON & B. B. FREDHOLM. 1992. Adenosine and brain ischemia. Cerebrovasc. Brain Metab. Rev. **4:** 346–369.
5. VON LUBITZ, D. K. J. E. & P. J. MARANGOS. 1992. Self-defense of the brain: adenosinergic strategies in neurodegeneration. In Emerging Strategies in Neuroprotection. P. J. Marangos and H. Lal, Eds. 151–186. Birkhauser. Boston.

6. MARANGOS, P. J. & J. P. BOULENGER. 1985. Basic and clinical aspects of adenosinergic neuromodulation. Neurosci. Biobehav. Rev. **9:** 421-430.
7. MATSUMOTO, K., R. GRAF, G. ROSNER, N. SCHIMADA & W. D. WEISS. 1992. Flow thresholds for extracellular purine catabolite elevation in rat focal ischemia. Brain Res. **579:** 309-314.
8. HOEHN, K. & T. D. WHITE. 1990. Role of excitatory amino acid receptors in $K^+$ and glutamate-evoked release of endogenous adenosine from rat cortical slices. J. Neurochem. **54:** 256-265.
9. HOEHN, K. & T. D. WHITE. 1990. $N$-methyl-D-aspartate, kainate and quisqualate release endogenous adenosine from rat cortical slices. Neurosci. **39:** 441-450.
10. BENVENISTE, H., J. DREJER, A. SCHOUSBOE & N. H. DIEMER. 1984. Elevation of the extracellular concentrations of glutamate and aspartate in rat hippocampus during transient cerebral ischemia monitored by intracerebral microdialysis. J. Neurochem. **43:** 1369-1374.
12. ANDINÉ, P., O. ORWAR, I. JACOBSON, M. SANDBERG & H. HAGBERG. 1991. Changes in extracellular amino acids and spontaneous neuronal activity during ischemia and extended reflow in the CA1 of the rat hippocampus. J. Neurochem. **57:** 222-229.
13. PHILLIS, J. W., G. A. WALTER & R. E. SIMPSON. 1991. Brain adenosine and transmitter amino acid release from the ischemic rat cerebral cortex: effects of the adenosine deaminase inhibitor deoxycoformycin. J. Neurochem. **56:** 644-650.
14. VAN CALKER, D., M. MÜLLER & G. HAMPRECHT. 1979. Adenosine regulates via two different types of receptors the accumulation of cyclic AMP in cultured brain cells. J. Neurochem. **33:** 999-1005.
15. JACOBSON, K. A., P. J. M. VAN GALEN & M. WILLIAMS. 1992. Perspective, adenosine receptors: pharmacology, structure activity relationships, and therapeutic potential. J. Med. Chem. **35:** 407-422.
16. STILES, G. L. Adenosine receptors. J. Biol. Chem. **267:** 6451-6454.
17. JI, X-D., D. VON LUBITZ, M. E. OLAH, G. L. STILES & K. A. JACOBSON. 1994. Species differences in ligand affinity at central $A_3$ adenosine receptors. Drug Dev. Res. **33:** 51-59.
18. RAMKUMAR, V., J. R. BUMGARNER, K. A. JACOBSON & G. L. STILES. 1988. Multiple components of the $A_1$ adenosine receptor-adenylate cyclase system are regulated in rat cerebral cortex by chronic caffeine ingestion. J. Clin. Invest. **82:** 242-247.
19. JARVIS, M. F. & M. WILLIAMS. 1989. Adenosine in central nervous system function. *In* Adenosine and Adenosine Receptors. M. Williams, Ed. 423-474. Humana Press. Clifton.
20. JACOBSON, K. A., O. NIKODIJEVIĆ, D. SHI, C. GALLO-RODRIGUEZ, M. E. OLAH, G. L. STILES & J. W. DALY. 1993. A role for central adenosine $A_3$ receptors: mediation of behavioral depressant responses. FEBS Lett. **336:** 57-64.
21. COTMAN, C. W., D. T. MONAGHAN, O. P. OTTERSEN & J. STORM-MATHIESEN. 1987. Anatomical organization of excitatory amino acid receptors and their pathways. TINS **10:** 273-280.
22. DAVAL, J-L., D. K. J. E. VON LUBITZ, J. DECKERT, D. J. REDMOND & P. J. MARANGOS. 1989. Protective effect of cyclohexyladenosine on adenosine $A_1$ receptors, guanine nucleotide and forskolin binding sites following transient brain ischemia: a quantitative autoradiographic study. Brain Res. **491:** 212-226.
23. VAN WYLEN, D. G. L., V. M. SCIOTTI & H. R. WINN. 1991. Adenosine and the regulation of cerebral blood flow. *In* Adenosine and Adenine Nucleotides as Regulators of Cellular Function. J. W. Phillis, Ed. 191-202. CRC Press. Boca Raton.
24. FERRÉ S., K. FUXE, G. VON EULER, B. JOHANSSON & B. B. FREDHOLM. 1992. Adenosine-dopamine interactions in the brain. Neurosci. **51:** 501-512.
25. BARRACO, R. A., K. A. MARTENS, M. PARIZON & H. J. NORMILE. 1993. Adenosine $A_{2a}$ receptors in the nucleus accumbens mediate locomotor depression. Brain Res. Bull. **31:** 397-404.
26. KOSTOPOULOS, G. K. & J. W. PHILLIS. 1977. Purinergic depression of neurons in different areas of the brain. Exp. Neurol. **55:** 719-724.

27. DUNWIDDIE, T. V. & B. J. HOFFER. 1980. Adenine nucleotides and synaptic transmission in the *in vitro* rat hippocampus. Br. J. Pharmacol. **69:** 59–68.
28. WU, P. H., J. W. PHILLIS & D. L. THIERRY. 1982. Adenosine receptor agonists inhibit $K^+$ evoked $Ca^{2+}$ uptake by rat cortical synaptosomes. J. Neurochem. **39:** 700–708.
29. SCHUBERT, P., U. HEINEMANN & R. KOLB. 1986. Differential effect of adenosine on pre- and postsynaptic calcium fluxes. Brain Res. **376:** 382–386.
30. SCHUBERT, P., F. KELLER & K. A. RUDOLPHI. 1993. Depression of synaptic transmission and evoked NMDA $Ca^{2+}$ influx in hippocampal neurons by adenosine and its blockade by LTP or ischemia. Drug Dev. Res. **28:** 399–405.
31. HARMS, H. H., G. WARDEH & A. H. MULDER. 1978. Adenosine modulates depolarization-induced release of $^3$H-noradrenaline from slices of rat brain neocortex. Eur. J. Pharmacol. **49:** 305–308.
32. DOLPHIN, A. C. & E. R. ARCHER. 1983. An adenosine agonist inhibits and a cyclic AMP analogue enhances the release of glutamate but not GABA from slices of rat dentate gyrus. Neurosci. Lett. **43:** 49–54.
33. CORADETTI, R., G. LO CONTE, F. MORONI, M. B. PASSANI & G. PEPEU. 1984. Adenosine decreases aspartate and glutamate release from rat hippocampal slices. Eur. J. Pharmacol. **104:** 19–26.
34. FREDHOLM, B. B. & T. V. DUNWIDDIE. 1988. How does adenosine inhibit transmitter release? TIPS **9:** 130–134.
35. HAAS, H. L. & R. W. GREENE. 1984. Adenosine enhances afterhyperpolarization and accommodation in hippocampal pyramidal cells. Pflüg. Arch. **402:** 144–247.
36. GREENE, R. W. & H. L. HAAS. 1991. The electrophysiology of adenosine in the mammalian central nervous system. Progr. Neurobiol. **36:** 329–341.
37. THOMPSON, S. M., H. L. HAAS & B. H. GÄHWILER. 1992. Comparison of the actions of adenosine at pre- and postsynaptic receptors in the rat hippocampus *in vitro*. J. Physiol. **451:** 347–363.
38. SCHUBERT, P., S. FERRONI & R. MAGER. 1991. Pharmacological blockade of $Cl^-$ pumps and $Cl^-$ channels reduces the adenosine mediated depression of stimulation train-evoked $Ca^{2+}$ fluxes in rat hippocampal slices. Neurosci. Lett. **124:** 174–177.
39. GERBER, U., R. W. GREENE, H. L. HAAS & D. R. STEVENS. 1989. Characterization of inhibition mediated by adenosine in the hippocampus of the rat *in vivo*. J. Physiol. **417:** 567–578.
40. DUNWIDDIE, T. V. 1985. The physiological role of adenosine in the central nervous system. Int. Rev. Neurobiol. **27:** 64–139.
41. DUNWIDDIE, T. V. 1980. Endogenously released adenosine regulates excitability in the *in vitro* hippocampus. Epilepsia **21:** 541–548.
42. SEBASTIAO, A. M. & J. A. RIBEIRO. 1992. Evidence for the presence of $A_2$ adenosine receptors in the rat hippocampus. Neurosci. Lett. **138:** 41.
43. SPIGNOLI, G., F. PEDATA & G. C. PEPEU. 1984. $A_1$ and $A_2$ adenosine receptors modulate acetylcholine release from brain slices. Eur. J. Pharmacol. **97:** 341–342.
44. O'REGAN, M. H., R. E. SIMPSON, L. M. PERKINS & J. W. PHILLIS. 1992. The selective adenosine $A_2$ receptor agonist CGS 21680 enhances excitatory transmitter amino acid release from the ischemic rat cerebral cortex. Neurosci. Lett. **138:** 169–172.
45. MAYFIELD, R. D., F. SUZUKI & N. ZAHNISER. 1993. Adenosine $A_{2a}$ receptor modulation of electrically evoked endogenous GABA release from slices of rat globus pallidus. J. Neurochem. **60:** 2334–2337.
46. SCHIFFMANN, S. N., P. HALLEUX, R. MENU & J-J. VANDERHAEGHEN. 1993. Adenosine $A_{2a}$ receptor expression in striatal neurons: implications for basal ganglia pathophysiology. Drug Dev. Res. **28:** 381–385.
47. FERRÉ, S., P. SNAPRUD & K. FUXE. 1993. Opposing actions of an adenosine $A_2$ and a GTP analogue on the regulation of dopamine $D_2$ receptors in rat neostriatal membranes. Eur. J. Pharmacol. Mol. Pharmacol. Sect. **244:** 311–315.
48. FERRÉ, S., G. VON EULER, B. JOHANSSON, B. B. FREDHOLM & K. FUXE. 1991. Stimulation of high affinity adenosine A-2 receptors decreases the affinity of dopamine D-2 receptors in rat striatal membranes. Proc. Natl. Acad. Sci. USA **88:** 7238–7241.
49. ABBRACCHIO, M. P., G. P. FOGLIATTO, A. M. PAOLETTI, E. ROVATI & F. CATTABENI.

1992. Prolonged *in vitro* exposure of rat brain slices to adenosine analogues: selective desensitization of adenosine $A_1$ but not $A_2$ receptors. Eur. J. Pharmacol. Mol. Pharmacol. Sect. **227:** 317–324.
50. VON LUBITZ, D. K. J. E., R. C-S. LIN, P. POPIK, M. F. CARTER & K. A. JACOBSON. 1994. Adenosine $A_3$ receptor stimulation and cerebral ischemia. Eur. J. Pharmacol. In press.
51. VON LUBITZ, D. K. J. E., S. I. DEUTSCH, M. F. CARTER, R. C-S. LIN, J. MASTROPAOLO & K. A. JACOBSON. 1994. The effects of adenosine $A_3$ receptor stimulation on seizures in mice. Eur. J. Pharmacol. In press.
52. EVANS, M. C., J. H. SWAN & B. S. MELDRUM. 1987. An adenosine analogue, 2-chloroadenosine, protects against long term development of ischaemic cell loss in the rat hippocampus. Neurosci. Lett. **83:** 287–292.
53. VON LUBITZ, D. K. J. E., J. M. DAMBROSIA & O. KEMPSKI. 1986. Postischemic application of cyclohexyladenosine (CHA): improvement of survival and of preservation of selectively vulnerable areas in gerbil. Abstr. X Int. Congr. Neuropathol., Stockholm: 108.
54. VON LUBITZ, D. K. J. E., J. M. DAMBROSIA & D. J. REDMOND. 1989. Protective effect of cyclohexyl adenosine in treatment of cerebral ischemia in gerbils. Neuroscience **2:** 451–457.
55. DRAGUNOW, M. 1991. Adenosine and epileptic seizures. *In* Adenosine and Adenine Nucleotides as Regulators of Cellular Function. J. W. Phillis, Ed. 367–379. CRC Press. Boca Raton.
56. HVIDBERG, A., M. H. RASMUSSEN, N. J. CHRISTENSEN & J. HILSTED. 1994. Theophylline enhances glucose recovery after hypoglycemia in healthy man and in type I diabetic patients. Metabolism **43:** 776–781.
57. FREDHOLM, B. B., K. LINDSTROM & A. WALLMAN-JOHANSSON. 1994. Propentophylline and other adenosine transport inhibitors increase the efflux of adenosine following electrical and metabolic stimulation of rat hippocampal slices. J. Neurochem. **62:** 563–573.
58. RAICHLE, M. 1983. The pathophysiology of brain ischemia. Ann. Neurol. **13:** 9–10.
59. SIESJÖ, B. K. & F. BENGTSSON. 1989. Calcium fluxes, calcium antagonists, and calcium-related pathology in brain ischemia, hypoglycemia, and spreading depression: a unifying hypothesis. J. Cereb. Blood Flow Metab. **9:** 127– .
60. CHOI, D. W. 1992. Excitotoxic cell death. J. Neurobiol. **9:** 1261–1276.
61. HANSEN, A. J. 1985. Effect of anoxia on ion distribution in the brain. Physiol. Rev. **65:** 101–148.
62. BEAL, M. F. 1992. Mechanisms of excitotoxicity in neurologic disease. FASEB J. **6:** 3338–3344.
63. HANSEN, A. J. 1990. Ion homeostasis in cerebral ischemia. *In* Cerebral Ischemia and Resuscitation. A. Schurr & B. M. Rigor, Eds. 77–87. CRC Press. Boca Raton.
64. BALESTRINO, M., P. AITKEN & G. SOMJEN. 1989. Spreading depression-like hypoxic depolarization in CA1 and facia dentata of hippocampal slices: relationship to selective vulnerability. Brain Res. **497:** 102–107.
65. LEE, K. S. & T. LOWENKOPF. 1993. Endogenous adenosine delays the onset of hypoxic depolarization in the rat hippocampus *in vitro* via an action at $A_1$ receptors. Brain Res. **609:** 313–315.
66. SIMPSON, R. E., M. H. O'REAGAN, L. M. PERKINS & J. W. PHILLIS. 1992. Excitatory transmitter amino acid release from the ischemic rat cerebral cortex. Effects of adenosine agonists and antagonists. J. Neurochem. **58:** 1683–1690.
67. CANTOR, S. L., M. H. ZORNOW, L. P. MILLER & T. L. YAKSH. 1992. The effect of cyclohexyladenosine on the periischemic increases of hippocampal glutamate and glycine in the rabbit. J. Neurochem. **59:** 1884–1892.
68. KLECKNER, N. W. & R. DINGLEDINE. 1988. Requirement for glycine in activation of NMDA-receptors expressed in Xenopus oocytes. Science **241:** 835–837.
69. GILL, R. & G. N. WOODRUFF. 1990. The neuroprotective actions of kynurenic acid and MK-801 in gerbils are synergistic and not related to hypothermia. Eur. J. Pharmacol. **176:** 143–149.

70. VON LUBITZ, D. K. J. E., R. C-S. LIN, R. J. MCKENZIE, T. M. DEVLIN, P. SKOLNICK & R. T. MCCABE. 1992. A novel treatment of global cerebral ischemia with a glycine partial agonist. Eur J. Pharmacol. **219:** 153–158.
71. BENGTSSON, F. & B. K. SIESJÖ. 1990. Cell damage in cerebral ischemia: physiological, biochemical, and structural aspects. *In* Cerebral Ischemia and Resuscitation. A. Schurr & B. M. Rigor, Eds. 215–233. CRC Press. Boca Raton.
72. ANDERSON, K. J., B. NELLGÅRD & T. WIELOCH. 1993. Ischemia-induced upregulation of excitatory amino acid transporters. Brain Res. **622:** 93–98.
73. SCHMIDT, W., G. WOLF, K. GRUNGREIFF & K. LINKE. 1993. Adenosine influences the high affinity uptake of transmitter glutamate and aspartate under conditions of hepatic encephalopathy. Metab. Brain Dis. **8:** 73–80.
74. PHILLIS, J. W., M. H. O'REGAN & G. A. WALTER. 1988. Effects of deoxycoformycin on adenosine, inosine, hypoxanthine, xanthine, and uric acid release from the hypoxaemic rat cerebral cortex. J. Cereb. Blood Flow Metab. **8:** 733–741.
75. KIRINO, T. & K. SANO. 1984. Selective vulnerability in the gerbil hippocampus following transient ischemia. Acta Neuropathol. (Berlin) **62:** 201–208.
76. RUDOLPHI, K. A., M. KEIL & H. J. HINZE. 1987. Effect of theophylline on ischemically induced hippocampal damage in Mongolian gerbils: a behavioural and histopathological study. J. Cereb. Blood Flow Metab. **7:** 74–81.
77. HERRON, C. E., R. J. LESTER, E. J. COAN & G. L. COLLINGRIDGE. 1986. Frequency-dependent involvement of NMDA receptors in the hippocampus: a novel synaptic mechanism. Nature **322:** 265–268.
78. SCHUBERT, P. 1988. Physiological modulation by adenosine selective blockade of $A_1$ receptors with DPCPX enhances stimulus train-evoked neuronal Ca influx in rat hippocampal slices. Brain Res. **458:** 162–165.
79. SCHUBERT, P. & R. MAGER. 1991. The critical input frequency for NMDA-mediated neuronal $Ca^{2+}$ frequency depends on endogenous adenosine. Int. J. Purine Pyrimidine Res. **2:** 11–25.
80. SEGAL, M., M. A. ROGAWSKI & J. L. BARKER. 1984. A transient potassium conductance regulates the excitability of cultured hippocampal and spinal neurons. J. Neurosci. **4:** 604–609.
81. TRUSSEL, L. O. & B. J. JACKSON. 1987. Dependence of an adenosine activated postassium current on GTP-binding protein in mammalian neurons. J. Neurosci. **7:** 3306–3316.
82. MAGER, R., S. FERRONI & P. SCHUBERT. 1990. Adenosine modulates a voltage-dependent chloride conductance in cultured hippocampal neurons. Brain Res. **532:** 58–62.
83. THOMPSON, S. M. & B. H. GÄHWILER. 1989. Activity dependent disinhibition. 1. Repetitive stimulation reduces IPSP driving force and conductance in rat hippocampus *in vitro*. J. Neurophysiol. **61:** 501–511.
84. CHESSELET, M-F., C. GONZALES, C-S. LIN, K. POLSKY & B-K. JIN. 1990. Ischemic damage in the striatum of adult gerbils: relative sparing of somatostatinergic and cholinergic interneurons contrasts with loss of efferent neurons. Exp. Neurol. **110:** 209–218.
85. GLOBUS, M. Y. T., R. BUSTO, W. D. DIETRICH, E. MARTINES, I. VALDES & M. D. GINSBERG. 1988. Intra-ischemia extracellular release of dopamine is associated with striatal vulnerability to ischemia. Neurosci. Lett. **91:** 36–40.
85. GLOBUS, M. Y. T., R. BUSTO, E. MARTINEZ, I. VALDES, W. D. DIETRICH & M. D. GINSBERG. 1991. Comparative effect of transient global ischemia on extracellular levels of glutamate, glycine, and γ-aminobutyric acid in vulnerable and nonvulnerable brain regions in the rat. J. Neurochem. **57:** 470–478.
85. CRAIN, B. J., W. D. WESTERKAM, A. H. HARRISON & J. V. NADLER. 1988. Selective neuronal death after transient forebrain ischemia in the Mongolian gerbil: a silver impregnation study. Neuroscience **27:** 387–402.
86. CHANG, C. J., H. ISHII, H. YAMAMOTO, T. YAMAMOTO & M. SPATZ. 1993. Effects of cerebral on regional dopamine release and $D_1$ and $D_2$ receptors. J. Neurochem. **60:** 1483–1490.
87. PRADO, R., R. BUSTO & M. Y. T. GLOBUS. 1992. Ischemia-induced changes in extracel-

88. CEPEDA, N. A. BUCHWALD & M. S. LEVINE. 1993. Neuromodulatory actions of dopamine in the neostriatum are dependent upon the excitatory amino acid receptor subtypes activated. Proc. Natl. Acad. Sci. **90:** 9576–9580.
lular levels of striatal cyclic AMP: role of dopamine neurotransmission. J. Neurochem. **59:** 1581–1584.
89. DIEMER, N. H. & E. SIEMKOWICZ. 1981. Regional neuronal damage after cerebral ischemia in normo- and hypoglycemic rats. Neuropathol. Appl. Neurobiol. **7:** 217–227.
90. ARAKI, T., H. KATO & K. KOGURE. 1989. Selective neuronal vulnerability following transient cerebral ischemia in the gerbil: distribution and time course. Acta Neurol. Scand. **80:** 548–553.
91. MARTINEZ-MIR, M. I., A. PROBST & J. M. PALACIOS. 1991. Adenosine $A_2$ receptors: selective localization in the human basal ganglia and alterations with disease. Neuroscience **42:** 697–706.
92. SCHIFFMANN, S. N. & J-J. VANDERHAEGHEN. 1993. Adenosine $A_2$ receptors regulate the gene expression of striatopallidal and striatonigral neurons. J. Neurosci. **13:** 1080–1087.
93. FORRESTER, T., A. M. HARPER, E. T. MACKENZIE & E. M. THOMPSON. 1979. Effect of adenosine triphosphate and some derivatives on cerebral blood flow and metabolism. J. Physiol. **296:** 343–355.
94. CRONSTEIN, B. N., R. I. LEVIN, J. BELANOFF, G. WEISSMANN & R. HIRSCHHORN. 1986. Adenosine: an endogenous inhibitor of neurtrophil-mediated injury to endothelial cells. J. Clin. Invest. **78:** 760–770.
95. SOLLEVI, A. 1986. Cardiovascular effects of adenosine in man: possible clinical implications, Progr. Neurobiol. **27:** 319–349.
96. BORN, G. V. R. & M. J. CROSS. 1963. The aggregation of blood platelets. J. Physiol. **168:** 178–195.
97. CUSACK, N. J. & S. M. O. HOURANI. 1991. Adenosine, adenine nucleotides, and platelet functions. *In* Adenosine and Adenine Nucleotides as Regulators of Cellular Function. J. W. Phillis, Ed. 121–131. CRC Press. Boca Raton.
98. CRONSTEIN, B. N. 1991. Purines and inflamation: neutrophils possess $P_1$ and $P_2$ purine receptors. *In* Adenosine and Adenine Nucleotides as Regulators of Cellular Function. J. W. Phillis, Ed. 133–140. CRC Press. Boca Raton.
99. GRISHAM, M. B., L. A. HERNANDEZ & D. N. GRANGER. 1989. Adenosine inhibits ischemia-reperfusion-induced leukocyte adherence and extravasation. Am. J. Physiol. **257:**H 1334–1339.
100. DRAGUNOW, M. & R. L. M. FAULL. 1988. Neuroprotective effects of adenosine. TIPS **9:** 193–194.
101. PHILLIS, J. W. 1990. Adenosine, inosine, and the oxypurines in cerebral ischemia. *In* Cerebral Ischemia and Resuscitation. A. Schurr & B. M. Rigor, Eds. 189–204. CRC Press. Boca Raton.
103. ROUSSEL, S., E. PINARD & J. SEYLAZ. 1991. Focal cerebral ischemia in chronic hypertension: no protection by (R)-phenylisopropyladenosine. Brain Res. **545:** 171–174.
103. LEE, K. S., W. TETZLAFFAND & G. W. KREUTZBERG. 1986. Rapid downregulation of hippocampal adenosine receptors following brief anoxia. Brain Res. **380:** 155–158.
104. ONODERA, H. & K. KOGURE. 1990. Calcium antagonist, adenosine $A_1$ and muscarine bindings in rat hippocampus after transient ischemia. Stroke **21:** 771–776.
105. LEE, K. S., P. SCHUBERT, M. REDDINGTON & G. W. KREUTZBERG. 1983. Regulation of strength of adenosine modulation in the hippocampus by a differential distribution of the density of $A_1$ receptors. Brain Res. **260:** 156–159.
106. VON LUBITZ, D. K. J. E., R. C-S. LIN, N. MELMAN, X-D. JI, M. F. CARTER, & K. A. JACOBSON. 1994. Chronic administration of adenosine $A_1$ receptor agonist or antagonist in cerebral ischemia. Eur. J. Pharmacol. **256:** 161–167.
107. GAO, Y. & J. W. PHILLIS. 1994. CGS 15943, an adenosine $A_2$ receptor antagonist, reduces cerebral ischemic injury in the Mongolian gerbil. Life Sci. **55:** 61–65.
107. BUSTO, R., W. D. DIETRICH, M. Y. T. GLOBUS & M. D. GINSBERG. 1989. The importance of brain temperature in cerebral ischemic injury. Stroke **20:** 1113–1114.

108. GOLDBERG, M. P., H. MONYER, J. H. WEISS & D. W. CHOI. 1988. Adenosine reduces cortical neuronal injury induced by oxygen and glucose deprivation *in vitro*. Neurosci. Lett. **89:** 323–327.
109. WAUQUIER, A., H. L. EDMONDS, JR. & G. H. C. CLINCKE. 1987. Cerebral resuscitation: pathophysiology and therapy. Neurosci. Biobehav. Rev. **11:** 287–306.
110. MILLER, J. T. 1983. Head injury and brain ischemia—implications for therapy. Br. J. Anaesth. **57:** 120–130.
111. VON LUBITZ, D. K. J. E. & P. J. MARANGOS. 1990. Cerebral ischemia in gerbils: postischemic administration of cyclohexyladenosine and 8-sulphophenyl-theophylline. J. Mol. Neurosci. **2:** 53–59.
112. RUDOLPHI, K. A., M. KEIL, J. FASTBOM & B. B. FREDHOLM. 1989. Ischaemic damage in gerbil hippocampus is reduced following upregulation of adenosine $A_1$ receptors by caffeine treatment. Neurosci. Lett. **103:** 275–280.
113. VON LUBITZ, D. K. J. E., I. A. PAUL & K. A. JACOBSON. 1993. Effects of $N^6$-cyclopentyl adenosine and 8-cyclopentyl-1,3 dipropylxanthine on $N$-methyl-D-aspartate induced seizures in mice. Eur. J. Pharmacol. **249:** 265–270.
114. VON LUBITZ, D. K. J. E., I. A. PAUL, R. T. BARTUS & K. A. JACOBSON. 1993. Effects of chronic administration of adenosine A1 receptor agonist and antagonist on spatial learning and memory. Eur. J. Pharmacol. **249:** 271–280.
115. VON LUBITZ, D. K. J. E., I. A. PAUL, X-D. JI, M. CARTER & K. A. JACOBSON. 1994. Chronic adenosine $A_1$ receptor agonist and antagonist: effect on receptor density and $N$-methyl-D-aspartate induced seizures in mice. Eur. J. Pharmacol. **253:** 95–99.
116. GEORGIEV, V., B. JOHANSSON & B. B. FREDHOLM. 1993. Long-term caffeine treatment leads to decreased susceptibility to NMDA-induced clonic seizures in mice without changes in adenosine $A_1$ receptor number. Brain Res. **612:** 271–277.
117. MAGISTRETTI, P. J., P. R. HOFF & J. L. MARTIN. 1986. Adenosine stimulates glycogenolysis in mouse cerebral cortex: a possible coupling mechanism between neuronal activity and energy metabolism. J. Neurosci. **6:** 2558–2562.
118. BOURKE, R. S., H. K. KIMELBERG & M. A. DAZE. 1978. Effects of inhibitors and adenosine on ($HCO^-/CO_2$) stimulated swelling and $Cl^-$ in brain slices and cultured astrocytes. Brain Res. **154:** 196–202.
119. PHILLIS, J. W. 1994. Adenosine metabolites may provide a primary source of oxygen free radicals in ischemic/reperfused rat brain. Drug. Dev. Res. **31:** 308.
120. PARSONS, W. J. & G. L. STILES. 1987. Heterologous desensitization of inhibitory adenosine $A_1$ receptor adenylate cyclase system in rat adipocytes. J. Biol. Chem. **262:** 841–847.
121. RAMKUMAR, V., G. L. STILES, M. A. BEAVEN & H. ALI, JR. 1993. The $A_3$ adenosine receptor is the unique adenosine receptor which facilitates release of allergic mediators in mast cells. J. Biol. Chem. **268:** 16887–16890.
122. SHI, D., O. NIKODIJEVIĆ, K. A. JACOBSON & J. W. DALY. 1993. Chronic caffeine alters the density of adenosine, adrenergic, cholinergic, GABA, and serotonin receptors and calcium channels in mouse brain. Cell. Mol. Neurobiol. **13:** 247–261.
123. LONGBAUGH, J. P., J. DIDSBURY, A. SPIEGEL & G. STILES. 1989. Modification of the rat adipocyte $A_1$ adenosine receptor-adenylate cyclase system during chronic exposure to an $A_1$ receptor agonist: alterations in the quantity of $G_{S\alpha}$ and $G_{i\alpha}$ are not associated with changes in their mRNAs. J. Pharmacol. Exp. Ther. (Mol. Pharmacol.) **36:** 681–688.

# Dexamethasone and the Prevention of Neonatal Hypoxic-Ischemic Brain Damage

URSULA I. TUOR

*Biosystems*
*Institute for Biodiagnostics*
*National Research Council of Canada (NRC)*
*435 Ellice Avenue*
*Winnipeg, Manitoba R3B 1Y6, Canada*

## INTRODUCTION

Glucocorticoids, which have been available clinically for decades, have been a class of potential neuroprotective agents widely investigated for their ability to reduce brain damage due to cerebral ischemia. In general, studies in adults have demonstrated that pretreatment or posttreatment with glucocorticoids is ineffective in ameliorating the extent of brain damage caused by either focal or global ischemia.[1-3] In some cases chronic increased levels of glucocorticoids were actually observed to have deleterious effects, particularly in the hippocampus.[4,5] Thus, the consensus was that glucocorticoids were ineffective for the treatment of stroke,[2] although high doses of glucocorticids such as methylprednisolone were more recently shown to be of benefit in the treatment of spinal cord injury.[6]

In neonates, the effect of glucocorticoids on hypoxic-ischemic brain damage has been studied less extensively. One study in neonatal rats demonstrated that immediate pretreatment with high doses of dexamethasone were not beneficial and might actually be harmful by increasing mortality.[7] Due to the increased clinical use of glucocorticoids in neonates,[8-11] we originally investigated dexamethasone's effects on hypoxic-ischemic brain damage in immature rats with the concern that it may exacerbate damage. It was a surprise when we discovered that cerebral damage in 7-day-old rats could be prevented by the administration of dexamethasone prior to cerebral hypoxia-ischemia.[12] Since then we have performed many additional experiments, some of which are described below. The results have provided some insight into the characteristics of the response and the mechanisms whereby dexamethasone may be acting to prevent damage. However, the exact way in which dexamethasone provides protection still remains to be elucidated.

### *Model of Hypoxia-Ischemia*

A well established neonatal model of hypoxia-ischemia was used in the studies described below.[12-15] Immature Wistar rats born in the animal facility were subjected to hypoxia-ischemia on the seventh day of life. These animals were anesthetized with halothane and the right carotid artery was isolated and ligated with 5-0 silk suture. A three-hour recovery period with the dam was followed by 3 hours in a hypoxic chamber (8% oxygen / 92% nitrogen at 37°C). This consistently produced neuronal damage with infarction of the striatum, thalamus, hippocampus and overlying cortex ipsilateral to the ligation.

The experimental design involved randomly assigning the rats to various treatment groups so that animals within any one group originated from at least four different litters. The rats were normally weighed several times including when they were injected with a drug, on the day of hypoxia-ischemia and on the day of perfusion-fixation. In subgroups of animals, blood glucose was measured using a drop of blood from the tail vein using glucose oxidase reagent strips (Chemstrip bG, Boehringer Mannheim, Germany).

## Assessment of Pathological Damage

Cerebral pathology was assessed in animals surviving two to seven days after hypoxia-ischemia.[12,16-18] Animals were anesthetized with pentobarbital and the brains were perfusion-fixed with 10% buffered formalin. The brains were removed and placed in formalin for several days. The presence or absence of gross cortical infarction was noted upon inspection of the brains at the time of removal. The cerebrum was sliced into 3 equal blocks, embedded in paraffin, sectioned with a microtome and the coronal sections were stained with hematoxylin and eosin. The extent of pathological damage was quantitated by an investigator blinded to the treatment group using an image analysis system (MCID, Imaging Research Inc, St. Catherine's, Ont).

## Dose and Time Dependence of the Response

Our initial experiments demonstrated that 0.5 mg/kg of dexamethasone administered in multiple doses 48, 24 and 0 hr prior to the hypoxia-ischemia prevented infarction in neonatal animals.[12] Unfortunately, posttreatment with multiple doses of dexamethasone at 0, 24 and 48 hr *after* the hypoxia was not effective. With posttreatment, all animals receiving either dexamethasone (0.5 mg/kg/day) or vehicle (0.1 ml/day) had a major infarct ipsilateral to the occlusion.[12]

In order to investigate the dose dependence of the protective effect, we systematically decreased the amount of dexamethasone administered. Growth in these animals was inhibited in a dose-dependent manner with body weight being significantly less in dexamethasone-treated animals (10.7–11.5 g) than controls (13–13.5 g).[12] With respect to pathological outcome, these experiments showed that even 0.01 mg/kg/day of dexamethasone administered prior to the hypoxia-ischemia prevented infarction (TABLE 1). The fact that such relatively low doses of dexamethasone are effective suggests that this synthetic glucocorticoid is acting at a physiologically relevant dose of glucocorticoid. This is in contrast to the very high pharmacological doses that have been reported to provide protection against spinal cord injury in the adult—possibly via a membrane stabilization or free radical scavenging effect.[6]

TABLE 1. Effect on Pathological Outcome of Various Doses of Dexamethasone Administered Daily[a] prior to Hypoxia-Ischemia[b] in Neonatal Rats

| Dose of Dexamethasone (mg/kg/day) | Incidence of Infarction (Total n) | Blood Glucose[c] (mM) |
|---|---|---|
| 0 | 79% (49) | 3.7 ± 0.6 |
| 0.0001 | 67% (13) | 1.8 ± 0.3 |
| 0.001 | 58% (13) | 6.0 ± 1.1 |
| 0.01 | 0% (8)[d] | 8.3 ± 0.6[d] |
| 0.1 | 0% (10)[d] | 12 ± 1[d] |
| 0.5 | 0% (22)[d] | — |

[a] 48, 24 and 0 hr prior to hypoxia-ischemia.
[b] Right carotid artery occlusion and 3 hr of hypoxia (8% oxygen).
[c] At the end of hypoxia. Data presented as mean ± SEM.
[d] $p < 0.05$, different from vehicle or 0 mg/kg/day dose.

In order to examine the time dependence of the response, we varied the interval between the dexamethasone administration and the hypoxic-ischemic insult. These studies showed that a single injection of dexamethasone (0.1 mg/kg, ip) 24 hr or 6 hr before hypoxia-ischemia prevents infarction, whereas the administration of dexamethasone either 3 hr or 0 hr prior to the hypoxia-ischemia is ineffective (FIG. 1).[12,18] Recently, we also examined the effect of injecting dexamethasone

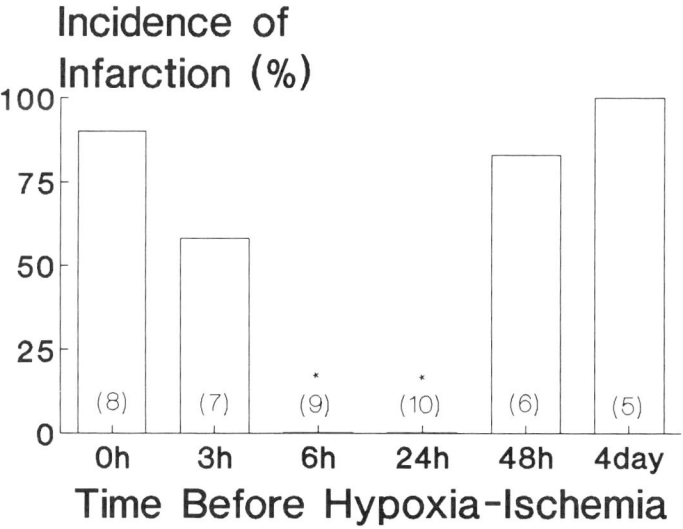

FIGURE 1. Time dependence of the neuroprotection produced by dexamethasone. A single injection of dexamethasone (0.1 mg/kg, ip) was administered at various times prior to hypoxia-ischemia in 7-day-old rats. Cerebral hypoxia-ischemia was produced by unilateral carotid artery occlusion and exposure to 3 hr of hypoxia (8% oxygen). The incidence of infarction is presented as a percentage of the total number of animals (n) with damage. Infarction was markedly reduced to 0% in animals treated with dexamethasone 24 to 6 hr prior to the hypoxia. *$p < 0.05$, different from vehicle-treated animals; Fisher's exact test.

either 4 days or 48 hr prior to the hypoxia-ischemia (unpublished results) and infarction was observed in a majority of these animals (FIG. 1). Thus, the protective effect of dexamethasone did not extend beyond 24–48 hr despite the fact that protection for several days was considered possible. Tolerance against ischemic damage had been shown to be produced by a heat stress or a sublethal ischemic insult, even if this stress was administered several days before the final ischemic insult.[19–22]

An important aspect of the time dependence of the response was that there was a delay of between 3–6 hr before the beneficial effects od dexamethasone became apparent. This delay suggests that dexamethasone is modifying gene expression. Of the two classes of receptors binding glucocorticoids, dexamethasone has a high affinity for the type II (glucocorticoid) receptor. These receptors are present either on membranes or within the cytosol. Membrane receptor-mediated effects are evident within seconds to minutes. Effects mediated through cytosolic receptors have a delayed response, since the soluble hormone receptor complex must translocate to the nucleus. There it interacts with a hormone response element on the DNA which regulates gene expression in either a positive or negative manner resulting in the inhibition or induction of a protein or enzyme.[23–25]

### *Hypothermia and Hypoxic-Ischemic Damage in the Neonate*

Body temperature is of crucial importance in determining the extent of damage incurred by an ischemic insult.[26] In this neonatal model of hypoxia-ischemia, full protection similar to that observed with dexamethasone was attained if temperature was reduced by 6–7°C from 37°C, whereas more moderate reductions in brain damage occurred if temperature was reduced to 34°C.[27,28] No beneficial effect was observed if body temperature was reduced after the hypoxia-ischemia.[27] Clearly, the presence of hypothermia in dexamethasone-treated animals could explain the neuroprotective effects observed. However, when we measured body temperature we found that thermoregulation was equivalent in dexamethasone- and vehicle-treated animals.[12] Thus, a reduction in body temperature with dexamethasone treatment does not explain dexamethasone's effects.

### *Dexamethasone and Altered Cerebral Perfusion*

The infarction observed in our model of hypoxia-ischemia is associated with a reduction in local cerebral blood flow ipsilateral to the side of the carotid artery occlusion.[29,30] Thus, another obvious way for dexamethasone to ameliorate the ischemia occurring during the hypoxia is to produce either a reduction in cerebrovascular resistance or an elevation in perfusion pressure. Indeed 'high'-dose dexamethasone therapy has been associated with hypertension and bradycardia in human infants,[8,31,32] although heart rate was not altered significantly by dexamethasone in our experiments.[12] High doses of glucocorticoids have also been reported to reduce cerebrovascular resistance and increase blood flow in injured spinal cord and in cerebral tumors.[33–36] However, others have also observed no change in cerebral blood flow,[37] a decrease in blood flow,[38] or a reduced pial vessel reactivity to hypercapnia[39] occurring following dexamethasone treatment. Adrenalectomy has also recently been shown to increase blood flow in the hippocampus, with corticosterone replacement preventing these elevations in flow.[40]

Since it was possible that dexamethasone provided neuroprotection simply by improving cerebral perfusion, we measured local cerebral blood flow using techniques similar to that developed by Lyons *et al.* for the 7-day-old rat.[41] Neonatal rats were treated with either vehicle or dexamethasone (0.1 mg/kg,ip) 24 hrs prior to hypoxia-ischemia and cerebral blood flow was measured with $^{14}$C-iodoantipyrine autoradiography after either 2 or 3 hr of hypoxia-ischemia.[16] Local cerebral blood flow was reduced ipsilateral to the carotid ligation in the distribution of the middle cerebral artery territory in both vehicle- and dexamethasone-treated animals. Indeed, absolute flow values were equivalent in animals treated with vehicle or dexamethasone at either 2 or 3 hours of hypoxia.[16] Since some of the interanimal variability in absolute flow may have obscured subtle ipsilateral-contralateral differences in flow between treatment groups, we also examined the effect of treatment on left-right differences in flow (FIG. 2). Comparison of these left-right differences in flow demonstrated further convergence rather than a divergence in the similarity of the results between groups. Thus, similar ischemic levels of cerebral blood flow occur irrespective of treatment, and dexamethasone must provide protection by affecting the brain and its metabolism rather than its blood supply.

### *Antioxidant Enzymes and Hypoxic-Ischemic Damage in the Neonate*

Antioxidant enzymes are important defences against free radicals which are generally considered to be generated during ischemia and/or cerebral reperfusion. These free radicals are also considered to mediate cellular damage via peroxidation of membrane phospholipids or oxidation of cellular proteins and nucleic acids.[42–44] Although the majority of information on free radicals has been obtained in adult animal models, there is evidence supporting a role for free radical-mediated damage during hypoxia-ischemia in the perinatal period.[44–48] Furthermore, in the neonatal rat model an oxygen free radical scavenger and xanthine oxidase inhibitor—allopurinol—reduces hypoxic-ischemic damage.[47]

Evidence is also available to suggest that glucocorticoids may induce antioxidant enzyme activity which would improve the brain's defence against free radical formation and thereby could potentially explain at least some of dexamethasone's neuroprotective mechanism of action. In the lung, glucocorticoids accelerate the ontogenic increases in the activities of the antioxidant enzymes—catalase and glutathione peroxidase.[49] In the brain, similar developmental increases in antioxidant enzyme activity occur during late fetal development in the guinea pig and during early postnatal development in the rat.[50,51] Indeed, antioxidant enzyme activity in the rat increases markedly (>100%) for catalase and CuZn-superoxide dismutase and moderately for glutathione peroxidase between postnatal days 0 and 40.[51] Also of interest is the observation that the administration of thyroid hormone in 10-day-old rats increases the cerebral activity of superoxide dismutase by approximately 40%.[52]

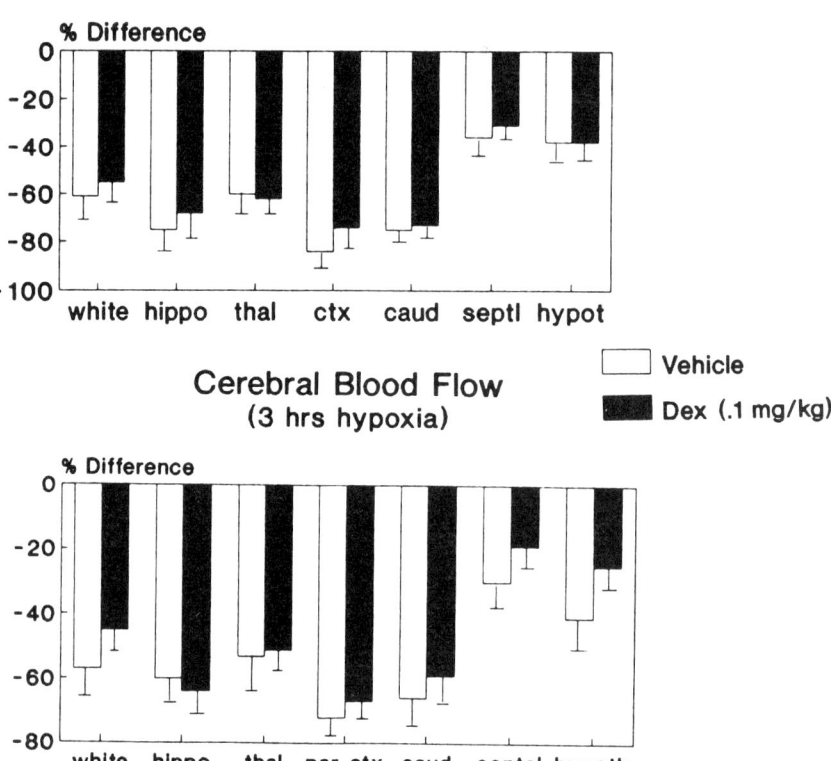

**FIGURE 2.** Local cerebral blood flow in 7-day-old rats subjected to unilateral carotid artery occlusion plus hypoxia. Cerebral blood flow was measured after either 2 hours (*upper panel*, n = 17) or 3 hours (*lower panel*, n = 15) of hypoxia using $^{14}C$-iodoantipyrine autoradiography. Cerebral blood flow is presented as a percentage of blood flow in the hemisphere contralateral to the occlusion. Relative reductions in flow ipsilateral to the occlusion were similar in vehicle- and dexamethasone-treated animals. (Data presented as mean ± SEM. All differences not significant statistically, Student *t* test.) Abbreviations: white - corpus callosum, hippo - hippocampus, thal - ventrolateral thalamus, ctx - parietal cortex, caud - caudate nucleus septl - septal nucleus, hypoth - hypothalamus.

Thus, to test whether dexamethasone induces antioxidant enzymes or modifies their activity during hypoxia-ischemia, we measured the activities of the enzymes catalase, glutathione peroxidase and CuZn- or Mn-superoxide dismutase within brains of animals treated with dexamethasone or vehicle.[17] Pretreatment with dexamethasone had no effect on endogenous antioxidant enzyme activities. Glutathione peroxidase, catalase, CuZn-superoxide dismutase and Mn-superoxide dismutase activities were similar in brains of animals treated with either dexamethasone or vehicle. In addition, exposure to 3 hr of hypoxia-ischemia had no effect on the enzyme activities of glutathione peroxidase or CuZn- and Mn-superoxide dismutase in the brains of either dexamethasone- or vehicle-treated animals (data not shown). Catalase activity tended to be less on the occluded side in dexamethasone-treated animals, but this difference was not significant statistically. This lack of effect of hypoxia-ischemia on antioxidant enzyme activity is similar to the observation that piglets subjected to ischemia and 30 min of reperfusion had no differences compared to controls in the activities of superoxide dismutase, catalase, glutathione peroxidase, glutathione reductase or glucose-6-phosphate dehydrogenase.[53] Thus, this group of experiments did not support the possibility that dexamethasone provides neuroprotection by improving the defense against free radical formation.

### Dexamethasone Compared to Other Potential Neuroprotective Agents

More recently we compared dexamethasone to several other potential neuroprotective agents and found it to be highly effective in preventing hypoxic-ischemic damage.[18] Similar to the adult, excessive calcium influx into cells is thought to play a pivotal role in the cascade of events leading to cell death due to hypoxia-ischemia.[44,54] Flunarizine is a piperazine derivative that inhibits voltage-sensitive calcium channels (L, T and N types) as well as inhibiting veratridine-sensitive sodium channels.[55,56] We confirmed that flunarizine given after the carotid artery occlusion and 30 min prior to the hypoxia (15 + 15 mg/kg, ip) is effective in reducing hypoxic-ischemic damage in this neonatal model[57,58] (FIG. 3). The exact mode of action of flunarizine is not clear but a combination of vasoactive and neuroprotective effects is possible. An antagonism of L-type calcium channels is unlikely since nimodipine, which antagonizes these channels, was ineffective in providing neuroprotection in this model (FIG. 3).

Lipid peroxidation with free radical formation has also been proposed as one of the lethal processes in cells subjected to hypoxia-ischemia.[43] The 21-aminosteroids are a group of drugs which have an increased capacity to inhibit lipid peroxidation but lack glucocorticoid effects. Despite such 21-aminosteroids reducing cerebral and spinal damage in various animal models of ischemia and trauma,[59-62] the administration of U-74689F (10 mg/kg pre- and posttreatment) failed to ameliorate damage in our neonatal model of hypoxia-ischemia (FIG. 3).[18] Similarly, U-74389F failed to provide protection against purely hypoxic brain damage in neonatal rats.[63] Even in adults, the effectiveness of 21-aminosteroids as neuroprotective agents is not universal.[64]

### Blood Glucose and Cerebral Hypoxic-Ischemic Damage in the Neonate

Hyperglycemia is a well documented effect of dexamethasone treatment[10,11] and is also known to influence pathological outcome following an episode of cerebral ischemia.[65] Our initial experiments demonstrated that infant rats treated with dexamethasone at doses which are protective, had elevated levels of blood glucose at the end of hypoxia-ischemia[12] (TABLE 1). In adult animals hyperglycemia during

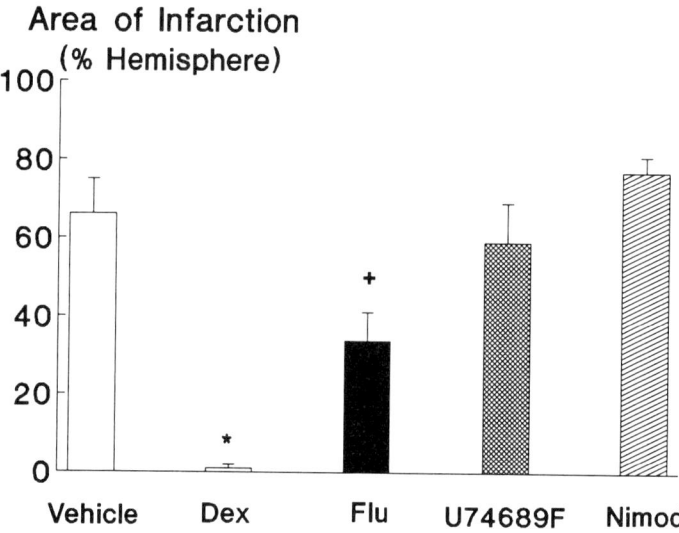

**FIGURE 3.** Comparison of the neuroprotective effect of dexamethasone with other potential therapies. Seven-day-old rats were subjected to unilateral carotid artery occlusion and 3 hours of hypoxia (8% oxygen). The area of infarction ipsilateral to the occlusion was measured as a % of the hemisphere in coronal sections at the level of the anterior hippocampus and thalamus. Dexamethasone (0.1 mg/kg, n = 9) administered 6 hr prior to hypoxia-ischemia produced marked reductions in the area of infarction compared to vehicle-treated animals (n = 38; 10 dexamethasone vehicle + 10 flunarizine vehicle + 10 nimodipine vehicle + 8 U74389F vehicle). The area of infarction was also reduced by flunarizine, a calcium and sodium antagonist, administered as 15 mg/kg after the carotid artery occlusion and another 15 mg/kg 30 min prior to the hypoxia (n = 14). Administration of the calcium antagonist nimodipine (0.5 mg/kg 1 hr prehypoxia, n = 12) or the 21-aminosteroid U74389 (10 mg/kg 30 min prior to and after hypoxia, n = 12) did not affect pathological outcome. (Data presented as mean ± SEM. *$p$ <0.05 different from vehicle-treated animals, + different from vehicle- and dexamethasone-treated animals.)

cerebral ischemia generally results in an augmentation of cerebral edema and/or pathology.[65] In contrast, hyperglycemia appears to be of benefit to neonatal animals during an episode of hypoxia and/or cerebral ischemia. Newborn rats and mice treated with glucose better survived anoxia or hypoxia-ischemia.[66,67] Hyperglycemic newborn lambs have also been shown to have an improved recovery of cerebral metabolism after a period of asphyxia,[68] and hyperglycemic fetal lambs have a better maintained electroencephalogram during ischemia.[69] In neonatal rats, glucose administered immediately after hypoxia-ischemia (bilateral carotid artery occlusion + 1 hr occlusion) reduced the volume of neocortical infarction, whereas high doses of glucose administered prior to and one hour after hypoxia prevented brain damage in immature rats subjected to hypoxia-ischemia (unilateral occlusion + 2 hr hypoxia).[70,71]

To test whether the moderate degree of hyperglycemia associated with dexamethasone treatment could prevent damage due to hypoxia-ischemia in neonatal

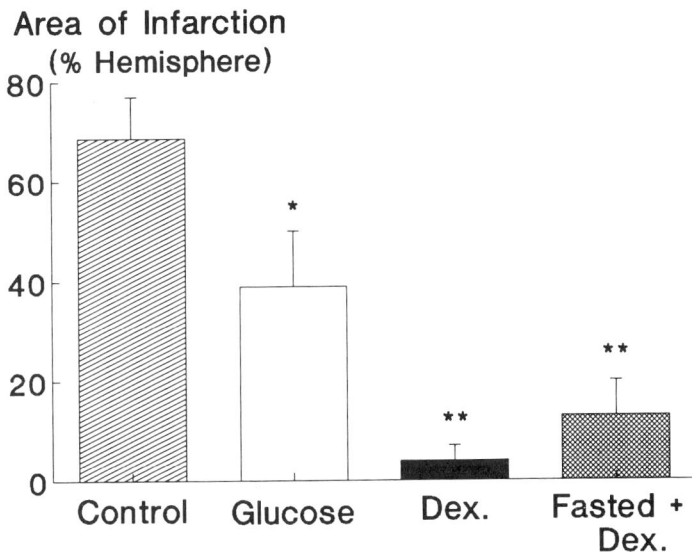

FIGURE 4. Effect of altering blood glucose on the neuroprotection provided by dexamethasone. Seven-day-old rats were subjected to unilateral carotid artery occlusion and 3 hr of hypoxia (8% oxygen). The area of infarction ipsilateral to the occlusion was measured as a % of the hemisphere in coronal sections at the level of the anterior hippocampus and thalamus. Dexamethasone (0.1 mg/kg, n = 28) administered 24 hr prior to hypoxia-ischemia produced marked reductions in the area of infarction independent of whether the animals had been fasted (n = 15) when compared to that in control animals (n = 13; 5 glucose vehicle + 8 dexamethasone vehicle). Repeated administration of d-glucose (10%, 0.1 ml/kg) at 0, 1, 2 and 3 hr of hypoxia (n = 13) resulted in a moderate reduction in the area of infarction. (Data presented as mean ± SEM. $*p$ <0.05, $**p$ <0.01, different from control.)

brain we maintained infant rats relatively hyperglycemic during hypoxia-ischemia by repeatedly administering 10% glucose (10 ml/kg, ip) at 0, 1, 2 and 3 hr of hypoxia.[17] The extent of damage in these animals was compared to that of immature rats receiving equivalent doses of saline or either vehicle or dexamethasone (0.1 mg/kg ip) 24 hr prior to hypoxia. Despite similar elevations in blood glucose at the end of hypoxia, glucose-treated animals had greater damage than dexamethasone-treated animals, and both of these groups had less damage than controls (FIG. 4). Infarction was evident in only 8% of the dexamethasone-treated animals compared with 54% of the glucose-treated animals and 95% of the control animals. Recently, we examined the effect of fasting on the effectiveness of dexamethasone (unpublished data). The results of these experiments showed that in fasted animals treated with dexamethasone, blood glucose values during hypoxia were similar to those of vehicle-treated animals. However, there was markedly less damage in these fasted animals than in the controls (FIG. 4). Thus, the relative hyperglycemia may contribute partially to the protection observed with dexamethasone treatment. However, this hyperglycemia is not essential for dexamethasone to provide protection, and additional or alternate mechanisms of action must be involved.

## Dexamethasone Effects on Glucose Utilization

Since the level of cerebral blood flow needed to maintain tissue viability is related to the local metabolic requirements of the tissue, a decrease in cerebral oxidative metabolism may reduce the susceptibility of the brain to ischemic damage. Previous examples of this are barbiturate anesthesia and hypothermia, which are considered to ameliorate ischemic damage, at least in part, by reducing cerebral oxidative metabolism.[72,73] Evidence is available to support such a mechanism of action for dexamethasone's beneficial effects. Local cerebral glucose utilization has been observed to be decreased following acute treatment with high doses of dexamethasone,[74-76] and electrophysiological studies indicate that glucocorticoids tend to inhibit neural activity within the central nervous system (CNS).[77]

To test whether dexamethasone provides protection by reducing energy requirements in brain, local cerebral glucose utilization was measured with autoradiographic techniques adapted for the 7-day-old rat.[78] Animals were treated with either vehicle or dexamethasone (0.1 mg/kg) 24 hr prior to the measurement of glucose utilization.[79] Local cerebral glucose utilization was measured in three groups of animals consisting of controls (no hypoxia) and animals subjected to hypoxia-ischemia, with measurements being made at the start or towards the end of the hypoxia-ischemia. In control animals, local cerebral glucose utilization was reduced in dexamethasone compared with vehicle-treated animals. However, during the first 90 min of hypoxia-ischemia, glucose utilization in both treatment groups increased compared to controls. The increase in glucose utilization was greater on the occluded side, particularly in dexamethasone-treated animals. In contrast, during the last 90 min of hypoxia, local cerebral glucose utilization in vehicle-treated animals declined 20–75% on the occluded side but remained elevated in the dexamethasone group resulting in a marked difference between groups (FIG. 5). In vehicle-treated animals, anaerobic glycolysis likely has not been adequate to maintain energy requirements resulting in a depletion of high energy phosphate reserves and subsequently a loss of ion pump homeostasis and electrical failure. Thus, the present results are consistent with the hypothesis that dexamethasone produces a reduction in basal metabolism which then extends the period for which anaerobic metabolism is able to maintain tissue viability. Additional experiments are required to determine the extent to which these changes actually contribute to dexamethasone's neuroprotective effects.

## Age Dependence of Glucocorticoid Effects

It would not be unexpected that the neuroprotection observed with dexamethasone is dependent on the age of the animal. There are major developmental changes in endogenous glucocorticoids, their receptors and the response of the hypothalamic-pituitary axis, all of which are rather complex and still being elucidated.[80-87] Endogenous levels of glucocorticoids vary throughout development and are considered important in inducing the differention of many different tissues including those within the CNS. Glucocorticoid levels increase towards the end of gestation and during labor in many species including sheep, rat and human,[88-92] although

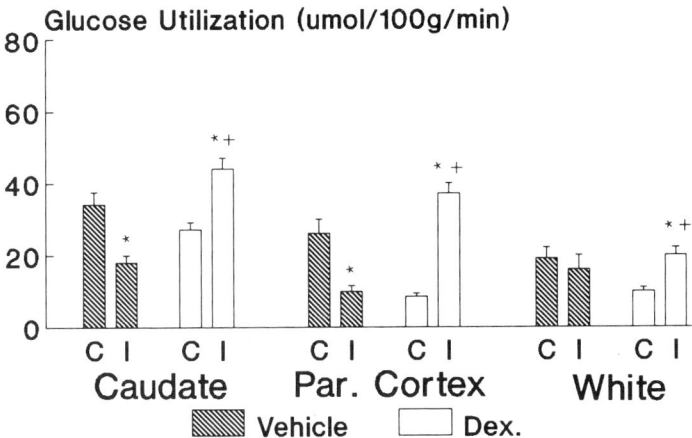

**FIGURE 5.** Effect of dexamethasone treatment on local cerebral glucose utilization during hypoxia-ischemia. Seven-day-old rats were subjected to hypoxia-ischemia (unilateral carotid artery occlusion + 3 hr of hypoxia) and treated with dexamethasone (0.1 mg/kg) 24 hr prior to hypoxia. Local cerebral glucose utilization was measured using $^{14}$C-2-deoxyglucose autoradiography during the last 90 min of hypoxia. Compared to the contralateral unoccluded side (C), glucose utilization was increased ipsilaterally (I) in dexamethasone-treated animals but decreased in vehicle-treated animals. (Data presented as mean ± SEM. *$p$ <0.05 different from contralateral; $^+p$ <0.05 different from vehicle.)

there are important differences between species.[90] In the rat, endogenous levels of glucocorticoids remain very low between approximately postnatal day 2 and 12 to 15, after which glucocorticoid levels increase reaching another maximum at about day 24.[91,92] The period when endogenous glucocorticoid levels are low (P2-P12) is correlated with a period when the hypothalamic-pituitary axis is hyporesponsive to stressful stimuli when compared to the adult.[81] In the adult, glucocorticoid (type II) binding sites are widely distributed in the body and CNS and are present in high concentrations in hypothalamus, hippocampus, septum, and amygdala and in moderate concentrations in cortex and caudate putamen.[81,93] During development, type II receptors are present at birth and gradually increase to adult levels by day 20.[94,95] Autoregulation of glucocorticoid receptors (*i.e.*, a downregulation of receptors by high glucocorticoid levels) occurs in adult and 2-week-old rats but not in neonatal rats.[96,97]

We examined the age dependence of the response by investigating whether dexamethasone provides cerebroprotection in older animals, *i.e.*, those 2 weeks and 4 weeks of age. Rats were treated with either dexamethasone or vehicle and subjected to an episode of hypoxia-ischemia which involved unilateral carotid artery occlusion plus 1 hr or 30 min of hypoxia in 2-week- and 4-week-old animals, respectively. The amount of infarction was markedly less in 2-week-old animals treated with dexamethasone compared to those treated with vehicle (FIG. 6). However, in 1-month-old animals, pretreatment with dexamethasone was of no benefit. Thus, dexamethasone is effective in reducing hypoxic-ischemic damage in young

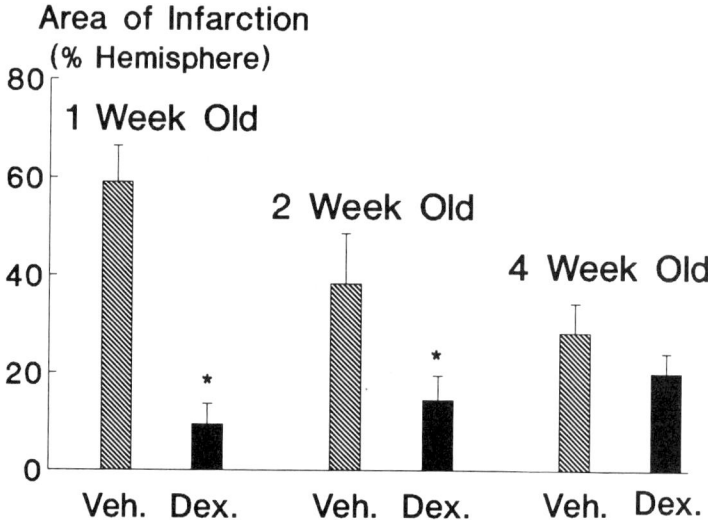

**FIGURE 6.** Age dependence of the response. Dexamethasone (0.1 mg/kg) was administered prior to hypoxia-ischemia in rats which were 1, 2 or 4 weeks of age. One-week-old rats received a single injection 24 hr prior to hypoxia-ischemia, whereas older animals received dexamethasone 24 and 5 hr prior to hypoxia-ischemia. Hypoxia-ischemia was produced by unilateral carotid artery occlusion and exposure to 3 hr, 1 hr and 30 min of hypoxia (8% oxygen) in rats aged 1, 2 and 4 weeks, respectively. The area of infarction ipsilateral to the occlusion was measured as a % of the hemisphere in coronal sections at the level of the anterior hippocampus and thalamus. Dexamethasone produced marked reductions in infarction in 1-week- and 2-week-old animals but not in 4-week-old rats. ($p < 0.05$, different from vehicle.)

but not in old rats, and this is consistent with previous experimental and clinical results in adults showing a lack of beneficial effect of glucocorticoids.[1-5] Clearly, developmental differences in the actions of dexamethasone and/or in the mechanisms of neuronal injury are important in the cerebroprotective effects of this synthetic glucocorticoid.

## REFERENCES

1. NORRIS, J. W. & V. C. HACHINSKI. 1986. High dose steroid therapy in cerebral infarction. Br. Med. J. **292:** 21–23.
2. GOLDSTEIN, M., H. J. M. BARNETT, J. M. ORGOGOZO, N. SARTORIUS, L. SYMON & N. V. VERESCHAGIN. 1989. Recommendations on stroke prevention, diagnosis and therapy: report of the WHO task force on stroke and other cerebrovascular disorders. Stroke **20:** 1407–1431.
3. JASTREMSKI, M., K. SUTTON-TYRELL, P. VAAGENES, N. ABRAMSON, D. HEISELMAN & P. SAFAR. 1989. (The brain resuscitation clinical trial I study group) Glucocorticoid treatment does not improve neurologic recovery following cardiac arrest. J. Am. Med. A. **262:** 3427–3430.
4. SAPOLSKY, R. M. & W. A. PULSINELLI. 1985. Glucocorticoids potentiate ischemic injury to neurons: therapeutic implications. Science **229:** 1397–1400.

5. KOIDE, T., T. W. WIELOCH & B. K. SIESJO. 1986. Chronic dexamethasone pretreatment aggravates ischemic neuronal necrosis. J. Cereb. Blood Flow Metab. **6:** 395–404.
6. HALL, E. D. 1992. The neuroprotective pharmacology of methylprednisolone. J. Neurosurg. **76:** 13–22.
7. ALTMAN, D. I., R. S. K. YOUNG & S. K. YAGEL. 1984. Effects od dexamethazone in hypoxic-ischemic brain injury in the neonatal rat. Biol. Neonate **46:** 149–156.
8. CUMMINGS, J. J., D. B. D'EUGENIO & S. J. GROSS. 1989. A controlled trial of dexamethasone in preterm infants at high risk for bronchopulmonary dysplasia. N. Engl. J. Med. **320:** 1505–1510.
9. AVERY, G. B., A. B. FLETCHER, M. KAPLAN & D. S. BRUDNO. 1985. Controlled trial of dexamethasone in respirator-dependent infants with bronchopulmonary dysplasia. Pediatrics **75:** 106–111.
10. HARKAVY, K. L., J. W. SCANLON, P. K. CHOWDHRY & L. J. GRYLACK. 1989. Dexamethasone therapy for chronic lung disease in ventilator- and oxygen-dependent infants: a controlled trial. J. Pediatr. **115:** 979–983.
11. OHLSSON, A., S. CALVERT, M. HOSKING & A. SHERMAN. 1989. Randomized controlled trial of dexamethasone treatment in very low birth weight infants with ventilatory-dependent chronic lung disease. Pediatr. Res. **25:** 1333.
12. BARKS, J. D. E., M. POST & U. I. TUOR. 1991. Dexamethasone prevents hypoxic-ischemic brain damage in the neonatal rat. Pediatr. Res. **29:** 558–563.
13. RICE, J. E., R. C. VANNUCCI & J. B. BRIERLEY. 1981. The influence of immaturity on hypoxic-ischemic brain damage in the rat. Ann. Neurol. **9:** 131–141.
14. Johnston, M. V. 1983. Neurotransmitter alterations in a model of perinatal hypoxic-ischemic brain injury. Ann. Neurol. **13:** 511–518.
15. TOWFIGHI, J., J. Y. YAGER, C. HOUSMAN & R. C. VANNUCCI. 1991. Neuropathology of remote hypoxic-ischemic damage in the immature rat. Acta Neuropathol. (Berlin) **81:** 578–587.
16. TUOR, U. I., C. S. SIMONE, J. D. E. BARKS & M. POST. 1993. Dexamethasone prevents cerebral infarction without affecting cerebral blood flow in neonatal rats. Stroke **24:** 452–457.
17. TUOR, U. I., C. S. SIMONE, R. ARELLANO, K. TANSWELL & M. POST. 1993. Glucocorticoid prevention of neonatal hypoxic-ischemic damage: role of hyperglycemia and antioxidant enzymes. Brain Res. **604:** 165–172.
18. CHUMAS, P. D., M. R. DEL BIGIO, J. M. DRAKE & U. I. TUOR. 1993. A comparison of the protective effect of dexamethasone to other potential prophylactic agents in a neonatal rat model of cerebral hypoxia-ischemia. J. Neurosurg. **79:** 414–420.
19. KUWABARA, K., M. TAGAYA, T. OHTSUKI, R. HATA, H. UEDA, N. HANDA, K. KIMURA & T. KAMADA. 1991. 'Ischemic tolerance' phenomenon detected in various brain regions. Brain Res. **561:** 203–211.
20. LIU, Y., H. KATO, N. NAKATA & K. KOGURE. 1992. Protection of rat hippocampus against ischemic neuronal damage by pretreatment with sublethal ischemia. Brain Res. **586:** 121–124.
21. SIMON, R. P., M. NIIRO & R. GWINN. 1993. Prior ischemic stress protects against experimental stroke. Neurosci. Lett. **163:** 135–137.
22. KATO, H., Y. LIU, T. ARAKI & K. KOGURE. 1994. Temporal profile on the effects of pretreatment with brief cerebral ischemia on the neuronal damage following secondary ischemic insult in the gerbil: cumulative damage and protective effects. Brain Res. **553:** 238–242.
23. VENKATESH, V. C. & P. L. BALLARD. 1991. Glucocorticoids and gene expression. Am. J. Respir. Cell Mol. Biol. **4:** 301–303.
24. BEATO, M. 1989. Gene regulation by steroid hormones. Cell **56:** 335–344.
25. MCEWEN, B. S. 1991. Non-genomic and genomic effects of steroids on neural activity. TIPS **12:** 141–147.
26. GINSBERG, M. D., L. L. STERNAU, M. Y-T. GLOBUS, W. D. DIETRICH & R. BUSTO. 1992. Therapeutic modulation of brain temperature: relevance to ischemic brain injury. Cerebrovasc. Brain Metab. Rev. **4:** 189–225.

27. YAGER, J., J. TOWFIGHI & R. C. VANNUCCI. 1994. Influence of mild hypothermia on hypoxic-ischemic brain damage in the immature rat. Pediatr. Res. **34:** 525–529.
28. SAEED, D., B. W. BOETZMAN & S. M. GOSPE. 1993. Brain injury and protective effects of hypothermia using triphenyltetrazolium chloride in neonatal rat. Pediatr. Neurol. **9:** 263–267.
29. SILVERSTEIN, F., K. BUCHANAN & M. V. JOHNSTON. 1984. Pathogenesis of hypoxic brain injury in perinatal rodent model. Neurosci. Lett. **49:** 271–277.
30. VANNUCCI, R. C., D. T. LYONS & F. VASTA. 1988. Regional cerebral blood flow during hypoxia-ischemia in immature rats. Stroke **19:** 245–250.
31. OHLSSON, A. & E. HEYMAN. 1988. Dexamethasone-induced bradycardia. Lancet **11:** 1074.
32. PUNTIS, J. W. L., M. E. I. MORGAN & G. M. DURBIN. 1988. Dexamethasone-induced bradycardia. Lancet **11:** 1372.
33. ANDERSON, D. K., E. D. MEANS, T. R. WATERS & E. S. GREEN. 1982. Microvascular perfusion and metabolism in injured spinal cord after methylprednisolone treatment. J. Neurosurg. **56:** 106–113.
34. HALL, E. D. & J. M. BRAUGHLER. 1982. Glucocorticoid mechanisms in acute spinal cord injury: a review and therapeutic rationale. Surg. Neurol. **18:** 320–327.
35. YOUNG, W. & E. S. FLAMM. 1982. Effect of high dose corticosteroid therapy on blood flow, evoked potentials and extracellular calcium in experimental spinal injury. J. Neurosurg. **57:** 667–673.
36. BUTTINGER, C., A. HARTMANN, R. VON KUMMER & J. MENZEL. 1982. *In* Treatment of Cerebral Edema. A. Hartmann & M. Brock, Eds. 132–138. Springer-Verlag. Berlin.
37. MENDELOW, A. D., B. H. EIDELMAN & T. A. MCCALDEN. 1978. The effect of intracarotid infusion of dexamethasone and 5-hydroxytryptamine on cerebral blood flow and metabolism in baboons. J. Neurosurg. **48:** 594–600.
38. LEENDERS, K. L., R. P. BEANEY, D. J. BROOKS, A. A. LAMMERTSMA, J. D. HEATHER & C. G. MCKENZIE. 1985. Dexamethasone treatment of brain tumor patients: effects on regional cerebral blood flow, blood volume, and oxygen utilization. Neurology **35:** 1610–1616.
39. WAGERLE, L. C., P. A. DEGIULIO, O. P. MISHRA & M. DELIVORIA-PAPADOPOULOS. 1991. Effect of dexamethasone on cerebral prostanoid formation and pial arteriolar reactivity to $CO_2$ in newborn pigs. Am. J. Physiol. **260:** H1313–H1318.
40. ENDO, Y., J-I. NISHIMURA & F. KIMURA. 1994. Adrenalectomy increases local cerebral blood flow in the rat hippocampus. Pflugers Arch. **426:** 183–188.
41. LYONS, D. T., F. VASTA & R. C. VANNUCI. 1987. Autoradiographic determination of regional cerebral blood flow in the immature rat. Pediatr. Res. **21:** 471–476.
42. WATSON, B. D. & M. D. GINSBERG. 1989. Ischemic injury in the brain. Role of oxygen radical-mediated processes. Ann. N.Y. Acad. Sci. **559:** 269–281.
43. SIESJO, B. K., C-D. AGARDH & F. BENGTSSON. 1989. Free radicals and brain damage. Cerebrovasc. Brain Metab. Rev. **1:** 165–211.
44. VANNUCCI, R. C. 1990. Experimental biology of cerebral hypoxia-ischemia: relation to perinatal brain damage. Pediatr. Res. **27:** 317–356.
45. ARMSTEAD, W. M., R. MIRRO, D. W. BUSIJA & C. W. LEFFLER. 1988. Postischemic generation of superoxide anion by newborn pig brain. Am. J. Physiol. **225:** H401–H403.
46. POURCYROUS, M., C. W. LEFFLER, R. MIRRO & D. W. BUSIJA. 1990. Brain superoxide anion generation during asphyxia and reventilation in newborn pigs. Pediatr. Res. **28:** 618–621.
47. PALMER, C., R. C. VANNUCCI & J. TOWFIGHI. 1990. Reduction of perinatal hypoxic-ischemic brain damage with allopurinol. Pediatr. Res. **27:** 332–336.
48. ROSENBERG, A. A., E. MURDAUGH & C. W. WHITE. 1989. The role of oxygen free radicals in post asphyxia cerebral hypoperfusion in newborn lambs. Pediatr. Res. **26:** 215–219.
49. FRANK, L., P. L. LEWIS & I. R. S. SOSENKO. 1985. Dexamethasone stimulation of fetal rat lung antioxidant enzyme activity in parallel with surfactant stimulation. Pediatrics **75:** 569–574.

50. MISHRA, O. P. & M. DELIVORIA-PAPADOPOULOS. 1988. Anti-oxidant enzymes in fetal guinea pig brain during development and the effect of maternal hypoxia. Brain Res. **470:** 173–179.
51. MEVELLI, I., A. RIGO, R. FEDERICO, M. R. CICIOLO & G. ROTILLO. 1982. Superoxide dismutase, glutathione peroxidase and catalase in developing rat brain. Biochem. J. **204:** 535–540.
52. PETROVIC, V. M., M. SPASIC, Z. SAICIC, B. MILIC & R. RADOJICIC. 1982. Increase in superoxide dismutase activity induced by thyroid hormones in the brains of neonate and adult rats. Experientia **38:** 1355–1356.
53. MISHRA, O. P., M. DELIVORIA-PAPADOPOULOS & L. C. WAGERLE. 1990. Anti-oxidant enzymes in the brain of newborn piglets during ischemia followed by reperfusion. Neuroscience **35:** 211–215.
54. ESPINOZA, M. I. & J. T. PARER. 1991. Mechanisms of asphyxial brain damage, and possible pharmacologic interventions, in the fetus. Am. J. Obstet. Gynecol. **164:** 1582–1591.
55. COHAN, S. L. 1990. Pharmacology of calcium antagonists: clinical relevance in neurology. Eur. Neurol. Suppl. **2:** 28–30.
56. PAUWELS, P. J., J. E. LEYSEN & P. A. JANSSEN. 1991. Minireview: $Ca^{++}$ and $Na^+$ channels involved in neuronal cell death. Protection by flunarizine. Life Sci. **48:** 1881–1893.
57. GUNN, A. J., T. MYDLAR, L. BENNETT et al. 1989. The neuroprotective actions of a calcium antagonist, flunarizine, in the infant rat. Pediatr. Res. **6:** 573–576.
58. SILVERSTEIN, F. S., K. BUCHANAN, C. HUDSON et al. 1986. Flunarizine limits hypoxia-ischemia induced morphologic injury in immature rat brain. Stroke **17:** 477–482.
59. HALL, E. D., K. E. PAZARA, J. M. BRAUGHLER, K. L. LINSEMAN & E. J. JACOBSEN. 1990. Nonsteroidal lazaroid U78517F in models of focal and global ischemia. Stroke **21**(Suppl 3): III83–III87.
60. BRAUGHLER, J. M., E. D. HALL & E. J. JACOBSEN. 1989. The 21-aminosteroids: potent inhibitors of lipid peroxidation for the treatment of central nervous system trauma and ischemia. Drugs Future **14:** 143–152.
61. XUE, D., A. SLIVKA & A. M. BUCHAN. 1992. Tirilazad reduces cortical infarction after transient but not permanent focal cerebral ischemia in rats. Stroke **23:** 894–899.
62. YOUNG, W., J. C. WOJEK & V. DECRESCITO. 1988. 21-aminosteroid reduces ion shifts and edema in the rat middle cerebral artery occlusion model of regional ischemia. Stroke **19:** 1013–1019.
63. RAO, K. V. S. & A. SNACHEZ. 1992. The role of U74389F in hypoxic injury of the newborn rat brain. Pediatr. Res. **31:** 352A.
64. BUCHAN, A. M., B. BRUEDERLIN, E. HEINICKE & H. LI. 1992. Failure of the lipid peroxidation inhibitor, U74006F, to prevent postischemic selective neuronal injury. J. Cereb. Blood Flow Metab. **12:** 250–256.
65. MARIE, C. & J. BRALET. 1991. Blood glucose level and morphological brain damage following cerebral ischemia. Cerebrovasc. Brain Metab. Rev. **3:** 29–38.
66. THURSTON, J. H., R. E. HAUHART & E. M. JONES. 1974. Anoxia in mice: reduced glucose in brain with normal or elevated glucose in plasma an increased survival after glucose treatment. Pediatr. Res. **8:** 238–243.
67. VANNUCCI, R. C. & S. J. VANNUCCI. 1978. Cerebral carbohydrate metabolism during hypoglycemia and anoxia in newborn rats. Ann. Neurol. **4:** 73–79.
68. ROSENBERG, A. A. & E. MURDAUGH. 1990. The effect of blood glucose concentration on postasphyxia cerebral hemodynamics in newborn lambs. Pediatr. Res. **27:** 454–459.
69. CHAO, C. R., A. R. HOHIMER & J. M. BISSONNETTE. 1989. The effect of elevated blood glucose on the electroencephalogram and cerebral metabolism during short-term brain ischemia in fetal sheep. Am. J. Obstet. Gynecol. **161:** 221–228.
70. HATTORI, H. & C. G. WASTERLAIN. 1990. Posthypoxic glucose supplement reduces hypoxic-ischemic brain damage in the neonatal rat. Ann. Neurol. **28:** 122–128.
71. VANNUCCI, R. C. 1992. Cerebral carbohydrate and energy metabolism in perinatal hypoxic-ischemic brain damage. Brain Pathol. **2:** 229–234.

72. SPETZLER, R. T. & M. N. HADLEY. 1989. Protection against cerebral ischemia: the role of barbiturates. Cerebrovasc. Brain Metab. Rev. **1:** 212–229.
73. GINSBERG, M. D. 1990. Local metabolic responses to cerebral ischemia. Cerebrovasc. Brain Metab. Rev. **2:** 58–93.
74. PHILLIPS, P. C., C. A. BERGER & D. A. ROTTENBERG. 1987. High-dose dexamethasone decreases regional cerebral glucose metabolism in the rat. Neurology 37(Suppl. 1): 248.
75. DORMER, F. R., K. MORI, C. A. DINARELLO & L. SOKOLOFF. 1988. Effects of leukocytic pyrogen (interleukin-1) on local cerebral glucose utilization in rats with and without premedication with indomethacin or dexamethasone. J. Cereb. Blood Flow Metab. **8:** 173–178.
76. KADEKARO, M., M. ITO & P. M. GROSS. 1988. Local cerebral glucose utilization is increased in acutely adrenalectomized rats. Neuroendocrinology **47:** 329–334.
77. JOËLS, M. & E. R. DE KLOET. 1992. Control of neuronal excitability by corticosteroid hormones. TINS **15:** 25–30.
78. VANNUCCI, R. C., M. A. CHRISTENSEN & D. T. STEIN. 1989. Regional cerebral glucose utilization in the immature rat: effect of hypoxia-ischemia. Pediatr. Res. **26:** 208–214.
79. TUOR, U. I. 1994. Prevention of neonatal hypoxic-ischemic damage with dexamethasone: local cerebral glucose utilization is affected prior to and during hypoxia. Stroke **25:** 261.
80. MEANEY, M. J., V. VIAU, S. BHATNAGAR, K. BETITO, L. J. INY, D. O'DONNELL & J. B. MITCHELL. 1991. Cellular mechanisms underlying the development and expression of individual differences in the hypothalamic-pituitary-adrenal stress response. J. Steroid Biochem. Mol. Biol. **39:** 265–274.
81. DE KLOET, E. R., P. ROSENFELD, A. M. VAN EEKELEN, W. SUTNATO & S. LEVINE. 1988. Stress, glucocorticoids and development. Prog. Brain Res. **73:** 101–120.
82. REUL, J. M. H. M., J. ROTHUIZEN & E. R. DE KLOET. 1991. Age-related changes in the dog hypothalamic-pituitary-adrenocortical system: neuroendocrine activity and corticosteroid receptors. J. Steroid Biochem. Mol. Biol. **40:** 63–69.
83. VAN EEKELEN, J. A. M., N. Y. ROTS, W. SUTANTO, M. S. OITZL & E. R. DE KLOET. 1991. Brain corticosteroid receptor gene expression and neuroendocrine dynamics during aging. J. Steroid Biochem. Mol. Biol. **40:** 679–683.
84. LAWSON, A., R. AHIMA, Z. KROZOWSKI & R. HARLAN. 1991. Postnatal development of corticosteroid receptor immunoreactivity in the rat hippocampus. Dev. Brain Res. **62:** 69–79.
85. LAWSON, A., R. S. AHIMA, Z. KROZOWSKI & R. E. HARLAN. 1992. Postnatal development of corticosteroid receptor immunoreactivity in the rat cerebellum and brain stem. Neuroendocrinology **55:** 695–707.
86. YANG, K., G. L. HAMMOND & J. R. G. CHALLIS. 1992. Characterization of an ovine glucocorticoid receptor cDNA and developmental changes in its mRNA levels in the fetal sheep hypothalamus, pituitary gland and adrenal. J. Mol. Endocrinol. **8:** 173–180.
87. ALEXIS, M. N., E. KITRAKI, K. SPANOU, F. STYLIANOPOULOU & C. E. SEKERIS. 1990. Ontogeny of the glucocorticoid receptor in the rat brain. Adv. Exp. Med. Biol. **265:** 269–276.
88. OKAMOTO, E., T. TAKAGI, T. MAKINO, H. SATA, I. IWATA, E. NISHINO, N. MITSUDA, N. SUGITA, Y. OTSUKI & O. TANIZAWA. 1989. Immunoreactive corticotropin-releasing hormone, adrenocorticotropin and cortisol in human plasma during pregnancy and delivery and postpartum. Horm. Metab. Res. **21:** 566–572.
89. PHOCAS, I., A. SARANDAKOU & D. RIZOS. 1990. Maternal serum total cortisol levels in normal and pathologic pregnancies. Int. J. Gynaecol. Obstet. **31:** 3–8.
90. Brooks, A. N. & J. R. G. Challis. 1988. Regulation of the hypothalamic-pituitary-adrenal axis in birth. Can. J. Physiol. Pharmacol. **66:** 1106–1112.
91. HENNING, S. J. 1978. Plasma concentrations of total and free corticosterone during development in the rat. Am. J. Physiol. **235:** E451–E456.
92. SAPOLSKY, R. M. & M. J. MEANEY. 1986. The maturation of the adrenocortical response in the rat. Brain Res. Rev. **11:** 65–76.

93. MAGARIÑOS, A. M., M. FERRINI & A. F. DE NICOLA. 1989. Corticosteroid receptors and glucocorticoid content in microdissected brain regions: correlative aspects. Neuroendocrinology **50:** 673–678.
94. SARRIEAU, A., S. SHARMA & M. J. MEANEY. 1988. Postnatal development and environmental regulation of hippocampal glucocorticoid and mineralocorticoid receptors. Dev. Brain Res. **43:** 158–162.
95. ROSENFELD, P., W. SUTANTO, S. LEVINE & E. R. DE KLOET. 1988. Ontogeny of type I and type II corticosteroid receptors in the rat hippocampus. Dev. Brain Res. **42:** 113–118.
96. MEANEY, M. J., D. H. AITKEN, S. R. BODNOFF, L. J. INY, J. E. TATAREWICZ & R. M. SAPOLSKY. 1985. Early postnatal handling alters glucocorticoid receptor concentrations in selected brain regions. Behav. Neurosci. **99:** 765–770.
97. MEANEY, M. J., R. M. SAPOLSKY & B. S. MCEWEN. 1985. The development of glucocorticoid receptor system in the rat limbic brain. I. Ontogeny and autoregulation. Dev. Brain Res. **18:** 159–164.

# Discussion

D. K. J. E. VON LUBITZ (*National Institute of Diabetes and Digestive and Kidney Diseases, NIH, Bethesda, MD*): The effects of elevated $Mg^{2+}$ are easily explained by its action at A1/A2 receptors. Trevor Stone demonstrated that $Mg^{2+}$ potentiates effects of A1/A2 receptor activation, and the protection shown by you may result from A2 receptor-mediated stabilization of cerebral blood flow (CBF) and A1-mediated effect on $Ca^{2+}$ overload and neurotransmitter release. Cotreatment with dipyridamole (adenosine turnover modifier, uptake blocker) would probably push your results into the statistically significant range due to sustained elevation of extracellular adenosine and potentiation of its effect by $Mg^{2+}$.

K. W. MUIR (*Western Infirmary, Glasgow*): The possible inducement of adenosine in mediating magnesium's actions at a cellular level is an interesting observation. However, as I have outlined, Mg has multiple potential actions including *N*-methyl-D-aspartate (NMDA) ion-channel blockade and block of voltage-sensitive calcium channels which are likely to be independent of adenosine effects. Cardiovascular effects have been shown to be probably due to stimulation of endothelial prostacyclin release. While there is a need for further mechanistic studies, experience with pre-eclampsia shows that there is therapeutic potential which need not await a clearly defined cellular mechanism for clinical studies. Incidentally, I do not feel that there is any prospect of demonstrating efficacy in a clinical study of this size on the basis of our current methodology, regardless of the pharmacological potency of the therapeutic agent.

S. GOLDIN (*Cambridge NeuroScience*): For RS 87476 (lifarizine), how would you rate behavioral effects in relation to blockers of presynaptic release or postsynaptic actions of glutamate?

K. R. LEES (*Western Infirmary, Glasgow*): From my personal observation and from the results of the study in the other centers, there is no doubt that behavioral effects were virtually absent. In particular there were no hallucinations with lifarizine.

M. MARIEN (*Pierre Fabre Research, France*): In young adult rats, a single dose of dexamethasone, in a dose range similar to that which you have shown to be neuroprotective in your model, and with a similar time course, increases the expression of mRNA of nerve growth factor in the cerebral cortex (by 2–3-fold) and to a lesser extent in the hippocampus. Would you care to speculate on the possible role of growth factors in the neuroprotective action of dexamethasone in your study?

U. TUOR (*Hospital for Sick Children, Toronto*): The 4–6-hr delay between the administration of dexamethasone and its ability to prevent hypoxic-ischemic damage in the neonatal rat suggests a genomic mechanism of action, which would be consistent with the induction of some neuroprotective protein(s), and, nerve growth factor would be an attractive potential candidate. Intracerebral administration of various growth factors such as basic fibroblast growth factor (bFGF) and insulin-like growth factor (IGF) have been shown to provide some protection against cerebral ischemic damage in various models and thus, the induction of

# DISCUSSION

nerve growth factor may contribute to dexamethasone's effects in the neonate. However, I believe that dexamethasone likely has a range of actions which in combination act to produce the rather dramatic prevention of infarction observed, and the induction of a single growth factor is unlikely to be able to produce the effects observed.

R. BULLOCK (*Medical College of Virginia*): What is the relationship between serum extracellular fluid (ECF) $Mg^{2+}$ levels, and what is the optimal protective level? How safe is the therapeutic index? Side effects (several) have been reported in eclampsia studies.

LEES: The dose-response relationship for neuroprotection has not yet been adequately established. Further studies in standard animal models would be very helpful in this respect. We were not able to measure cerebrospinal fluid (CSF) concentrations of magnesium in our patients, but it has been shown that intravenous magnesium sulfate given to pre-eclamptics significantly raises CSF magnesium. The therapeutic index for magnesium is wide. Only transient and nonsignificant effects have been reported in studies of pre-eclampsia, and in intervention studies after acute myocardial infarction, which used very similar doses to ours. An approximate doubling of serum Mg levels (to 2 $mmolL^{-1}$) results from such doses, and is associated only with transient facial flushing. Tendon reflexes become suppressed from plasma levels of 6 $mmolL^{-1}$, with neuromuscular blockade at higher doses. However, serum levels of 6 $mmolL^{-1}$ have been survived in pre-eclampsia. The therapeutic index probably compares favorably with other pharmacological interventions.

D. BONHAUS (*Syntex Research, Palo Alto, CA*): Given that the pilot study with lifarizine showed a trend to efficacy, what would be the required size of the study to show statistical significance?

LEES: Not yet determined.

GOLDIN: You mentioned that several patients in the lifarizine-treated group were withdrawn from treatment due to cardiovascular abnormalities, and one had a treatment-related seizure. How were these withdrawals dealt with in the statistical analysis of improvement in Rankin and Barthel scores?

LEES: Patients who fulfilled the criteria for 'evaluable patients,' *i.e.*, who had a diagnosis of ischemic stroke confirmed, were included for efficacy analysis.

A. J. MERCER (*Wellcome Research Laboratories, Beckenham, UK*): How was the dose of lifarizine used decided upon?

LEES: I believe this was based on volunteer studies, aiming to select the maximal dose which did not appear likely to produce cardiovascular effects.

BULLOCK: Do you think if you had given high doses, you would have seen the effects you wanted?

LEES: We were not disappointed with the results of this study. We found trends in favor of benefit with magnesium. With a pilot study of this size we would not expect to demonstrate statistically significant effects on outcome with magnesium or with any other neuroprotective compound in patients with acute stroke.

# Risk Assessment Strategies for Neuroprotective Agents

WILLIAM SLIKKER, JR. AND DAVID W. GAYLOR

*Divisions of Neurotoxicology and Biometry & Risk Assessment
National Center for Toxicological Research
Food and Drug Administration
Jefferson, Arkansas 72079-9502*

## DEFINITION OF TERMS

### Neurotoxicity

Neurotoxicity may be defined as any adverse effect on the structure or function of the central and/or peripheral nervous system by a biological, chemical, or physical agent. Neurotoxic effects may be permanent or reversible, produced by neuropharmacological or neurodegenerative properties of a neurotoxicant, or the result of direct or indirect actions on the nervous system. Adverse effects can include both unwanted effects and any alteration from baseline that diminishes the ability of an organism to survive, reproduce, or adapt to its environment. A multidisciplinary approach is necessary for the assessment of neurotoxicity because of the complexity and diverse functions of the nervous system. Many effects relevant to the neurotoxicologist can be measured directly by neurochemical, neurophysiological, and neuropathological techniques, whereas, others must be inferred from observed behavior (FIG. 1). The research approach consists of the following three steps: 1) gathering information from all available endpoints or disciplines and using it to generate a neurotoxicity profile; 2) correlating structural, neurochemical and neurophysiological data with overt behavioral manifestations of neurotoxicity; 3) developing a pharmacokinetic/metabolic basis to aid in data interpretation and for interspecies extrapolation. Future approaches for neurotoxicity assessments may include additional disciplines and approaches such as molecular biology and psychology (FIG. 2). To allow for successful interspecies extrapolation, physiologically-based pharmacokinetic modeling (PBPk) may be used to predict target tissue exposure to an agent in several species including humans.

### Assessing Human Neurotoxicity

Because of technical and ethical considerations, neurotoxicity in humans is primarily measured by noninvasive neurophysiological and neurobehavioral methods. Clinical neurology and neuropsychology approaches have been used extensively to evaluate neurological diseases, and these same methods have been used to assess patients suspected of having neurotoxic insults.[1] In addition, many neu-

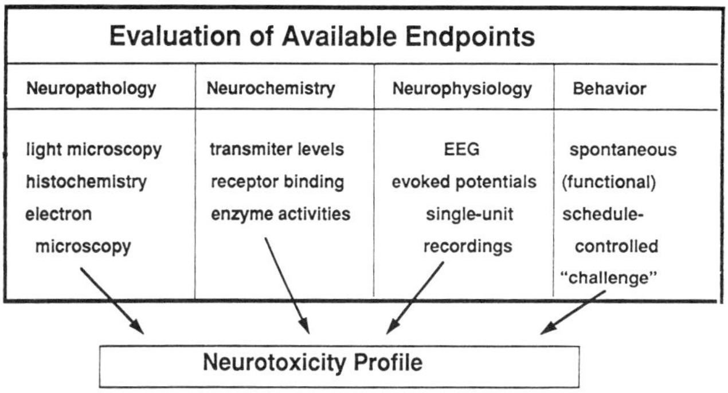

Evaluation of Available Endpoints
Neuropathology
Neurochemistry
Neurophysiology
Behavior
light microscopy
histochemistry
electron microscopy
transmiter levels
receptor binding
enzyme activities
EEG
evoked potentials
single-unit recordings
spontaneous (functional)
schedule-controlled
"challenge"
Neurotoxicity Profile

**FIGURE 1.** Description of research approach including endpoints that may be evaluated to generate a neurotoxicity profile for a given agent.

Psychological
Behavioral
Physiological
Morphological
Neurochemical
Molecular

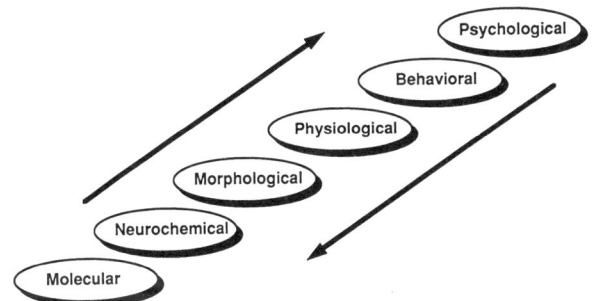

**FIGURE 2.** Description of the discipline-continuum approach for the evaluation of agents. Initial studies of an agent begin within any discipline on the continuum and additional studies may follow within other disciplines. Data generated from the various disciplines or from different species may be integrated with the use of pharmacokinetics.

robehavioral methods have been proposed or used to assess neurobehavioral function in humans (TABLE 1). In recent years, imaging techniques including magnetic resonance imaging (MRI) and computerized tomography (CT), and computerized brain electrical activity mapping, as well as operant behavioral assessments have provided noninvasive and quantitative methods for human neurotoxicity assessment. Epidemiological approaches, including retrospective and prospective studies provide the means for evaluating the effects of neurotoxic substances in human populations.[1]

### *Animal Models*

While human data are available from clinical trials for therapeutics such as neuroprotective agents, initial preclinical studies to determine dose, pharmacokinetic and safety parameters are usually performed in animal models. *In vivo* animal studies currently serve as the principal approach for detecting and characterizing

TABLE 1. Some Human Neurobehavioral Methods

| Neurobehavioral Function | Test |
|---|---|
| Sensation | flicker fusion |
| | lanthony (color vision) |
| Motor/dexterity | pursuit aiming |
| | finger tapping |
| | postural stability |
| | reaction time |
| | Santa Ana peg board |
| Cognition | Benton visual retention |
| | continuous performance task |
| | digit-symbol |
| | digit span |
| | dual tasks |
| | paired-associate |
| | symbol-digit task |
| | Wechsler Adult Intelligence Scale—Revised® (components) |
| | Wechsler Memory Scale® |
| Affect | profile of mood states (POMS) |

neurotoxic hazards and helping to identify factors affecting susceptibility to neurotoxicity. *In vitro* tests have been proposed as a means of complementing whole animal tests and, when properly developed, may be less time consuming and more cost effective than *in vivo* assessments.[1] The currently used *in vitro* tests, however, have certain limitations including the inability to model neurobehavioral effects (*e.g.*, memory, learning, or sensory dysfunction). Validation of animal models, whether *in vivo* or *in vitro*, is of paramount importance and may include measures of construct, criterion, and predictive validity. Despite the biological similarity of humans and many animal models, differential susceptibility to toxicants is well documented between species. Predictive capability or concordance between human and animal models after exposure to human neurotoxicants has frequently been reported.[1,2,3] These comparable outcomes provide a firm foundation for the use of animal models in neurotoxicity risk assessment.

## *Neurotoxicity Endpoints*

Examples of neurotoxicity endpoints for each of the four major disciplines of neurotoxicity are shown in TABLES 2–5.[1]

TABLE 2. Neuropathological or Structural Endpoints[a]

| |
|---|
| Accumulation, proliferation or rearrangement of structural elements |
| Breakdown of cells |
| Glial fibrillary acidic protein (GFAP) increases (adult) |
| Gross changes in morphology, including brain weight |
| Discoloration of nerve tissue |
| Hemorrhage in nerve tissue |

[a] From Reiter *et al.*[1] Reprinted from the *Federal Register*.

TABLE 3. Neurochemical Endpoints

Alterations in synthesis, release, uptake, degradation of neurotransmitters
Alterations in second messenger-associated signal transduction
Alterations in membrane-bound enzymes regulating neuronal activity
Decreases in brain acetylcholinesterase (AChE)
Neurotoxic esterase (NTE)
Altered developmental patterns of neurochemical systems
Altered proteins (c-fos, substance P)

TABLE 4. Neurophysiological Endpoints

Change in velocity, amplitude or refractory period of nerve conduction
Change in latency or amplitude of sensory-evoked potential
Change in electroencephalogram (EEG) pattern or power spectrum

TABLE 5. Behavioral Endpoints

Absence or altered occurrence, magnitude or latency of sensorimotor reflex
Altered magnitude of neurological measurements, such as grip strength or hindlimb splay
Increases or decreases in motor activity
Changes in rate, temporal patterning, or accuracy of schedule-controlled behavior
Changes in motor coordination, weakness, paralysis, abnormal movement or posture, tremor, ongoing performance
Changes in touch, sight, sound, taste, or smell sensations
Changes in learning and/or memory
Occurrences of seizures
Altered temporal development of behaviors or reflex responses
Autonomic signs

## *Risk Assessment/Risk Management*

Risk assessment is an empirically-based process used to estimate the risk that exposure of an individual or population to a chemical, physical, or biological agent will be associated with an adverse or abnormal effect. The risk assessment process usually involves four steps: hazard identification, dose-response assessment, exposure assessment, and risk characterization.[4] Risk assessment should not be confused with risk management, a process whereby information, concerning the benefits as well as the risks of exposure (treatment) are considered to determine whether, or at what dose, an individual agent should be used. Most often, risk assessments are performed by researchers, whereas risk management is often conducted by regulatory agencies as directed by legislative bodies via legislation or by physician/patient interactions focused on risk/benefit considerations for the individual in need of treatment.

## CURRENTLY USED RISK ASSESSMENT APPROACHES

### *Safety-Factor Approach*

The most frequently used approach for risk assessment of neurotoxicants and other noncancer endpoints is the uncertainty or safety-factor approach.[5,6] Within

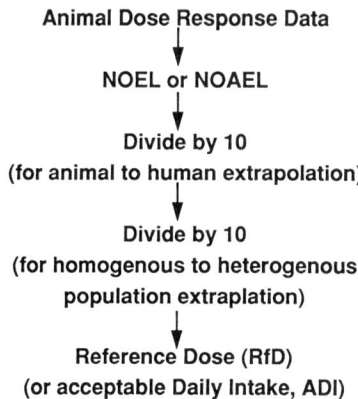

**FIGURE 3.** Description of the use of safety factors in deriving a reference dose. NOEL = no observed effect level, NOAEL = no observed adverse effect level.

the Environmental Protection Agency (EPA), for example, this approach involves the determination of reference doses (RfDs) by dividing a no observed adverse effect level (NOAEL) by uncertainty factors that presumably account for interspecies and intraspecies differences in sensitivity.[5] Generally, an uncertainty factor of 10 is used to allow for the presumed greater sensitivity in humans than in animals and another uncertainty factor of 10 is used to allow for variability in sensitivity among humans. In this case, the RfD is equal to the NOAEL divided by 100 (FIG. 3). If the NOAEL cannot be established, it is replaced by the lowest observed adverse effect level (LOAEL) in the RfD calculation and an additional uncertainty factor of 10 is generally introduced (*i.e.*, the RfD equals the LOAEL divided by 1000).

*Limitations and Assumptions*

There are several features of this RfD or safety factor approach which deserve consideration. First, the method assumes a theoretical threshold dose below which no biological effects of any type are observed in a heterogeneous population. Not only is the determination of a threshold dose influenced by the sensitivity of the analytical methods employed, but the theoretical bases of a threshold dose may be questioned. Unfortunately, less sensitive experiments can result in higher RfDs. If, due to normal variation in cellular function an adverse effect can occur in untreated control subjects, then endogenous or exogenous factors may already be supplying a stimulus which is equivalent to a dose above the threshold dose. If exposure to an agent augments this stimulus, then an addiitional risk is expected and no threshold dose exists for that agent.[7] Second, the magnitudes of the safety factors used to determine RfDs [interspecies extrapolation (10) and intraspecies extrapolation (10)] are based more on best estimates than actual data.[1,8]

The RfD approach relies on a single experimental observation (the NOAEL

TABLE 6. Quantitative Risk Assessment

---
Establish mathematical relationship between biological effect (or biomarker) and dose of chemical administered
Determine the distribution of individual measurements of biological effects about the dose-response curve
Define an adverse (or abnormal) level of a biological effect in an untreated population
Combine all the above information to estimate the risk (proportion of individuals exceeding an adverse level) as a function of dose

---

or LOAEL), instead of using complete dose-response curve data in the calculation of risk estimates. Because chemical interactions with biological systems are often specific, stereoselective, and/or saturable, a chemical's dose-response curve may not be linear. Examples include enzyme-substrate binding leading to substrate metabolism, transport, and receptor-binding, any or all of which may be a requirement for an agent's effect or toxicity. The certainty of low-dose extrapolation has been determined to be markedly affected by the shape of the dose-response curve.[9] Therefore, the use of dose-response curve data should enhance the certainty of risk estimations when thresholds are not assumed or determined.

## QUANTITATIVE, DOSE-RESPONSE-BASED RISK ASSESSMENT APPROACHES

### Dose-Response Models

Dose-response models have generated considerable interest and are seen by many to be more appropriate (and quantitative) than the safety-factor approach to risk assessment. Rather than routinely applying a "fixed" safety factor to the NOAEL (which is based on a single dose) to estimate a "safe" dose, these approaches use data from the entire dose-response curve.[1]

Two fundamentally different approaches in the use of dose-response data to estimate risk have been developed. Dews and co-workers[10-12] and Crump[13] have demonstrated an approach in which they use information on the shape of the dose-response curve to estimate levels of exposure associated with relatively small effects (*i.e.*, a 1, 5, or 10 percent change in a biological endpoint). Both Dews and Crump fit a mathematical function to the data and provide an estimate of the variability in exposure levels associated with a relatively small effect.

In another approach developed by Gaylor and Slikker,[7,14] a mathematical relationship is first established between the average biological effect and the dose of a given chemical. A second step determines the distribution (variability) of individual measurements of biological effects about the dose-response curve. The third step statistically defines an adverse or "abnormal" level of a biological effect in an untreated population. The fourth step estimates the probability of an adverse or abnormal level as a function of dose utilizing the information from the first three steps. The advantages of these dose-response models are that they encourage the generation and use of data needed to define a complete dose-response curve (TABLE 6) and provide an estimate of risk and/or changes in the average response as a function of dose.

TABLE 7. General Assumptions That Underlie Traditional Risk Assessment

---
A threshold dose exists for noncancer endpoints
NOAEL/LOAEL[a] uncertainty- or safety-factor approaches are reasonable
Variability in the toxic response to the chemical exposure is not due to a heterogeneous population response
Average dose or total dose is a reasonable measure of exposure when doses are not equivalent in time, rate, or route of administration and the average (or total) dose is proportional to adverse effect
Structure-activity correlations can be used to predict human toxicity
The mechanism of action is the same at all doses for all species

---

[a] NOAEL, no observed adverse effect level; LOAEL, lowest observed adverse effect level.

## Biologically-Based Risk Assessment

The development of quantitative risk assessment approaches depends, in part, on the availability of information on the mechanism of action and pharmacokinetics of the agent in question. In the development of a biologically-based, dose-response model for the psychoactive agent, methylenedioxymethamphetamine (MDMA), Slikker and Gaylor[15] considered several factors, including the pharmacokinetics of the parent chemical, the target tissue concentrations of the parent chemical or its bioactivated proximate toxicant, the uptake kinetics of the parent chemical or metabolite into the target cell and membrane interactions, and the interaction of the chemical or metabolite with presumed receptor site(s). Because these theoretical factors contain a saturable step due to limited amounts of required enzyme, reuptake, or receptor site(s), a nonlinear, saturable dose-response curve was predicted. In this case of neurochemical effects of MDMA in the rodent, saturation mechanisms were hypothesized and indeed saturation curves provided relatively good fits to the experimental results. Some of the advantages of the biologically-based, quantitative approaches over the currently used RfD risk assessment procedures include the ability to 1) utilize continuous data, 2) utilize all the dose-response curve data, 3) incorporate biological information into the dose-response model, and 4) provide an actual risk of exposure to a given dose.[8] The conclusion was that use of dose-response models based on plausible biological mechanisms provides more validity to prediction than purely empirical models.

## Generic Assumptions

Risk assessment for neurotoxicity shares many common features with other noncancer toxicities such as developmental toxicity and immunotoxicity. As such, there are several generic assumptions that apply to all traditional, noncancer endpoint risk assessment procedures.[16] Despite their diversity, these assumptions share the attribute of being partially replaceable by factual information (TABLE 7). Many assumptions remain, however, and uncertainty reduction by filling knowledge gaps will ultimately require greater understanding of the biological mechanisms underlying neurotoxicity.

TABLE 8. Biomarkers of Neurotoxicity

| Biomarkers of Exposure | Agents | Time of Exposure |
|---|---|---|
| Blood or dentine concentration | lead | pre- or postnatal |
| Cerebral spinal fluid Concentrations of Dopamine Metabolites | MPTP[a] | postnatal |
| Cerebral spinal fluid Concentrations of a serotonin Metabolites | MDMA[b] | postnatal |
| Serum esterase | organophosphates | postnatal |

[a] MPTP, 1-methyl-4-phenyl-1,2,3,6-tetrahydropyridine.
[b] MDMA, methylenedioxymethamphetamine.

TABLE 9. Biomarkers of Neurotoxicity

| Biomarkers of Effect | Agents | Time of Exposure |
|---|---|---|
| Neurotransmitters | reserpine, MDMA[c] | pre- and postnatal |
| Receptors | reserpine | prenatal |
| Uptake sites | MDMA[c] | postnatal |
| Enzymes | | |
| Neurotransmitter synthesis | methamphetamine, MDMA[c] | postnatal |
| Metabolites (OCD[a]) | methylmercury, TMT[d] | pre- and postnatal |
| Neuropathology/ neurohistology | TMT,[d] MDMA[c] | postnatal |
| Proteins (GFAP[b]) | TMT,[d] MPTP[e] | postnatal |
| Neurophysiological | lead | pre- and postnatal |
| Behavior | cocaine, diazepam | pre- and postnatal |

[a] ODC orotidine-5-phosphate decarboxylase.
[b] GFAP, glial fibrillary acidic protein.
[c] MDMA, methylenedioxymethamphetamine.
[d] TMT, trimethyltin.
[e] MPTP, 1-methyl-4-phenyl-1,2,3,6-tetrahydropyridine.

*Biological Markers*

The appropriate selection and use of biological markers or biomarkers is fundamental for the conduct of risk assessments, for neurotoxicants and biomarkers can be used to reduce knowledge gaps and minimize assumptions. Biomarkers may be defined as indicators signaling events in a biological system and are classified into three categories, those of exposure, effect, and susceptibility.[16] Exposure biomarkers involve the quantitation either of exogenous agents or the complex of endogenous substances with exogenous agents within the system (TABLE 8). Biomarkers of effect are measures of an endogenous component of the biological system that is recognized as an alteration or disease (TABLE 9). A biomarker of susceptibility (TABLE 10) is an indicator that demonstrates that a particular biologi-

TABLE 10. Biomarkers of Neurotoxicity

| Biomarkers of Susceptibility | Agents | Time of Exposure |
|---|---|---|
| δ-Aminolevulinic acid dehydratase | lead | postnatal |
| Glucose-6-phosphate dehydrogenase | lead | postnatal |

cal system is especially vulnerable to toxic insult by an exogenous agent.[17] While the application of biomarkers to neurotoxicity risk assessment has not been widespread, biomarkers have been used for hazard identification or to investigate the mechanism of action of neurotoxicants.[18]

A single risk assessment model may not be adequate for all conditions of exposure, for all endpoints, or for all agents. Risk assessment models of the future may well include biomarkers of both effect and exposure as well as biologically-based mechanistic and pharmacokinetic considerations derived from both epidemiologic and experimental test system data.

## CONCLUSION

Although neuroprotective agents represent a special class of therapeutics designed specifically for certain beneficial effects, there remains the possibility that their use may also be accompanied by untoward effects. Quantitative risk assessment procedures can be used not only to identify those untoward effects or hazards but to determine the risk of adverse or abnormal outcome at any dose selected. Armed with quantitative information derived from biologically-based risk assessment procedures, informed risk management decisions can be made by regulators or physicians and their patients. Both the risk along with the uncertainty of risk and expected benefit of an agent can be weighed separately and balanced against each other. The greater the certainty of the risk of a given dose of neuroprotective agent, the greater the confidence in the final risk management decision.

## SUMMARY

Neurotoxicity may be defined as any adverse effect on the structure or function of the central and/or peripheral nervous system by a biological, chemical, or physical agent. Neurotoxic effects may be permanent or reversible, produced by neuropharmacological or neurodegenerative properties of a neurotoxicant, or the result of direct or indirect actions on the nervous system. A multidisciplinary approach is necessary to assess neurotoxicity because of the complexity and diverse functions of the nervous system. Many of the relevant effects can be measured directly by neurochemical, neurophysiological, and neuropathological techniques, whereas, others must be inferred from observed behavior. Some neurotoxicological data can be derived directly from humans. Neurotoxicity in humans is most commonly measured by relatively noninvasive neurophysiologic and neurobehavioral methods that assess cognitive, affective, sensory, and motor function. For most toxicological assessments, however, it is necessary to rely on information derived from animal models.[2,3] There are many approaches that can be used to assess neurotoxicity, including whole animal (*in vivo*) and tissue/cell culture (*in vitro*) testing. Neurotoxicity can be described at multiple levels of organization, including neurochemical, anatomical, physiological, and behavioral.

An important aspect of neurotoxic endpoint evaluation involves risk assessment procedures. Risk assessment may be defined as an empirically-based process used to determine the probability that adverse or abnormal effects are associated with exposure to a chemical, physical or biological agent. Risk management, on the other hand, is the process that applies information obtained through the risk assessment process to determine whether the assessed risk should be reduced and, if so, to what extent. For chemicals such as neuroprotective agents and other drugs designed to provide therapeutic benefits, information concerning these benefits is considered during the risk management phase. The risk assessment process usually involves four steps: hazard identification, dose-response assessment, exposure assessment, and risk characterization. Neurotoxicity risk assessment models of the future may well include biomarkers of both effect and exposure as well as biologically-based mechanistic and pharmacokinetic considerations derived from both epidemiologic and experimental data.

## REFERENCES

1. REITER, L. W., H. A. TILSON, J. DOUGHERTY, G. J. HARRY, C. J. JONES, S. MCMASTER, W. SLIKKER, JR. & T. J. SABOTKA. 1993. Final report: Principles of neurotoxicity risk assessment. Fed. Reg. **59**(158): 42360–42404.
2. SLIKKER, W., JR. 1994. Principles of developmental neurotoxicology. Neurotoxicology **15**(1): 11–16.
3. SLIKKER, W., JR. 1994. Placental transfer and pharmacokinetics of developmental neurotoxicants. *In* Principles of Neurotoxicology. L. Chang, Ed. 659–680. Marcel Dekker, Inc. New York.
4. NATIONAL RESEARCH COUNCIL (NRC). 1983. Risk assessment in the Federal Government. National Academy Press. Washington, DC.
5. BARNES, D. G. & M. DOURSON. 1988. Reference dose (RfD): description and use in health risk assessments. Reg. Toxicol. Pharmacol. **8**: 471–486.
6. KIMMEL, C. A. 1990. Quantitative approaches to human risk assessment for noncancer health effects. Neurotoxicology **11**: 189–198.
7. GAYLOR, D. W. & W. SLIKKER, JR. 1990. Risk assessment for neurotoxic effects. Neurotoxicology **11**: 211–218.
8. SLIKKER, W., JR. & D. W. GAYLOR. 1995. Concepts on quantitative risk assessment of neurotoxicants. *In* Neurotoxicology: Approaches and Methods. L. W. Chang & W. Slikker, Jr., Eds. 771–776. Academic Press. San Diego.
9. FOOD AND DRUG ADMINISTRATION ADVISORY COMMITTEE ON PROTOCOLS FOR SAFETY EVALUATION. 1971. Panel on carcinogenesis report on cancer testing in the safety evaluation of food additives and pesticides. Toxicol. Appl. Pharmacol. **20**: 419–438.
10. DEWS, P. B. 1986. On the assessment of risk. *In* Developmental Behavioral Pharmacology. N. Krasnegor, J. Gray & T. Thompson, Eds. 53–65. Lawrence Erlbaum Associates. Hillsdale, NJ.
11. GLOWA, J. R. & P. B. DEWS. 1987. Behavioral toxicology of volatile organic solvents. IV. Comparison of the behavioral effects of acetone, methyl ethyl ketone, ethyl acetate, carbon disulfide, and toluene on the responding of mice. J. Am. Coll. Toxicol. **6**: 461–469.
12. GLOWA, J. R., J. DEWESSE, M. E. NATALE & J. J. HOLLAND. 1983. Behavioral toxicology of volatile organic solvents. I. Methods: acute effects. J. Am. Coll. Toxicol. **2**: 175–185.
13. CRUMP, K. S. 1984. A new method for determining allowable daily intakes. Fund. Appl. Toxicol. **4**: 854–871.
14. GAYLOR, D. W. & W. SLIKKER, JR. 1992. Risk assessment for neurotoxicants. *In* Neurotoxicology. H. Tilson & C. Mitchell, Eds. 331–343. Raven Press. New York.
15. SLIKKER, W., JR. & D. W. GAYLOR. 1990. Biologically based dose-response model for neurotoxicity risk assessment. Korean J. Toxicol. **6**: 204–213.

16. SHEEHAN, D., J. F. YOUNG, W. SLIKKER, JR., D. W. GAYLOR & D. MATTISON. 1989. Workshop on risk assessment in reproductive and developmental toxicology: addressing the assumptions and identifying the research needs. Reg. Toxicol. Pharmacol. **10:** 110–122.
17. COMMITTEE ON BIOLOGICAL MARKERS OF THE NATIONAL RESEARCH COUNCIL. 1987. Biological markers in environmental health research. Environ. Health Perspect. **74:** 3–9.
18. SLIKKER, W., JR. 1991. Biomarkers of neurotoxicity: an overview. Recent advances on biomarker research. Biomed. Environ. Sci. **4:** 192–196.

# Discussion

D. BONHAUS (*Syntex Research, Palo Alto, CA*): Since a drug, or treatment scheme, which prevents death but does not improve quality of life (*i.e.*, marginally improves those who would otherwise die) may only be of questionable value, is it appropriate to use biologic markers that predict outcome in order to decide whom to withhold treatment from?

W. SLIKKER (*National Center for Toxicological Research, FDA, Jefferson, AR*): Biological markers (or biomarkers) may be defined as indicators signaling events in a biological system, and they are classified into three categories, those of exposure, effect, and susceptibility. Appropriate biomarkers of effect, for example, may be used for the conduct of risk assessments for nervous system active agents. The question you ask, however, is a risk management decision, *i.e.*, a decision made by the physician in this case based on both the risk of treatment and the benefit of treatment. The risk of a given treatment is determined by a risk assessment that might use biomarkers as an endpoint of toxicity. The benefit of a given treatment would be based on efficacy studies and/or clinical trials. Provided with the data, the physician in consultation with the patient or family members would make the risk management decision as to who would receive which treatment.

BONHAUS: Do we design our clinical trials to exclude those patients whose outcome will likely be poor from a quality of life standpoint, or is a decrease in mortality (irrespective of quality of life) a useful marker of drug efficacy?

SLIKKER: In reading reports concerning clinical trials, it would appear that enrollment is rigidly controlled to meet certain criteria. These criteria, including selection of endpoints to be evaluated, are determined by the study director in consultation with his/her coworkers and also, at least in part, by the goal of the study. Any endpoint including enhanced survival may be used.

# Neuroprotective Use-Dependent Blockers of Na$^+$ and Ca$^{2+}$ Channels Controlling Presynaptic Release of Glutamate[a]

STANLEY M. GOLDIN,[b,c,e] KATRAGADDA SUBBARAO,[b]
RAHUL SHARMA,[b] ANDREW G. KNAPP,[b] JAMES B. FISCHER,[b]
DEBORAH DALY,[b] GRAHAM J. DURANT,[b] N. LAXMA
REDDY,[b] LAIN-YEN HU,[b] SHARAD MAGAR,[b] MICHAEL E.
PERLMAN,[b] JUN CHEN,[d] STEVEN H. GRAHAM,[d] W. F. HOLT,[b]
DAVID BERLOVE,[b] AND LEE D. MARGOLIN[b]

[b]Cambridge NeuroScience
Cambridge, Massachusetts 02139
[c]Department of Biological Chemistry and Molecular
Pharmacology
Harvard Medical School
Boston, Massachusetts 02115
[d] Department of Neurology
University of California
and
Veterans Affairs Medical Center
San Francisco, California 94110

## SUMMARY

We have originated a family of N,N'-disubstituted guanidines that block the voltage-activated Ca$^{2+}$ and Na$^+$ channels governing glutamate release. These compounds, CNS 1237 (N-acenaphthyl-N'-methoxynaphthyl guanidine) and its analogues, are "use dependent" in their ability to attenuate neurotransmitter release: they block glutamate release with greater efficacy under conditions of persistent or repetitive depolarization, as would be encountered under pathophysiological circumstances, relative to their ability to block glutamate release elicited by brief, transient depolarizations more characteristic of normal physiological release events in nonischemic brain. Using electrophysiological and rapid kinetic methods, we have differentiated the use-dependent block of the relevant Na$^+$ and Ca$^{2+}$ channels governing neurotransmitter release from the mechanism of channel antagonism exhibited by, respectively, the substituted guanidine Na$^+$ channel blocker tetrodotoxin (TTX) and venom peptide Ca$^{2+}$ antagonists.

To characterize use-dependent Na$^+$ channel block by CNS 1237, we have

---

[a] This work was supported in part by NIH SBIR Grant No. R43-NS29597 (Cambridge NeuroScience/S. Goldin, P.I.).

[e] Address for correspondence: 10 Russell Road, Lexington, MA 02173.

employed whole-cell voltage-clamp recordings from a Chinese hamster ovary (CHO) cell line expressing cloned mammalian type II $Na^+$ channels. These experiments demonstrated that, in contrast to the actions of TTX under the same conditions, the potency of $Na^+$ channel block by CNS 1237 is greatly enhanced by depolarizing stimuli in a frequency-dependent manner. $Ca^{2+}$ channel-activated glutamate release from brain nerve terminal preparations was measured with ~300 msec time resolution over a 5-second period of high $K^+$-depolarization, using a rapid superfusion technique.[42] CNS 1237 and analogues, at 1–3 $\mu$M, accelerated the decay of glutamate release by 40–70%, reflecting depolarization-induced enhancement of block. In contrast, blockade of glutamate release by the $Ca^{2+}$ channel antagonist peptide toxins $\omega$-aga IV-A (from spider venom) and $\omega$-conotoxin M-VII-C (from cone snail venom) exhibited "reverse-use-dependence:" at concentrations of 0.3 $\mu$M, which blocked the initial amplitude of glutamate release by 40–60%, the decay time constant for glutamate release was significantly increased, indicating depolarization-induced relief of block.

These findings establish that CNS 1237 and other members of this compound series are use-dependent blockers of the voltage-activated ion channels governing glutamate release. Studies of CNS 1237 in the rat middle cerebral artery occlusion (MCAO) focal stroke model have indicated infarct size reduction comparable to that observed by the same investigators for the glutamate release blocker (BW 619C89 (Burroughs-Wellcome, now in clinical development). Maximal infarct size reduction is achieved with a 3-mg/kg bolus followed by a 4-hour infusion of 0.75 mg/kg/hr. Neuroprotective doses of CNS 1237 produced no significant reduction of blood pressure, and a modest dose-dependent reduction in heart rate. Maximal neuroprotection was maintained over a 4-fold dose range in the absence of significant reduction of blood pressure. We hypothesize that use-dependence channel block by CNS 1237, acting at a common site of shared homology between presynaptic $Ca^{2+}$ channels and type II neuronal $Na^+$ channels, is the mechanistic basis for its neuroprotective efficacy.

## INTRODUCTION

### Use-Dependent Blockers of the Postsynaptic Actions of Released Glutamate

Blockers of a key postsynaptic event resulting from glutamate release resulting from brain ischemia, namely, $Ca^{2+}$ entry through the ion channel associated with the $N$-methyl-D-aspartate (NMDA) subclass of glutamate receptors, are now in clinical trials for stroke and head trauma.[1] Such ion-channel blockers, among them the substituted guanidine CNS 1102 (aptiganel hydrochloride), exhibit "use-dependence" in their actions: sustained depolarization of the postsynaptic membrane, as occurs during an ischemic or traumatic insult to the brain, relieves block by extracellular $Mg^{2+}$ of the ion-channel of the NMDA receptor,[2] affording the opportunity for these drugs to block the channel. This property distinguishes ion-channel blockers from antagonists of the NMDA/glutamate receptor binding site such as CGS 19755, and these mechanistic differences between the two classes of agents may extend to their relative efficacy and safety as neuroprotectants.

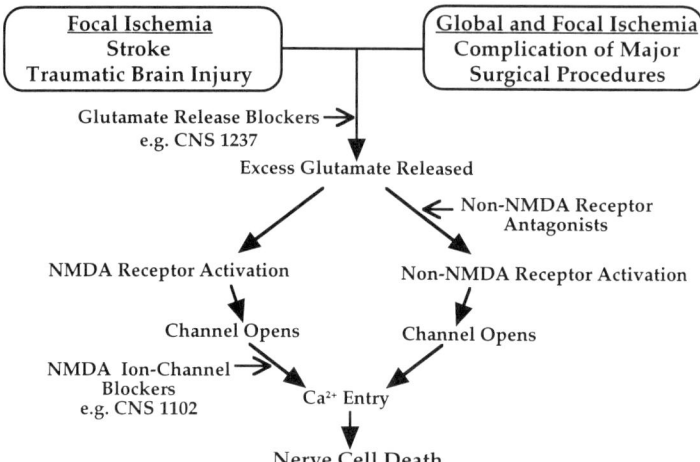

**FIGURE 1.** Diagram depicting a cascade of biological events initiated by brain ischemia and leading to nerve cell death. See text for further explanation.

Recent microdialysis studies of glutamate release in the brains of head trauma patients[3] indicate that within hours of injury, extracellular glutamate reaches levels (mean of 30 $\mu$M) sufficient to compete with glutamate receptor antagonists such as CGS 19755 for the glutamate binding site of the NMDA receptor. This raises the concern that the environment within injured brain tissue may attenuate the ability of such receptor antagonists to block NMDA receptor activation, creating a situation of *de facto* "reverse use-dependence." The results of ongoing clinical trials and further *in vivo* studies may, in the future, shed light on the degree to which differences in the mechanism of action between NMDA receptor antagonists and ion-channel blockers affect their relative efficacy and safety.

The direct demonstration of excessive glutamate release in brain-injured patients supports the hypothesis that blockers of glutamate release could be used as neuroprotective agents. This article focuses on our efforts to develop such a class of use-dependent neuroprotective agents: potent blockers of the voltage-activated $Ca^{2+}$ and $Na^+$ channels controlling the release of glutamate. Our own *in vitro* and *in vivo* findings are prefaced by an overview of the role of specific subclasses of voltage-activated $Ca^{2+}$ and $Na^+$ channels in regulation of glutamate release and metabolism in ischemic brain.

### *Glutamate Release Blockers as Neuroprotectants*

FIGURE 1 illustrates the generally accepted key steps in the cascade of events that lead to neuronal cell death in ischemia. NMDA antagonists prevent nerve cell death resulting from the events depicted in the lefthand limb of the diagram. Antagonists of non-NMDA receptors block cell death resulting from the events shown on the righthand limb of the diagram. NMDA antagonists are highly effective in animal models of focal cerebral ischemia,[4] but are reportedly less effective in models of global cerebral ischemia.[5,6] In contrast, non-NMDA antagonists such as 2,3-dihydroxy-6-nitro-7-sulphamoyl-benzo(f)-quinoxaline (NBQX) are highly effective in rat models of global cerebral ischemia,[7] but are apparently less effective in models of focal cerebral ischemia.[8]

A blocker of glutamate release, by acting at an earlier stage of the process, prevents excessive activation of *both* NMDA and non-NMDA receptor subclasses, and thus in theory combines the advantages of blockers of ion channel activity mediated by both NMDA and non-NMDA receptors. The anticipated efficacy of glutamate release blockers in both focal and global ischemia was recently demonstrated in *in vivo* studies of the glutamate release blocker BW 1003C87.[9,10]

Glutamate release blockers should be well suited to acute treatment of brain damage resulting from high risk cardiovascular surgery. For example, in coronary artery bypass surgery, subsequent neurological deficits have been attributed not only to interruption of the brain's blood supply from the heart, which constitutes a global ischemic insult, but also to small clots (microemboli) that product multiple focal cerebral lesions.[11]

### *Voltage-Activated $Na^+$ and $Ca^{2+}$ Channels Together Govern Presynaptic Glutamate Release*

Voltage-activated $Na^+$-channels in axons and nerve terminals initiate glutamate release by propagating a depolarizing stimulus to the sites of vesicular release.[12] Presynaptic voltage-activated $Ca^{2+}$ channels at the release sites are opened in response to this depolarization. The elevation of cytoplasmic $Ca^{2+}$ levels in the nerve terminal initiates the process of exocytosis of glutamate.[6,8]

### *Neuronal Voltage-Activated $Na^+$ Channels*

The following discussion serves to further explain the connection between block of neuronal $Na^+$ channels and inhibition of glutamate release. In focal ischemic situations such as stroke, sustained hypoxia in the "core region" results from occlusion of the blood supply by a clot.[13] As hypoxia develops, adenosine triphosphate (ATP) depletion leads to an inability of the active Na/K-ion pump, the Na,K-ATPase, to maintain the ion gradients which generate the normal membrane potential of resting nerve cells.[14] As the cell depolarizes and reaches the threshold for action potential firing, $Na^+$ channels are activated. Based on extrapolation of our understanding of the physiology and pathophysiology of brain function, hyperactivity of $Na^+$ channels appears to have at least two important pathophysiological consequences leading to excessive glutamate release:

a. Trains of action potentials may invade the penumbra from the core. This propagates the excessive glutamate release, and hence the neuronal damage, to regions well beyond the ischemic focus;

b.  Ion gradients in axons and nerve terminals are further depleted, generating an increased energy demand to reestablish $Na^+$ and $K^+$ gradients and, secondarily, for reuptake and resynthesis of neurotransmitters released as a result of hyperactivity. The resulting rise in intracellular $[Na^+]$ and concomitant membrane depolarization causes damaging levels of $Ca^{2+}$ to enter the neuron through reverse operation of the electrogenic $Na^+/Ca^{2+}$ exchanger. These secondary events can lead to further excessive release of glutamate.

Stys et al.[15] reported the development of $Na^+$ channel hyperactivity in anoxia of central white matter and demonstrated in vivo the neuroprotective effect of the $Na^+$ channel blockers tetrodotoxin (TTX) and saxitoxin (STX). Their experiments substantiate the pathophysiological role of mechanisms (a) and (b) described above.

The neuron-specific type II subclass of voltage-activated $Na^+$ channels, found in nerve axons and nerve terminals,[16,17] is claimed to be the most directly involved of all the $Na^+$ channels in initiating release of glutamate and other neurotransmitters.[18] Several antagonists of the neuron-specific type II subclass of voltage-gated $Na^+$ channels have been shown to be neuroprotective blockers of glutamate release.[9,15,19-22]

A particularly concrete demonstration of the neuroprotective efficacy of glutamate release inhibitors which act through blockade of type II $Na^+$ channels comes from recently published in vivo studies of the glutamate release blockers, BW 1003C87 and BW 619C89 (Burroughs-Wellcome), the latter now in human clinical trials as a neuroprotectant.[9,10,23,24]

*Presynaptic $Ca^{2+}$ Channel Subclasses: P-, Q-, and N-Type*

Regarding the involvement of presynaptic voltage-activated $Ca^{2+}$ channels in glutamate release, it is first useful to summarize the current state of knowledge of $Ca^{2+}$ channel diversity and pharmacology. It is generally accepted that there are at least four subclasses of $Ca^{2+}$ channels (T, N, P and L) that differ in their pharmacology, location in neuronal and nonneuronal tissues, and physiological properties.[25,26] Pharmacological criteria have been used to distinguish among these channel subclasses: L-type $Ca^{2+}$ channels are particularly sensitive to dihydropyridine $Ca^{2+}$ antagonists such as nifedipine and nimodipine, and N-type $Ca^{2+}$ channels are specifically blocked by the cone snail peptide, $\omega$-conotoxin G-VI-A.[27] Recently, a new subclass of presynaptic $Ca^{2+}$ channels controlling neurotransmitter release, termed "Q-type," was identified.[28] Q-type channels are closely related to P-type $Ca^{2+}$ channels: P- and Q-type $Ca^{2+}$ channels are insensitive to dihydropyridine $Ca^{2+}$ antagonists or $\omega$-conotoxin G-VI-A. However, both P- and Q-type channels are specifically blocked by the spider venom peptide $\omega$-aga IV-A, the former subclass being more sensitive to this toxin than the latter.

Recent evidence suggests that N-, P-, and Q-type channels all contribute to the presynaptic regulation of glutamate release in central neurons.[29,30] P- and/or Q-type $Ca^{2+}$ channels appear to play the dominant role in control of glutamate release from isolated nerve terminal preparations (synaptosomes) of mammalian

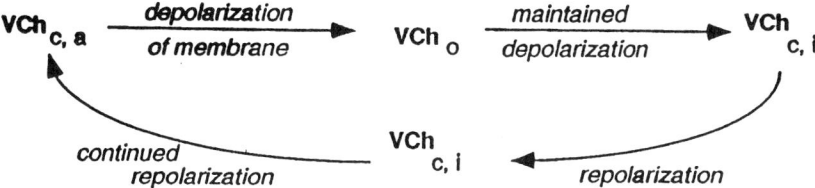

**FIGURE 2.** Conformational states correlated with particular functional states of voltage-activated $Ca^{2+}$ and $Na^+$ channels. $VCh_{c,a}$ = closed, activatable channel; $VCh_o$ = open channel; $VCH_{c,i}$ = inactivated channel.

brain, as shown below and by Turner et al.[31] Studies of glutamate release as measured by rapid superfusion have demonstrated[31,32] that the P-/Q-type $Ca^{2+}$ channel selective spider venom peptide ω-aga IV-A blocks glutamate release from rat brain synaptosomes. This establishes that the P- and/or Q-type $Ca^{2+}$ channel(s) constitute the presynaptic $Ca^{2+}$ channel subclass(es) controlling the $Ca^2$-dependent glutamate release which, as demonstrated below, is blocked by members of our novel compound series.

## Properties of Voltage-Activated Channels Controlling Presynaptic Glutamate Release

Use-dependence may be engineered into a blocker of voltage-activated channels controlling glutamate release by designing compounds which selectively interact with a particular functional state of the channel. Voltage-activated $Ca^{2+}$ and $Na^+$ channels cycle through a series of conformational states in response to changes in membrane potential, which occur during both normal and pathophysiological channel activity.[33,34] These conformational states, which correlate with particular functional states of the channels, are most simply schematized as in FIGURE 2.

In response to depolarization of the cell membrane to, typically, $-10$ to $+20$ mV, an ion channel is more likely to be found in the open state or in the closed, inactivated state. Ion channels in a metabolically "healthy" cell are most frequently found in the closed, activatable state at the cell's hyperpolarized, "resting" membrane potential of, typically, $-60$ to $-100$ mV.

Certain pathophysiological circumstances produce sustained and/or repetitive depolarization of the cell membrane. Excessive depolarization occurs in acute disorders, among them brain ischemia resulting from stroke and cardiac arrest[6,8] and head trauma.[35] Excessive depolarization has also been hypothesized to occur in chronic disorders, among them epilepsy,[36,37] amyotrophic lateral sclerosis (ALS),[38] and Huntington's disease.[39] Excessive and/or inappropriately timed depolarization of the cell membrane accelerates cellular $Ca^{2+}$ entry, which in turn elevates free cellular $Ca^{2+}$ levels to a degree that leads to cellular injury and destruction.[8,35,39]

## METHODS

### Electrophysiology

The ability of CNS 1237 to block voltage-activated type II $Na^+$ channels was determined electrophysiologically in a Chinese hamster ovary (CHO) cell line expressing cloned type II $Na^+$ channels (CNaIIA-1) derived from rat brain.[40] The experiments utilized the whole cell configuration of the voltage clamp recording technique,[41] which allows a direct measurement of inward $Na^+$ current. The protocol takes advantage of the fact that varying the timing of stimuli relative to the application $Na^+$ channel antagonists provides a means of distinguishing between tonic (resting state) and frequency-dependent (open state) blockade of $Na^+$ channels.

The CNaIIA-1 cells are grown in RPMI 1640 (MediaTech) supplemented with 5% fetal calf serum, G418, and proline. Trypsin (1:250) is used to split the cells 1 X per week and cells are seeded @ 1:100 into a T75 flask and 1:200–1:6400 into a 24-well plate containing glass coverslips. Cells whose passage number exceeds 20–25 were not used.

The external recording solution contains, in mM: 150 NaCl, 5 KCl, 1.5 $CaCl_2$, 1 $MgCl_2$, 5 glucose, 5 HEPES, pH 7.4. The internal pipette solution contains 150 CsF, 10 EGTA, 10 HEPES, pH 7.4 adjusted with CsOH. Whole cell currents are measured using an Axopatch 200A integrating patch clamp amplifier. Inward sodium currents are elicited by stepping from a holding potential of $-90$ mV to a test potential of 0 mV.

An experimental protocol was developed to differentiate between a compound's ability to induce tonic block (blockade of the resting state) and its ability to produce frequency-dependent block (block of the open and/or inactivated state) of sodium channels. Tonic and frequency-dependent block was determined by first recording a series of control whole-cell sodium currents evoked by stimuli delivered at a rate of 1 Hz (FIG. 3A). The drugs were then bath applied to the recording chamber at a rate of 2 ml/min for a period of 2 min in the absence of stimulation. A series of 10 stimuli was delivered (again at 1 Hz) in the presence of the drug. The drugs were then washed out and the cell allowed to fully recover. The entire regime was then repeated using trains of 40 stimuli at 10 Hz. The degree of tonic block was determined by dividing the current amplitude recorded from the first pulse of the test train ($I_{first}$) by the average current recording during the control train ($I_{ave.control}$). The degree of frequency-dependent block was determined by dividing all the current amplitudes of a given trial ($I_{pulse}$) by the largest amplitude of that trial ($I_{max\ pulse}$, usually the first) for frequency-dependent block (Eq. 2).

$$\text{Relative current}_{tonic} = (I_{first}/I_{ave.control}) \quad (1)$$

$$\text{Relative current}_{frequency\text{-}dependent} = (I_{pulse}/I_{max\ pulse}) \quad (2)$$

Relative current$_{frequency\text{-}dependent}$ was then plotted together as a function of time and the resulting graph was fitted by the single exponential function shown in Eq. 3.

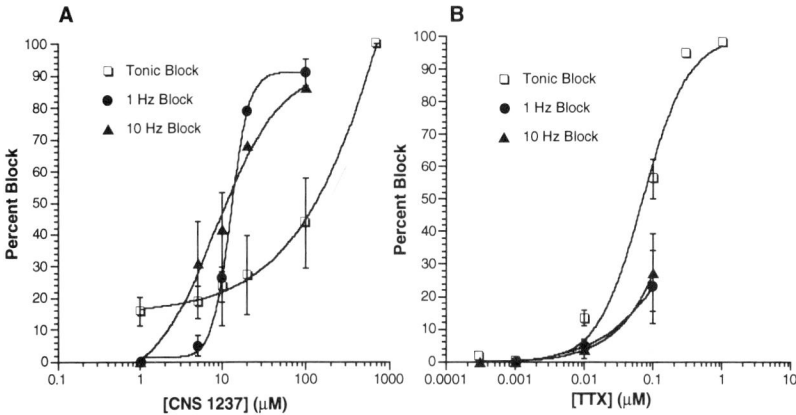

**FIGURE 3.** (A) Use-dependent enhancement of the potency of block by CNS 1237 of voltage-activated Na$^+$ channels expressed in a CNaIIA-1 cells. (B) Relative lack of use-dependence of the ability of TTX to block Na$^+$ channels, when subjected to the same protocol. See Methods and Results for further details.

$$y = ae^{(-x/t)} + b, \qquad (3)$$

where $t$ is the time constant of the onset of block and $b$ is the maximum degree of block.

### Rapid Superfusion

The rapid superfusion method has been described in detail elsewhere.[42]

### $^{45}Ca^{2+}$ Uptake

The uptake of $^{45}Ca^{2+}$ into brain synaptosomes was performed by an adaptation of the method of Nachsen and Blaustein[43] as previously described.[44] This method identifies a component of $^{45}Ca^{2+}$ uptake mediated by the voltage-activated calcium channels directly controlling neurotransmitter release.[43] The principle of the method involves opening ion permeation through synaptosomal calcium channels by high K$^+$-induced depolarization of the synaptosomal preparation. The rapid component of $^{45}Ca^{2+}$ uptake measured by this procedure is mediated by presynaptic calcium channels.

Briefly, synaptosomes were suspended in low potassium "LK" buffer (containing 3 mM KCl). Test compounds in LK buffer were added, and the mixture was preincubated for 5 minutes at room temperature. $^{45}Ca^{2+}$ uptake was then initiated by adding isotope in either LK or in buffer ("HK") containing high potassium (150 mM KCl). After 5 seconds, the $^{45}Ca^{2+}$ uptake was stopped by adding 0.9 ml quench buffer (LK + 10 mM EGTA). This solution was then filtered under vacuum

TABLE 1. Dosing Parameters for CNS 1237

| Group (# of Rats) | Bolus Dose, mg/kg @ Conc., mg/ml | 4-Hour Infusion Rate, mg/kg/hr @ Conc., mg/ml | 4-Hour Infusion Volume, ml/kg/hr |
|---|---|---|---|
| A (8) | none (vehicle) | 0 (vehicle) | 1.0 |
| B (8) | 3 @ 0.75 | 0.75 @ 0.75 | 1.0 |
| C (8) | 6 @ 1.5 | 1.5 @ 1.5 | 1.0 |
| D (8) | 12 @ 3.0 | 3.0 @ 3.0 | 1.0 |

and the filters washed. Net depolarization-induced $^{45}Ca^{2+}$ uptake was determined as the difference between $^{45}Ca^{2+}$ uptake in HK and LK buffers.

## Middle Cerebral Artery Occlusion

The middle cerebral artery occlusion (MCAO) model and infarct analysis have been described elsewhere.[9,23] Focal ischemia was induced in rats by occlusion of the MCA, using the technique of Shiraishi et al.[45] Male Sprague-Dawley rats (275–300 g) were induced with 5% isoflurane, intubated, and ventilated with 1.5% isoflurane. The femoral artery and vein were cannulated. Normothermia is maintained by heating the animals with an infrared heating lamp, which was thermostatically controlled to maintain contralateral temporalis muscle temperature at 37 ± 0.2°C. An incision was made over the temporal scalp, the temporalis muscle was retracted, and a portion of the maxilla was removed to expose the foramen ovale. The foramen ovale was enlarged to expose the origin of the MCA. The MCA was then coagulated under direct vision from its origin to the olfactory tract. Care was taken to coagulate the penetrating arteries that arise from the MCA and supply the lateral caudate at this level.

The operator and all assistants were blinded as to which animal received drug. CNS 1237, mesylate salt, was given as an i.v. bolus (slow push over 15') in 0.3 M mannitol, at the concentrations specified below. All surgery except electrocoagulation of the MCA and perforators was performed immediately before the bolus dose. Electrocoagulation, which takes 1–2 minutes, commenced 5 minutes following the push. This procedure helps make the onset of ischemia as uniform as possible with respect to dosing. The infusion was initiated immediately after the surgery. Four dose groups of 8 animals each were tested (TABLE 1).

Animals were euthanized with pentobarbital 24 hr after MCA occlusion. Brains were coronally sectioned at 2-mm intervals from the anterior limit of the caudate to the posterior hippocampus. Sections were rapidly immersed in 2% 2, 3, 5-triphenyltetrazolium chloride (TTC) in buffered Ringer's solution at pH 7.4 for 20 minutes at 37.5°C,[46] and sections were transferred to 4% formaldehyde buffer for 15 minutes prior to photography. Photographs of the 8 sections were analyzed by a blinded observer using a computerized image analysis system (MCID, St. Catherine, Ontario, Canada). Unstained tissue was classified as infarcted. Hemispheric infarct area in each section was calculated by subtracting the area of normally TTC staining brain in the ischemic hemisphere from the contralateral nonischemic hemisphere area. The volume of infarction for the total brain hemisphere was calculated by summing the infarct area in each section measured, and multiplying by the distance between sections.[46]

Blood pressure was monitored continuously during and for 4 hours following the surgery for selected animals. Heart rate was monitored continuously during the loading infusion, at 10-minute intervals for the first hour, and at 30-minute intervals thereafter.

## RESULTS AND DISCUSSION

### *Depolarization-Dependent Enhancement of Block of Voltage-Activated $Na^+$ Channels*

The CNaII CHO cell line was employed to assess the electrophysiological actions of CNS 1237 ($N$-$N'$-acenaphthyl-methoxynaphthyl-guanidine) in a manner that directly demonstrated its use-dependent block of cloned, expressed type II $Na^+$ channels. Channel block by CNS 1237 was examined using the whole-cell voltage clamp recording technique.

As illustrated (FIG. 3A), CNS 1237 is markedly more potent in its ability to block type II $Na^+$ channels when the channels are repetitively opened by trains of depolarizing impulses. The $IC_{50}$ for *tonic* blockade of this channel is ~100 $\mu$M, whereas the $IC_{50}$ for additional *frequency-dependent* blockade of this channel is at least tenfold lower. These effects are analogous to the actions of a number of antiarrhythmic drugs on cardiac $Na^+$ channels.[47] This supports the hypothesis that CNS 1237 interacts preferentially with open and/or inactivated states of the channel, relative to its actions on channels in the closed but activatable state favored in resting, hyperpolarized cells.

In contrast, tetrodotoxin (TTX) exhibits potent block of said $Na^+$ channels irrespective of whether the channels are repetitively opened by trains of depolarization of the cell membrane (FIG. 3B). The tonic block dose-response curve for TTX is shifted to the left of the frequency-dependent curves, which overlap each other. Therefore it is concluded that TTX is better at producing tonic block of $Na^+$ channels than it is at producing frequency-dependent block.

Repetitive depolarizing pulses accelerate the rate at which CNS 1237 blocks type II neuronal $Na^+$ channels, as illustrated in FIGURE 4A. Following an initial reduction of whole cell current due to tonic block (relative current is 0.85 at time = 0), blockade progresses in a use-dependent manner; that is, the attenuation of the remaining whole cell $Na^+$ current by CNS 1237 is enhanced by repetitive depolarization. As the stimulation rate is increased from 1 Hz to 10 Hz, the rate and magnitude of blockade is concomitantly increased. We hypothesize that this is due either to enhancement by repetitive depolarization of the rate of onset of block, and/or to an increase in the potency of the compound's ability to block $Na^+$ channels at steady state when equilibrium between the blocked and unblocked states of the channel at this stimulus frequency has been reached.

This characteristic is contrasted with the inability of TTX to produce the same phenomenon when tested as described: as shown (FIG. 4B), at concentrations of

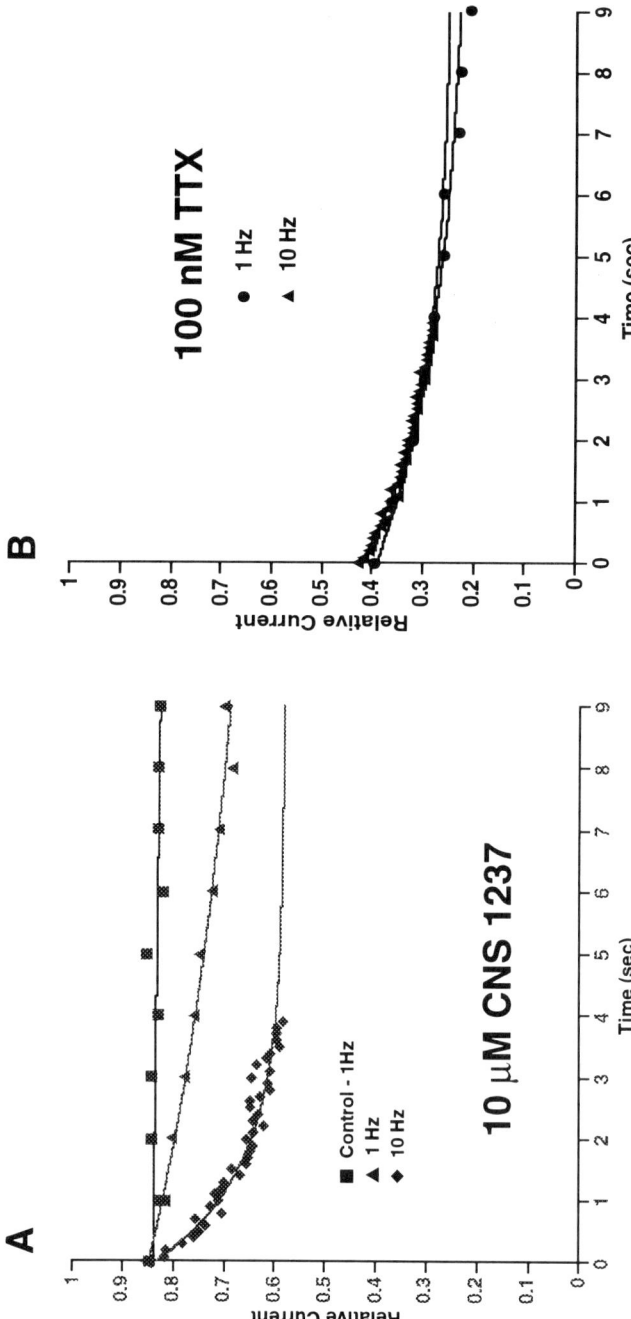

**FIGURE 4.** (**A**) Use-dependent acceleration of block by 10 μM CNS 1237 of voltage-activated Na$^+$ channels expressed in a CNaIIA-1 cells. Following an initial reduction of whole cell current due to tonic block (relative current is 0.85 at time = 0), blockade progresses in a use-dependent manner; that is, the attenuation of the remaining whole cell Na$^+$ current by CNS 1237 is enhanced by repetitive depolarization. As the stimulation rate is increased from 1 Hz to 10 Hz, the rate and magnitude of blockade is concomitantly increased. (**B**) The lack of depolarization-dependent enhancement of the rate of block of voltage-activated Na$^+$ channels by TTX, when subjected to the same protocol. See Methods and Results for further details.

tetrodotoxin (50 nM) sufficient to achieve ~40% tonic block, low levels of stimulation do not accelerate or potentiate additional block. Thus, in contrast to CNS 1237, TTX rapidly blocks type II $Na^+$ channels, in a manner largely independent of repetitive stimulation.

## Use-Dependent Block by CNS 1237 and Analogues of $Ca^{2+}$-Channel-Mediated Glutamate Release

We have employed a novel rapid superfusion system[42] to measure $^3$H-glutamate release from brain nerve terminals. The method involves first preloading rat brain synaptosomes with $^3$H-glutamate via the $Na^+$-dependent glutamate uptake system. The preloaded nerve terminals are retained in a superfusion chamber accessed by high-speed, solenoid-driven valves. Microcomputer-operated circuitry controls the timing of valve operation; the valves control the delivery under nitrogen pressure of depolarizing pulses of high $K^+$ buffer, $Ca^{2+}$, and/or drugs to the synaptosomes. The $^3$H-glutamate-containing effluent is continuously collected in a high speed fraction collector on a time scale as short as 30 msec. The high solution flow rate and minimal dead volume of the superfusion chamber, afford rapid solution changes and precise control of the chemical microenvironment of the nerve terminal preparation. This rapid superfusion method resolves a phasic $Ca^{2+}$-dependent component of glutamate release which decays with a time constant of ~100 msec, a more persistent $Ca^{2+}$-dependent component (time constant $\geq$ 1 sec), and a persistent $Ca^{2+}$-independent component of release.

The adaptation of rapid superfusion to drug discovery led to the creation of CNS 1237 and analogues: a family of substituted guanidines which selectively block the component of $Ca^{2+}$-dependent glutamate release mediated by persistent depolarization.[48] CNS 1237 and analogues exhibited use-dependent block of $Ca^{2+}$-dependent $^3$H-glutamate release, as revealed by further characterization of the kinetics of glutamate release inhibition. The decay of glutamate release, when measured at ~300 msec time resolution, can be fitted by a single exponential with a decay time constant of about one second (FIG. 5). This figure illustrates the ability of CNS 1237 to inhibit glutamate release and accelerate the decay of the $Ca^{2+}$-dependent release event: CNS 1237, at 1 $\mu$M, has little effect on the initial amplitude of the glutamate release event, but after 1–2 sec of sustained depolarization will reduce the rate of release by ~40–60%. This observation constituted the first line of evidence that this acceleration of decay was due to depolarization-dependent block of the presynaptic $Ca^{2+}$ channels controlling $Ca^{2+}$-dependent glutamate release. This property constituted a novel selection criterion, which has facilitated the creation of a variety of additional analogues of CNS 1237 which exhibit use-dependence (FIG. 6).

Such use-dependent block is a therapeutically attractive property for an antiischemic agent, as such an agent would be more effective in blocking persistent, excessive glutamate release activity observed in ischemia than the brief, transient responses characteristic of "normal" release events. This property of CNS 1237 and analogues is closely analogous to the "classical" observation of the acceleration of decay of action potentials by use-dependent ion channel antagonists such

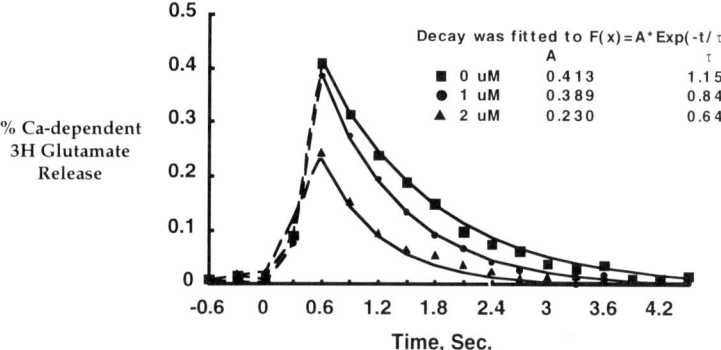

**FIGURE 5.** CNS 1237 reduces the amplitude and accelerates the decay of $Ca^{2+}$-dependent $^3$H-glutamate release. Rat brain nerve terminals, loaded with $^3$H-glutamate, were superfused with high-K buffer (55 mM K) with or without $Ca^{2+}$ (2.4 mM). Similar experiments were also done with 1 $\mu$M and 2 $\mu$M CNS 1237 in superfusion buffers. Experiments without $Ca^{2+}$ were subtracted from the corresponding experiments with $Ca^{2+}$ to obtain $Ca^{2+}$-dependent release. Release was expressed as % of specific $^3$H-glutamate uptake by nerve terminals. $Ca^{2+}$-dependent release was fitted to a single exponential decay equation. See Methods, Results, and Ref. 1 for further details. (From Goldin et al.[59] Reprinted by permission from the New York Academy of Sciences.)

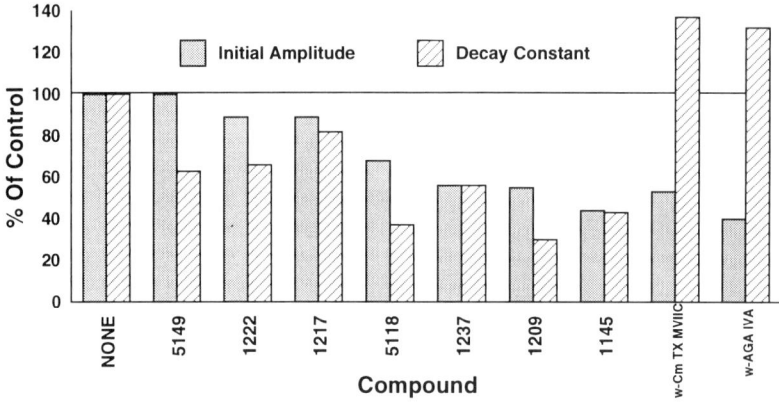

**FIGURE. 6.** Use-dependent actions of proprietary substituted guanidies on nerve terminal $Ca^{2+}$ channels, as manifested by the ability of the compounds to accelerate the decay of K-evoked, $Ca^{2+}$-dependent glutamate release from brain nerve terminals as measured by rapid superfusion. As shown, this is in contrast to prolongation of the decay constant of glutamate release by the peptide toxin blockers of presynaptic P- and Q-type channels, $\omega$-conotoxin M-VII-C and $\omega$-aga IV-A. Initial amplitudes and decay constants were calculated as in FIGURE 4. The results are from a minimum of 3 different experiments of each condition. CNS compounds were tested at 2 $\mu$M with the exception of 5149 (1 $\mu$M) and 5118 (3 $\mu$M). $\omega$-Aga IV-A and $\omega$-conotoxin M-VII-C were tested at 0.3 $\mu$M. See Methods, Results, and Ref. 1 for further details.

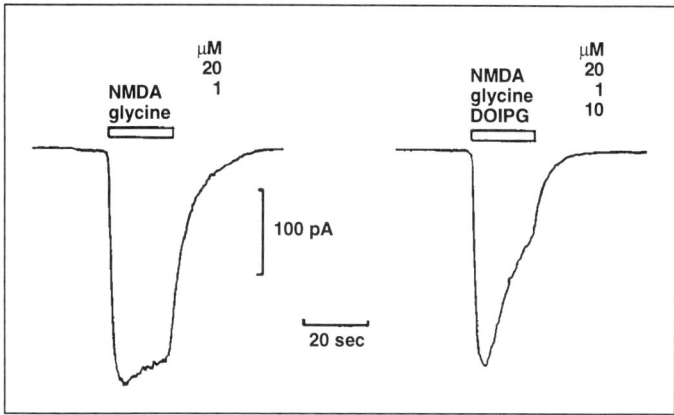

**FIGURE 7.** Use-dependent block of NMDA-activated ion channels by the NMDA antagonist $N,N'$-di-($o$-iodophenyl)guanidine (DOIPG), a structural and functional analogue of CNS 1102. Use dependence is manifested by the effect of 10 $\mu$M DOIPG on membrane currents induced by the application of 20 $\mu$M NMDA (plus 1 $\mu$M glycine) to a cultured rat hippocampal neuron. *Left:* control response to NMDA. *Right:* response generated when DOIPG was included with NMDA. Note the marked acceleration of the decay of the response induced by DOIPG. This behavior is due to block of open NMDA-activated channels by DOIPG. See Ref. 50 for further details. (From Keana *et al.*[50] Reprinted by permission from the National Academy of Sciences.)

as lidocaine,[49] and also bears relation to the effect of analogues of CNS 1102, which accelerate the decay of NMDA-induced postsynaptic currents in hippocampal neurons as a result of their use-dependent block of the ion channel associated with the NMDA receptor[50] (FIG. 7).

### $Ca^{2+}$-Dependent Glutamate Release Is Mediated by Presynaptic P-Q Type $Ca^{2+}$ Channels

Further evidence supports the hypothesis that depolarization-dependent block of $Ca^{2+}$-dependent $^3$H-glutamate release from brain nerve terminals by CNS 1237 is due to blockade of presynaptic $Ca^{2+}$ channels. We have confirmed the recent report[51] that $\omega$-aga IV-A blocks the uptake of radioisotopically labeled $Ca^{2+}$ ($^{45}Ca^{2+}$) into synaptosomes (TABLE 2), establishing additional direct evidence that P-type and/or Q-type $Ca^{2+}$ channels are found presynaptically and control the release of glutamate from brain nerve terminals. Notably, CNS 1237 and analogues

**TABLE 2.** Inhibition of $^{45}Ca^{2+}$ Uptake by the P-/Q-Type $Ca^{2+}$ Channel-Specific Spider Toxin, $\omega$-Aga IV-A

| Compound | IC$_{50}$, Block of $^{45}Ca^{2+}$ Uptake, $\mu$M |
|---|---|
| $\omega$-Aga IV-A | 152 |

**TABLE 3.** Inhibition of $^{45}Ca^{2+}$ Uptake through Presynaptic $Ca^{2+}$ Channels

| Compound No. | Name | $IC_{50}$, Block of $^{45}Ca^{2+}$ Uptake, $\mu M$ | Salt |
| --- | --- | --- | --- |
| CNS 1145 | $N,N^+$-bis(5-acenaphthyl)-guanidine | 1.1 | HBr |
| CNS 1209 | $N,N'$-bis(3-acenaphthyl)-guanidine | 11* | HBr |
| CNS 1222 | $N$-(5-(3)-acenaphthyl)-$N'$-(4-isopropylphenyl)-guanidine | 6.3* | HCl |
| CNS 1237 | $N$-(5-acenaphthyl)-$N'$-(4-methoxynaphthyl)-guanidine | 2.7 | mesylate |
| CNS 5088 | $N$-(5-acenaphthyl)-$N'$-(3-biphenyl)-guanidine | 1.4 | HCl |
| CNS 5118 | $N$-(5-acenaphthyl)-$N'$-(3-acenaphthyl)-guanidine | 8.6* | mesylate |

\* The $IC_{50}$ may be severalfold lower when corrected for partitioning of drug into synaptosomes. Other values noted have been corrected for drug partitioning.

which exhibit depolarization-dependent block of $^3$H-glutamate release from brain nerve terminal preparations also block the uptake of $^{45}Ca^{2+}$ into synaptosomes prepared by the same method (Table 3). The $IC_{50}$ for block of $^{45}Ca^{2+}$ uptake are in reasonable agreement with the concentrations of these compounds which attenuate $^3$H-glutamate release, as shown below.

### "Reverse Use-Dependence" of Venom Peptide Block of $Ca^{2+}$-Channel-Mediated Glutamate Release

It has been shown electrophysiologically that prolonged or repetitive depolarization relieves rather than potentiates block of voltage-activated $Ca^{2+}$ channels by $\omega$-aga IV-A and $\omega$-conotoxin M-VII-C.[31,52] This has also been shown to be the case for structurally related cone snail peptides $\omega$-conotoxin M-VII-A (SNX-111) and $\omega$-conotoxin G-VI-A.[53]

Our rapid superfusion measurements of the effects of $\omega$-aga IV-A and $\omega$-conotoxin M-VII-C on glutamate release confirm this observation: as shown in FIGURE 6, the decay constant for $Ca^{2+}$-dependent neurotransmitter release blocked by these venom peptides is prolonged rather than reduced, in direct contrast to the actions of CNS 1237 and analogues on $Ca^{2+}$-dependent $^3$H-glutamate release from brain nerve terminal preparations.

The aforementioned results indicate that presynaptic P- and/or Q-type $Ca^{2+}$ channels control $Ca^{2+}$-dependent $^3$H-glutamate release and are the targets of use-dependent blockade by CNS 1237 of $K^+$-stimulated, $Ca^{2+}$-dependent $^3$H-glutamate release from brain synaptosomes.

### Neuroprotective Efficacy and Cardiovascular Safety of CNS 1237 in a Rat MCAO Model

The evidence above indicates that CNS 1237 blocks, at comparable concentrations, both the presynaptic $Ca^{2+}$ channels and the neuronal $Na^+$ channels corresponding to those which control glutamate release *in vivo*. Block occurs in a use-

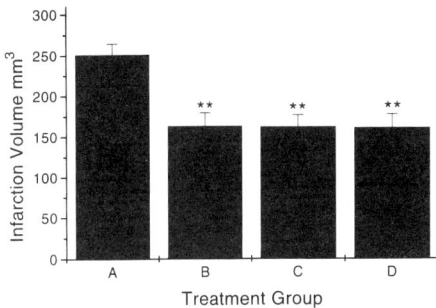

**FIGURE 8.** Infarction volumes in rat MCAO after drug treatment (B-D) vs control (A). All 3 treatment groups had significantly reduced infarction volumes ($\geq 35\%$) compared to control. *Error bars* denote SEM values. See Methods for details of protocol and dosing groups.

dependent manner suggesting a potentially attractive profile of efficacy and safety for this compound. Acceptable pharmacokinetic properties and blood/brain barrier penetrability of this compound enabled a test of this hypothesis by examining its neuroprotective efficacy in the rat MCAO model, generally regarded as a realistic model of focal ischemic brain damage as occurs in stroke.

This study established that, in anesthetized rats, CNS 1237 offers substantial neuroprotection in the MCAO stroke model (FIG. 8). At the doses tested, the dose-response curve was flat at 35–36% reduction of infarct volume: there was no statistically significant difference between degree of protection at the highest vs the lowest dose. The degree of protection is comparable to that seen by the same investigators, employing the same MCAO procedure, in recently published studies of BW 619C89, a $Na^+$ channel-selective glutamate release blocker now in clinical trials.[23] Maximal protection occurs at doses of CNS 1237 (3 mg/kg bolus plus a 4-hour infusion of 0.75 mg/kg) severalfold lower than that required for maximal protection by BW 619C89. The reduction of infarct volume is, however, lower than that reported for BW 619C89 by Leach *et al.*[54] and Swan *et al.*[24] in MCAO studies of Fischer 344 rats.

Neuroprotective doses of CNS 1237 produced no significant reduction of blood pressure, except for a transient, mild decrease in blood pressure 2 minutes after bolus infusion in the highest dose tested (FIG. 9). Maximal neuroprotection was maintained over a 4-fold dose range in the absence of significant reduction of blood pressure. CNS 1237 produced a modest dose-dependent reduction in heart rate (FIG. 10). At the lowest dose tested of CNS 1237 the reduction of heart rate ($\leq 9\%$) is of borderline statistical significance.

## CONCLUDING REMARKS

The naturally occurring $Na^+$ channel blockers, TTX and STX[55] do not block $Na^+$ channels in a use-dependent manner as tested in our experimental protocol. The toxicity of TTX and STX, the most serious manifestation of which is respiratory paralysis,[56] precludes their therapeutic utility. Toxicity results from the tendency of these agents to indiscriminately block said ion channels whether or not they are in the open, activatable, or closed conformations.

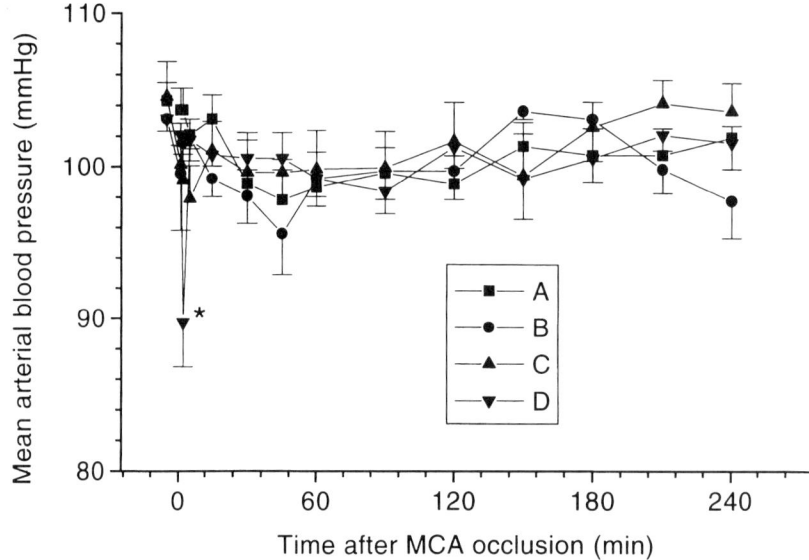

**FIGURE 9.** Effect of drug treatment upon mean arterial blood pressure. There were no significant alterations in blood pressure except for a transient mild decrease in mean arterial blood pressure (MABP) at 2 minutes after bolus injection of drug at the highest dose (group D). *Error bars* denote SEM values. See Methods for details of protocol and dosing groups.

Certain venom peptides which block N-type presynaptic $Ca^{2+}$ channels and result in block of neurotransmitter release, among them the cone snail peptide ω-conotoxin M-VII-A (SNX-111), have shown efficacy in animal models of transient global brain ischemia.[57] SNX 111 is currently in human clinical trials for prevention of global ischemic brain damage. SNX 111 demonstrates side effects, notably profound hypotension, which may seriously limit its use in treatment of focal ischemia.[58] N-channel block by SNX 111 exhibits "reverse use-dependence," *i.e.*, it is relieved rather than enhanced by repetitive depolarization, as revealed by brain slice studies.[53] It is not yet known whether these side effects are solely the consequence of blockade of N-type channels, or whether they are attributable to the tendacy of the peptide to block N-channels in a reverse use-dependent manner.

CNS 1237 presents an attractive profile of efficacy and cardiovascular safety in the rat MCAO focal ischemia model relative to that of other blockers of voltage-activated $Na^+$ and/or $Ca^{2+}$ channels discussed in this article and elsewhere in this volume. We hypothesize that positive use-dependence accounts at least in part for this efficacy and safety profile. Just as use-dependence has proved to be a desirable and possibly essential property for successful cardiovascular drugs which block voltage-activated cardiac $Ca^{2+}$ and/or $Na^+$ channels, it is our expectation that this is also the case for neuroprotective blockers of the voltage-activated ion channels controlling glutamate release.

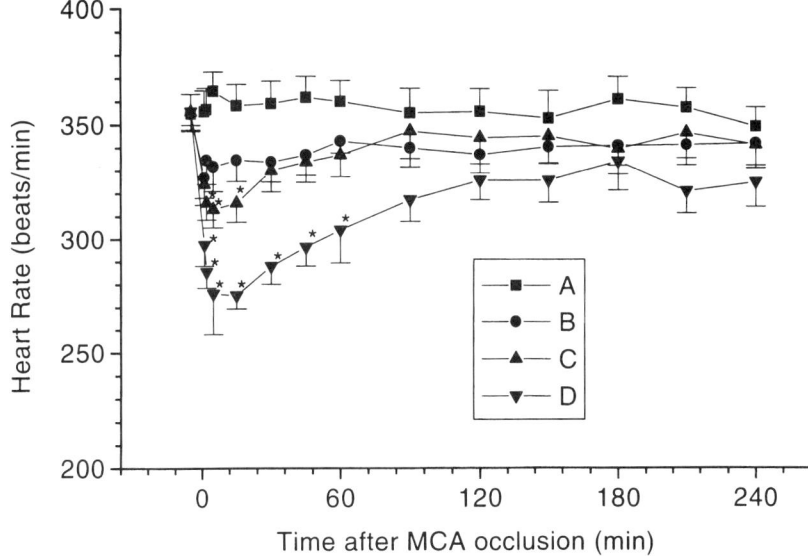

**FIGURE 10.** Effect of drug treatment upon heart rate. Treatment groups C and D had significantly lower heart rates than control (group A) during the first 30 minutes of drug infusion. The heart rate decrease for the lowest dose (group B) was below the level of statistical significance. *Error bars* denote SEM values. See Methods for details of protocol and dosing groups.

We hypothesize that the dual actions of CNS 1237 are due to interactions at a common site of shared homology between presynaptic $Ca^{2+}$ channels and type II neuronal $Na^+$ channels. Unpublished evidence indicates that this site is in the immediate vicinity of the SS1-SS2 segment, known as the "ion-selectivity filter domain" of type II neuronal $Na^+$ channels. We are currently exploring known characteristics of this site, revealed by the biophysical, structural and molecular biological analysis by site-directed mutagenesis of the cloned, expressed channel targets, as the basis for rational design of analogues of CNS 1237. We have created new analogues that are severalfold more potent than CNS 1237, and which also show promising preclinical indications of neuroprotective efficacy *in vivo*.

## ACKNOWLEDGEMENT

We thank Dr. Robert N. McBurney for his advice and support of this effort, and for critical review of the manuscript.

## REFERENCES

1. MUIR, K. *et al.* 1995. CNS 1102 clinical trials. This volume.
2. MAYER, M. L., G. L. WESTBROOK & P. B. GUTHRIE. 1984. Nature **309:** 261–263.

3. BULLOCK *et al.* 1995. Glutamate release from TBI patients. This volume.
4. ALBERS, G. W., M. P. GOLDBERG & D. W. CHOI. 1989. Ann. Neurol. **25:** 398–403.
5. BUCHAN, A., H. LI & W. A. PULSINELLI. 1991. J. Neurosci. **11:** 1049–1056.
6. CHOI, D. W. 1990. Cerebrovasc. Brain Metab. Rev. **2:** 105–147.
7. BUCHAN, A., H. LI, S. CHO & W. A. PULSINELLI. 1991. Neurosci. Lett. **132:** 255–258.
8. MELDRUM, B. S. 1990. Cerebrovasc. Brain Metab. Rev. **2:** 27–57.
9. GRAHAM, S. H., J. CHEN, F. H. SHARP & R. P. SIMON. 1993. J. Cereb. Blood Flow Metab. **13:** 88–97.
10. MELDRUM, B. S. *et al.* 1992. Brain Res. **593:** 1–6.
11. SHAW, P. J. *et al.* 1987. Stroke **18:** 700–707.
12. ZIVIN, J. A. & D. W. CHOI. 1991. Sci. Am. **265:** 36–43.
13. ZIVIN, J. A. 1990. *In* Protection of the Brain from Ischemia. P. R. Weinstein & A. I. Faden, Eds. 104–122. Williams and Wilkens. Baltimore.
14. SHIMIZU, H. *et al.* 1993. Brain Res. **605:** 33–42.
15. STYS, P. K., S. G. WAXMAN & B. R. RANSOM. 1992. J. Neurosci. **12:** 430–439.
16. WESTENBROOK, R. E. *et al.* 1989. Neuron **3:** 695–704.
17. CATTERALL, W. A. 1992. Physiol. Rev. **72:** S15–S41.
18. LEACH, M. J. *et al.* 1986. Epilepsia **27:** 490–497.
19. MELDRUM, B. S. *et al.* 1992. Brain Res. **593:** 1–6.
20. WAHL, F. *et al.* 1993. Eur. J. Pharmacol. **230:** 209–214.
21. LEACH, M. J. *et al.* 1986. Epilepsia **27:** 490–497.
22. BENOIT, E. & D. ESCANDE. 1991. Pflugers Arch. **419:** 603–609.
23. GRAHAM, S. H., J. CHEN, M. J. LEACH & R. P. SIMON. 1994. J. Pharmacol. Exp. Ther. **269:** 854–859.
24. SWAN *et al.* 1994. Rat MCAO studies of BW 619C89. This volume.
25. BEAN, B. P. 1989. Ann. Rev. Physiol. **51:** 367–384.
26. MINTZ, I. M., M. E. ADAMS & B. P. BEAN. 1992. Neuron **9:** 85–95.
27. BEAN, B. P. 1989. Ann. Rev. Physiol. **51:** 367–384.
28. ZHANG, J-F. *et al.* 1993. Neuropharmacology **32:** 1075–1088.
29. LUEBKE, J. I., K. DUNLAP & T. J. TURNER. 1993. Neuron **11:** 1–20.
30. WU, L-G. & P. SAGGAU. 1994. J. Neurosci. **14:** 5613–5622.
31. TURNER, T. J., M. E. ADAMS & K. DUNLAP. 1993. Proc. Natl. Acad. Sci. USA **90:** 9518–9522.
32. SUBBARAO, K. *et al.* 1993. Soc. Neurosci. Abstr. **19:** 1750.
33. TRIGGLE, D. *et al.* 1989. Med. Res. Rev. **9:** 123–180.
34. SIEGELBAUM, S. A. & J. KOESTER. 1991. *In* Principles of Neural Science, 3rd edit. E. R. Kandel *et al.*, Eds. 66–79. Appleton & Lange. Norwalk, CT.
35. MARSHALL, L. F. 1990. Curr. Opin. Neurol. Neurosurg. **3:** 4–9.
36. PORTER, R. J. 1989. Epilepsia **30**(Suppl 1): S29–S34.
37. ROGAWSKI, M. A. & R. J. PORTER. 1990. Pharmacol. Rev. **42:** 224–270.
38. APPEL, S. H. 1993. Trends Neurosci. **16:** 3–5.
39. CHOI, D. W. 1988. Neuron **1:** 623–634.
40. WEST, J. W., T. SCHEUER, L. MAECHLER & W. A. CATTERALL. 1992. Neuron **8:** 59–70.
41. HAMILL, O. P. *et al.* 1981. Pflugers Arch. **391:** 85–100.
42. TURNER, T. J., L. B. PEARCE, & S. GOLDIN. 1989. Anal. Biochem. **178:** 8–16.
43. NACHSEN, D. A. & M. P. BLAUSTEIN. 1982. J. Gen. Physiol. **79:** 1065–1087.
44. GOLDIN, S. *et al.* Patent application PCT/US92/01050.
45. SHIRASHI, K., F. R. SHARP & R. P. SIMON. 1989. J. Cereb. Blood Flow Metab. **9:** 765–773.
46. BEDERSON, J. B. *et al.* 1986. Stroke **17:** 1304–1308.
47. HILLE, B. 1992. Ionic Channels of Excitable Membranes, 2nd ed. 226–303. Sinauer Assoc. Sunderland, MA.
48. McBURNEY, R. N. *et al.* 1992. J. Neurotrauma. **9**(Suppl. 2), S531–S543.
49. BEAN, B. P., C. J. COHEN & R. W. TSIEN. 1983. J. Gen. Physiol. **81:** 613–642.
50. KEANA, J. F. W. *et al.* 1989. Proc. Natl. Acad. Sci. USA **86:** 5631–5635.
51. POCOCK, J. M., V. VENEMA & M. ADAMS. 1992. Neurochem. Int. **20:** 263–270.
52. MINTZ, I. M. & B. P. BEAN. 1993. Soc. Neurosci. Abstr. **19:** 1478.

53. WURSTER, S. & D. J. DOOLEY. 1993. Soc. Neurosci. Abstr. **19:** 1750.
54. LEACH, M J. *et al.* 1993. Stroke **24:** 1063–1067.
55. HILLE, B. 1992. Ionic Channels of Excitable Membranes, 2nd ed. 59–67. Sinauer Assoc. Sunderland, MA.
56. NARAHASHI, T. 1975. *In* The Nervous System, Vol. 2. D. B. Tower, Ed. 101–110. Raven Press. New York.
57. VALENTINO, K. *et al.* 1993. Proc. Natl. Acad. Sci. USA **90:** 7894–7897.
58. XUE, D. *et al.* 1993. Soc. Neurosci. Abstr. **19:** 1643.
59. GOLDIN, S. M. *et al.* 1993. Ann. N.Y. Acad. Sci. **710:** 271.

# Receptor Subtypes Linked to Metabotropic Glutamate Receptor Agonist-Mediated Limbic Seizures in Mice

JOSEPH P. TIZZANO,[a,c] KELLY I. GRIFFEY,[a] AND
DARRYLE D. SCHOEPP[b]

*[a]Toxicology Research Division*
*[b]Central Nervous System Division*
*Lilly Research Laboratories*
*Eli Lilly and Company*
*Indianapolis, Indiana 46285*

## INTRODUCTION

Glutamate is the major excitatory neurotransmitter in the central nervous system (CNS), and contributes excitatory input to most neurons throughout the brain and spinal cord. Numerous animal studies have shown that glutamatergic excitatory neurotransmission plays a critical role in brain function (*e.g.*, the regulation of neurotransmitter release, memory and learning, development, and synaptogenesis) as well as in dysfunction (*e.g.*, epilepsy, stroke, and neurodegenerative disorders).[1]

Metabotropic glutamate receptors (mGluRs) are a recently recognized novel family of excitatory amino acid (EAA) receptors.[2,3] In contrast to ion channel-linked (ionotropic) glutamate receptors, mGluRs are coupled to multiple cellular effectors via guanosine triphosphate (GTP)-binding proteins. Rat mGluRs that have been cloned fall into three groups based on their degree of sequence homology and similar pharmacology. Group 1 mGluRs include mGluR1 and mGluR5, which can be activated by (1S,3R)-1-aminocyclopentane-1,3-dicarboxylate (1S,3R-ACPD) and are linked to phosphoinositide hydrolysis when expressed in nonneuronal cells.[4] Group 2 mGluRs include mGluR2 and mGluR3. These receptors are also sensitive to 1*S*,3*R*-ACPD, but are negatively coupled to cyclic adenosine monophosphate (cAMP) formation when expressed. Group 2 mGluRs are most potently activated by (1S, 3S, 4S)-(carboxycyclopropyl)glycine (L-CCG1).[4] Rat mGluR4, mGluR6, and mGluR7 (group 3 mGluRs) are insensitive to 1S,3R-ACPD, but can be activated by L-2-amino-4-phosphonobutyrate (L-AP4), L-serine-O-phosphate (L-SOP).[4] In preparations that include brain slices and primary neuronal and glial cultures it has been demonstrated using the above-mentioned mGluR selective agonists that *in situ* mGluRs are also coupled to enhanced phos-

---

[c] Address correspondence to: Joseph P. Tizzano, Toxicology Research Division, Lilly Research Laboratories, Eli Lilly and Company, P.O. Box 708, Greenfield, IN 46140.

phoinositide hydrolysis and inhibition of adenylate cyclase.[5–7] Other effector systems are also coupled to mGluRs *in situ*, since mGluR agonists have been observed to activate phospholipase D,[1] increased cyclic AMP formation,[8] and modulate ion channels including voltage-sensitive calcium channels.[9,10] Current understanding of the functions of this diverse and heterogeneous class of glutamate receptors is in its infancy. However, it is clear that activation of mGluRs can both enhance and suppress the excitability of central neurons by actions at both pre- and postsynaptic sites.[11]

*In vivo* studies have suggested a role for mGluRs in epileptogenesis and neuronal injury. Injection of the mGluR selective agonist 1S,3R-ACPD into the rat or mouse brain leads to limbic seizures and selective neuronal injury.[12–14] Previous studies in mice have shown that pharmacologically, 1S,3R-ACPD induced limbic seizures can be attenuated by the mGluR partial agonist/antagonist L-2-amino-3-phosphonopropionate (L-AP3) and dantrolene, an inhibitor of intracellular calcium mobilization, but not by ionotropic glutamate receptor antagonists.[14] These data suggest a role for phosphoinositide-coupled mGluRs (mGluR1 and/or mGluR5?) in mediating this effect of 1S,3R-ACPD. The present investigation further examines the pharmacology of mGluR-agonist-mediated limbic seizures in mice. Specifically, the effects of mGluR agonists that act on negatively coupled cAMP-linked mGluRs were characterized in this seizure model.

## MATERIALS AND METHODS

All experiments were carried out in accordance with Eli Lilly and Co. animal care and use policy. Male CD-1 mice (20–25 g, Charles River Labs., Inc., Portage, MI) were physically restrained to allow unilateral intracerebral (I.C.) injections as described previously.[14] Briefly, I.C. injections were made using a 10 μl Hamilton microsyringe. The entry site was 2 mm lateral from bregma, with the syringe placed parallel to the midline angled 45° posterior and the injection was made to a depth of 3.7 mm. Animals received I.C. injections (5 μl) of (1S,3R)-1-aminocyclopentane-1,3-dicarboxylate (1S,3R-ACPD) (400 nmol), a dose which we showed previously to induce limbic seizures in 90–100% of treated mice.[14] In all experiments, various mGluR receptor agonists or antagonists or sterile water vehicle (controls) were given by contralateral I.C. injection 15 minutes before 1S,3R-ACPD. These included (1S, 3S, 4S)-carboxycyclopropyl)glycine (L-CCG1), L and D-2-amino-4-phosphonobutyrate (L- and D-AP4), L- and D-serine-O-phosphate (L- and D-SOP). All drugs were dissolved in sterile water and then neutralized with 5 N NaOH to a pH 7–8. Each dose group consisted of ten mice, and following drug administration, mice were observed in separate plastic enclosures over a 10-minute period.

## RESULTS AND DISCUSSION

Similar to our previous work,[14] the administration of 1S,3R-ACPD (400 nmols I.C.) in mice produced limbic seizures. Behaviors that preceded limbic seizures

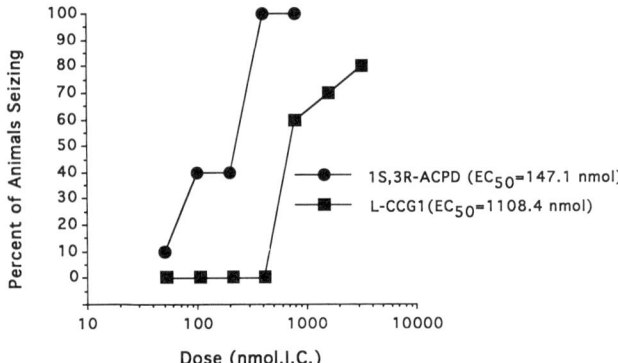

**FIGURE 1.** Dose-response for limbic seizures in mice induced by I.C. administration of 1S,3R-ACPD or L-CCG1. Mice were observed for limbic seizures over a 10-minute period following I.C. injection of 1S,3R-ACPD or L-CCG1. Ten animals were tested at each dose. The *vertical axis* represents the percentage of animals that exhibited limbic seizures at a particular dose of ACPD or L-CCG1.

included: increased scratching and face cleaning, ears pinned back, hunched posture, jumping, and head and tail extension. Limbic seizures in treated mice were characterized by the presence of at least one episode of clonic forelimb contractions followed by hindlimb rearing to a praying stance, then loss of balance and falling. The onset of these behaviors was within one minute following injection and lasted approximately 20 minutes in duration. Following injection of sterile water vehicle, all mice remained clinically normal during the observation period (TABLE 1).

To examine the *in vivo* consequence of activating group 2 mGluRs (see Introduction), animals were given an I.C. injection of L-CCG1. L-CCG1 induced limbic seizures that were qualitatively similar to those produced by 1S,3R-ACPD. However, L-CCG1 was considerably less potent in this regard (FIG. 1). Furthermore,

TABLE 1. Effects of L-CCG1 on 1S,3R-ACPD-induced Limbic Seizures in Mice[a]

| Treatment | | # Animals Seized/ # Animals Tested |
|---|---|---|
| Control | ($H_2O$, I. C. + $H_2O$, I.C.) | 0/10 |
| Control | ($H_2O$, I.C. + 1S,3R-ACPD, 400 nmol, I.C.) | 10/10 |
| L-CCG1 | 50 (nmol, I.C.) | 9/10 |
| | 100 (nmol, I.C.) | 8/10 |
| | 200 (nmol, I.C.) | 8/10 |
| | 400 (nmol, I.C.) | 4/10[b] |

[a] Animals were observed 10 minutes for limbic seizures following administration of 1S,3R-ACPD. Intracerebral injections of L-CCG1 or sterile water were given 15 minutes prior to 1S,3R-ACPD (400 nmol, I.C.).

[b] $p < 0.05$, when compared to sterile water vehicle injections, Fisher's exact probability test.

TABLE 2. Effects of L-AP4 and D-AP4 on 1S,3R-ACPD-induced Limbic Seizures in Mice[a]

| Treatment | | # Animals Seized/ # Animals Tested |
|---|---|---|
| Control | ($H_2O$, I.C. + $H_2O$, I.C.) | 0/10 |
| Control | ($H_2O$, I.C. + 1S,3R-ACPD, 400 nmol, I.C.) | 10/10 |
| L-AP4 | 200 (nmol, I.C.) | 7/10 |
|  | 400 (nmol, I.C.) | 5/10[b] |
|  | 800 (nmol, I.C.) | 1/10[b] |
| D-AP4 | 800 (nmol, I.C.) | 8/10 |

[a] Animals were observed 10 minutes for limbic seizures following administration of 1S,3R-ACPD. Intracerebral injections of L-AP4, D-AP4 or sterile water were given 15 minutes prior to 1S,3R-ACPD (400 nmol, I.C.).

[b] $p < 0.05$, when compared to sterile water vehicle injections, Fisher's exact probability test.

lower doses of L-CCG1, which do not induce limbic seizures, protected against seizures induced by 1S,3R-ACPD (TABLE 1). L-CCG1 most potently acts on group 2 mGluRs to decrease cAMP formation in brain tissues. However, this compound will also activate phosphoinositide-coupled mGluRs at higher concentrations.[15,16] This suggests that the group 2 mGluR activity of this compound may be suppressing the seizures evoked by activation of phosphoinositide-coupled mGluRs. One mechanism for this might be inhibition of glutamate release through the activation of presynaptic mGluRs (see FIG. 2 below).[17]

Studies over ten years ago demonstrated that the compound L-AP4 acts on presynaptic sites in the rodent brain to suppress excitatory synaptic transmission from limbic pathways that include the lateral entorhinal cortex.[18] These (as well as other) effects of L-AP4 are likely mediated by activation of the group 3 mGluRs. In our studies here, L-AP4 (800 nmol I.C.) did not induce limbic seizures in mice. In contrast, this compound blocked seizures induced by 1S,3R-ACPD ($ED_{50}$ = 335 nmol; TABLE 2). This protective effect of L-AP4 was stereoselective, since it

TABLE 3. Effects of L-SOP and D-SOP on 1S,3R-ACPD-induced Limbic Seizures in Mice[a]

| Treatment | | # Animals Seized/ # Animals Tested |
|---|---|---|
| Control | ($H_2O$, I.C. + $H_2O$, I.C.) | 0/10 |
| Control | ($H_2O$, I.C. + 1S,3R-ACPD, 400 nmol, I.C.) | 10/10 |
| L-SOP | 850 (nmol, I.C.) | 8/10 |
|  | 1600 (nmol, I.C.) | 6/10 |
|  | 3200 (nmol, I.C.) | 2/8[b] |
| D-SOP | 3200 (nmol, I.C.) | 8/10[b] |

[a] Animals were observed 10 minutes for limbic seizures following administration of 1S,3R-ACPD. Intracerebral injections of L-SOP, D-SOP or sterile water were given 15 minutes prior to 1S,3R-ACPD (400 nmol, I.C.).

[b] $p < 0.05$, when compared to sterile water vehicle injections, Fisher's exact probability test.

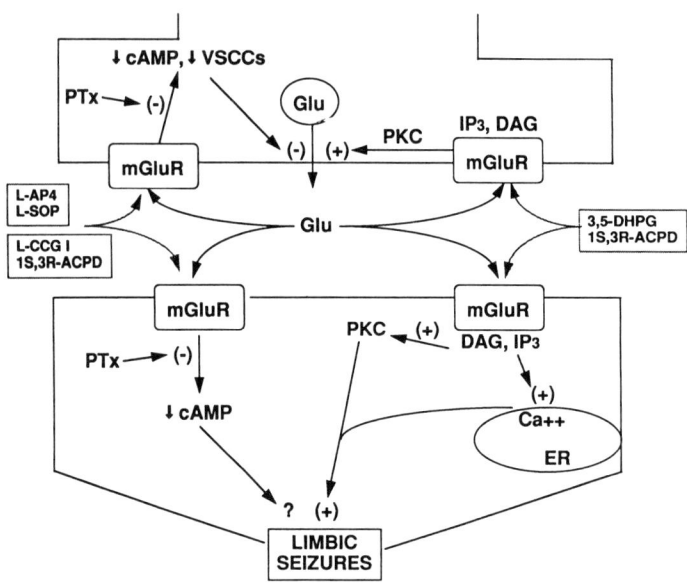

**FIGURE 2.** Hypothesized cellular mechanisms for induction or protection of mGluR agonist-induced limbic seizures in the mouse. Agonists which act on phosphoinositide coupled (group 1) mGluRs (3,5-DHPG and 1S,3R-ACPD) induce limbic seizures when injected I.C. in mouse. These agonists can act on postsynaptic mGluRs which couple to phospholipase C to form the second messengers inositol trisphosphate (IP$_3$) and diacylglycerol (DAG), which mobilize intracellular calcium and activate protein kinase C (PKC), respectively. Presynaptic mGluRs which are also coupled to phosphoinositide hydrolysis have also been shown to enhance the release of transmitter glutamate through a mechanism involving activation of protein kinase C.[19] Agonists that are selective for mGluR subtypes negatively linked to cAMP formation include L-CCG1, L-AP4, and L-SOP. These agonists block seizures induced by agonists acting on phosphoinositide coupled mGluRs. The cAMP-coupled mGluRs likely function as autoreceptors at presynaptic sites where they negatively modulate the release of transmitter glutamate. The mechanism for this effect may also involve inhibition of voltage-sensitive calcium channels.

was not mimicked by 800 nmol of D-AP4. Group 3 mGluRs are also selectively activated by L-SOP, and this compound also produced stereoselective antagonism of 1S,3R-ACPD induced seizures (ED$_{50}$ = 1841 nmol; TABLE 3). Similar to L-CCG1, it is possible that the protective mechanism of the agonists involves suppression of excitatory amino acid neuronal transmission by activation of L-AP4-sensitive presynaptic autoreceptors that negatively influence the release of glutamate (FIG. 2).

In summary, the *in vivo* activation of mGluRs with 1S,3R-ACPD leads to limbic seizures. We hypothesize that 1S,3R-ACPD seizures are likely mediated through the activation phosphoinositide coupled mGluRs, since they are blocked by agents which inhibit mGluR-mediated mobilization of intracellular calcium (FIGURE 2).[14] We have shown here that mGluR agonists which act on group 2 or group 3 mGluRs (those which decrease cAMP) suppress seizures induced by 1S,3R-ACPD. Thus, the convulsant potency of 1S,3R-ACPD is likely negatively influenced by the group 2 mGluR activity which is present in this compound (along with its group 1 mGluR activity). We would predict that a selective agonist for phosphoinositide mGluRs, with no activity at cAMP-linked mGluRs would be a particularly potent convulsant in this model. Preliminary studies with the compound 3,5-dihydroxyphenyl glycine (DHPG), which is highly selective for phosphoinositide-coupled mGluRs, supports this hypothesis (FIG. 2). The manifestation of limbic seizures subsequent to mGluR activation by compounds such as 1S,3R-ACPD and DHPG suggests a novel approach to understanding seizure states in animals and possibly epilepsy in humans. The ability of other mGluRs to suppress seizures states in this model also suggests possible strategies for the development of novel anticonvulsant agents.

## REFERENCES

1. MCDONALD, J. W. & M. V. JOHNSTON. 1990. Brain Res. Rev. **15:** 41–70.
2. CONN, P. J. & M. A. DESAI. 1991. Drug Dev. Res. **24:** 207–229.
3. SCHOEPP, D. D. & P. J. CONN. 1993. Trends Pharmacol. Sci. **14:** 13–20.
4. NAKANISHI, S. 1992. Science **258:** 597–603.
5. PALMER, E., D. T. MONAGHAN & C. W. COTMAN. 1989. Eur. J. Pharmacol. **166:** 585–587.
6. DESAI, M. A. & P. J. CONN. 1990. Neurosci. Lett. **109:** 157–162.
7. SCHOEPP, D. D., B. G. JOHNSON, R. A. TRUE & J. A. MONN. 1991. Eur. J. Pharmacol. Mol. Pharmacol. Sect. **207:** 351–353.
8. WINDER, D. G. & P. J. CONN. 1992. J. Neurochem. **59:** 375–378.
9. LESTER, R. A. J. & C. E. JAHR. 1990. Neuron **4:** 741–749.
10. CHARPAK, S. & B. H. GAHWILER. 1991. Proc. R. Soc. Lond. B. **243:** 221–226.
11. SCHOEPP, D. D., B. G. JOHNSON & J. A. MONN. 1992. J. Neurochem. **58:** 1184–1186.
12. SACAAN, A. I. & D. D. SCHOEPP. 1991. Neurosci. Lett. **259:** :1366–1370.
13. LIPARTITI, M., E. FADDA, G. SAVIONI, R. SILIPRANDI, J. SAUTTER, R. ARBAN & H. MANEV. 1993. Life Sci. **52:** 85–90.
14. TIZZANO, J. P., K. I. GRIFFEY, J. A. JOHNSON, A. S. FIX, D. R. HELTON & D. D. SCHOEPP. 1993. Neurosci. Lett. **162:** 12–16.
15. HAYASHI, Y., T. TANABE, I. ARAMORI, M. MASU, K. SHIMAMOTO, Y. OHFUNE & S. NAKANISHI. 1992. Br. J. Pharmacol. **107:** 539–543.
16. SCHOEPP, D. D. 1994. Neurochem. Int. **24:** 439–449.
17. LOMBARDI, G., M. ALESIANI, P. LEONARDI, G. CHERICI, R. PELLICCIARI & F. MORONI. 1993. Br. J. Pharmacol. **110:** 1407–1412.
18. KOERNER, J. F. & C. W. COTMAN. 1981. Brain Res. **216:** 192–198.
19. HERRERO, I., M. T. MIRAS-PORTUGAL & J. SANCHEZ-PRIETO. 1992. Nature **360:** 163–166.

# Neuroprotective Properties of the Uncompetitive NMDA Receptor Antagonist Remacemide Hydrochloride

GENE C. PALMER,[a,c] EDWARD F. CREGAN,[a] ALFONSO R. BORRELLI,[a] AND FRANCES WILLETT[b]

[a]Biology Department
Fisons Pharmaceuticals
P.O. Box 1710
Rochester, New York 14603
and
[b]Department of Medical Affairs
Fisons plc
Pharmaceutical Division
Research and Development Laboratories
Bakewell Road, Loughborough
Leicestershire LE 11 ORH, United Kingdom

## Background and Mechanism of Action of Remacemide Hydrochloride

Remacemide hydrochloride (HCl) or (±)-2-amino-$N$-(1-methyl-1,2-diphenylethyl)-acetamide HCl was profiled initially as an antiepileptic agent and for this indication clinical trials commenced. Original work revealed specificity regarding protection of rodents from tonic seizures elicited by maximal electroshock (MES). Follow-up investigations indicated efficacy against tonic convulsions in response to 4-aminopyridine and suppression of sound-induced seizures in DBA2 mice. An extensive effort showed that remacemide HCl possessed a good margin of acute safety and little incidence of toxicity following chronic (up to 1 year) administration. Human trials revealed the drug was effective and well tolerated in drug-resistant epileptics.[1,2]

Repeated attempts to discern a mechanism of action for remacemide HCl failed, until three major discoveries were made. First, a more pharmacologically active desglycinated metabolite (FPL 12495) was identified in all species studied.[1] Second, FPL 12495AA was found to be a potent inhibitor of sustained repetitive firing in cultured neurons, an event linked to the fast $Na^+$ channel.[3] Later work showed that both compounds possessed affinity at the batrachotoxin binding site on the $Na^+$ channel.[2] These two studies along with potency in the 4-aminopyridine seizure test[4] provided a link for anticonvulsant activity associated with seizure spread as predicted by the MES test.[5,6] Third, remacemide HCl and the desglycine metabolite protected mice from the convulsions/mortality following infusion of $N$-methyl-D,L-aspartic acid. Simultaneously, it was shown that the desglycine metab-

---

[c] Recipient of communications and requests for reprints.

TABLE 1. Remacemide Hydrochloride and the Desglycine Metabolite: Mechanisms of Action Associated with Neuroprotection[a]

| Description of Test | Remacemide Hydrochloride | Desglycine Metabolite |
|---|---|---|
| *In vitro* | | |
| $IC_{50}$ for MK-801 binding (rat brain synaptosomes) | 68 $\mu$M | 0.48 $\mu$M |
| $IC_{50}$ for NMDA currents (cultured neurons)[b] | 76–75 $\mu$M | 0.6-4 $\mu$M |
| $IC_{50}$ for NMDA depolarization (hippocampal slices) | >30 $\mu$M | 2 $\mu$M |
| $IC_{50}$ sustained repetitive firing (cultured neurons) | 8 $\mu$M | 0.8 $\mu$M |
| Kd batrachotoxin binding (rat brain synaptosomes) | 15.6 $\mu$M | 7.9 $\mu$M |
| *In vivo*, mice ip | | |
| $ED_{50}$ NMDA-induced seizures | 57 | 32 |
| $ED_{50}$ NMDA-induced mortality | 22 | 17 |
| $ED_{50}$ 4-aminopyridine-seizures | 18 | 18 |
| $ED_{50}$ MES | 22 | 17 |
| $ED_{50}$ kainate-induced seizures | 60 | IA |
| $ED_{50}$ kainate-induced mortality | 28 | IA |

[a] *In vivo* concentrations given as mg/kg, IA = inactive.
[b] Data for isomers;[8] remainder of data found in Refs. 1, 2.

olite exhibited a moderate degree of potency with respect to uncompetitive inhibition at the ionic channel/MK801 subsite on the NMDA (N-methyl-D-aspartic acid) receptor ($IC_{50} = 0.48$ $\mu$M vs 68 $\mu$M for remacemide HCl).[1,2] *In vitro* work demonstrated effectiveness of the desglycine metabolite to prevent NMDA-induced depolarization in rat hippocampal slices[7] and block NMDA currents in cultured neurons[8] (TABLE 1). The desglycine metabolite, especially in the *in vitro* experiments, was more potent than remacemide HCl. The data indicated that efficacy for remacemide HCl was manifested in part via metabolic conversion to a more active desglycine metabolite. Recently remacemide HCl and the desglycine metabolite were found to possess greater affinity for the cerebellar subtype of NMDA receptor than in the cortical subtype.[9] Furthermore, Rogawski[6] demonstrated that the less potent NMDA antagonists possess more rapid association/dissociation kinetics and has suggested that this action explains the better clinical tolerability for this class of compounds. In summary, the mechanism of action of remacemide HCl can best be described as that of a weak uncompetitive NMDA antagonist and a moderate inhibitor of the $Na^+$ channel, while the desglycine metabolite is a moderate uncompetitive NMDA antagonist and a potent inhibitor of the $Na^+$ channel. Of further interest, only remacemide HCl was capable of protecting mice from convulsions/mortality in response to kainate, an action mediated by yet another glutamate receptor subtype.[4]

In light of reports that antagonists of the NMDA subtype of glutamate receptors would afford neuroprotection in animal models of anoxia/ischemia—the so-called "excitotoxicity" hypothesis,[10–12] a series of investigations were planned to develop remacemide HCl as a candidate for clinical trials in stroke/neuroprotection. Common problems observed following acute administration of NMDA antagonists include: A propensity to inhibit learning and memory, induction of phencyclidine (PCP)-like behaviors, motor hyperactivity, enhanced startle to an auditory stimulus, and ataxia.[13,14] These parameters were not observed in rodents following administration of large doses of remacemide HCl.[1,2]

## Global Ischemia Models

Short periods of global ischemia (*e.g.*, cardiac arrest, coronary artery bypass) produce delayed cell death in specific brain areas exhibiting selective necrosis of neurons, namely the CA1, and to a lesser extent, the CA3 pyramidal neurons of the hippocampus, the medium-sized neurons in the striatum, cortical layers 3, 5 and 6, as well as the Purkinje cells of the anterior cerebellum.[15] There is some debate, depending upon the animal models used, as to whether NMDA receptor antagonists are capable of protecting laboratory animals from the consequences of global ischemia.[15] Some investigators argue that protection, if any, is achieved by drug-induced hypothermia,[16] an event particularly observed in gerbils,[17] while other investigators show protection in the face of maintaining body and/or brain temperature.[18-21] However, the following section reveals effectiveness of remacemide HCl in global ischemia models.

### Protection of Mice against Hypoxia

Anoxic/hypoxic conditions promote release of the excitatory amino acids, glutamate and aspartate. Immoderate stimulation of the receptor-operated ion channel leads to excess entrance of $Ca^{++}$ into the neurons and contributes to cell death.[10,18] Hypoxia is a useful screen to determine both potential and effective doses for evaluation of a compound in more labor-intensive global and focal ischemia models. In our study pretreatment with remacemide HCl to mice maintained in a thermoregulated environment led to an extension in the time to mortality following exposure to hypoxia. The respective intravenous and oral doses of remacemide HCl required to extend survival time by 50% were 14.3 and 55.5 mg/kg (TABLE 1). Incidentally, the respective $ED_{50}$s for protection of this substrain of CF1 mice (obtained from Harlan Laboratories) in the MES test are 19.1 (iv) and 58 (po) mg/kg[1,2] (TABLE 1).

### Global Ischemia: Rat 4-Vessel Occlusion (4-VO) Model

The rat 4-vessel occlusion technique for global ischemia was conducted as described,[22] taking care to maintain body and brain (1 study) temperature at 37°C. Three separate experiments were performed: 1) Thirty minutes of 4-VO with histological and electrophysiological verification of CA1 neuronal viability; 2) Pretraining rats to asymptote in the T-maze followed by 30 min 4-VO with memory retesting; and 3) Fifteen minutes of 4-VO followed by detailed analysis of CA1 neuronal damage using gross scoring, planimetry, and cell counting.

In the first study rats were given 30 min 4-VO and upon reflow were treated with remacemide HCl (20 mg/kg, ip) followed by another treatment 6 hr later and bid for 6 days with the brains removed on day 8. Alternating slices of hippocampus from the septal to the middle region were taken from both sides for electrophysiological and histological verification of CA1 neuronal viability. As shown in TABLE

TABLE 2. Effect of Remacemide Hydrochloride Given after 30 Min 4-VO on CA1 Neuronal Viability Assessed by Histological and Electrophysiological Techniques[a]

| Conditions (N) | CA1 Score Histology | Electrophysiology Score (Maximal Population Spike mV) | |
|---|---|---|---|
| | | Antidromic | Orthodromic |
| Sham-operated control (N = 8) | 0.0 ± 0 | 9.4 ± 0.8 | 9.0 ± 0.7 |
| Remacemide HCl ischemia (N = 11) | 1.5 ± 0.4* | 4.1 ± 1.4 | 3.4 ± 1.2 |
| Saline-ischemia (N = 10) | 2.6 ± 0.3 | 1.7 ± 0.8 | 1.5 ± 0.7 |

[a] Values are mean ± SE and include the combined scores from left and right sides, which did not differ significantly (ANOVA), the N = separate animals. Remacemide HCl was injected ip at 20 mg/kg at the time of reflow, 6 hr later and bid for 6 more days, with brains taken on day 8. Gross histology scoring was derived from 3 hippocampal slices from each side (ANOVA did not detect differences between sections, left vs right sides, or between raters): 0 = no damage, 1 = up to 33% damage, 2 = 34 to 66% damage, 3 = 67 to 100% damage.

* Difference compared to saline ischemia; ANOVA treatment effect $p = 0.02$.

2, remacemide HCl treatment significantly reduced pyramidal CA1 damage. The antidromic and orthodromic population spikes recorded from the CA1 exhibited a tendency to be greater than those observed from the ischemic rats receiving saline.[7] A closer histological inspection of the damaged CA1 regions revealed islands of viable pyramidal neurons. In retrospect, a more accurate determination of electrophysiology might have included recordings from at least 3 CA1 loci within an individual slice. However, we used the present technique successfully in the past and did obtain significant preservation of electrophysiological responses in the CA1 using FPL 13950, a structural analog of remacemide HCl (Palmer et al., submitted).

The CA1 neurons are a key link in the central circuits mediating the processes of short-term memory; hence patients recovering from stroke experience this syndrome.[23,24] In our study rats were first trained to asymptotic levels for memory and performance in the T-maze using a "win shift" strategy employing a discrete trial, paired run, contingently reinforced (food), alternation procedure with memory delays of 10, 90 and 180 sec. Upon completion of training, rats received 30 min 4-VO, a circumstance previously shown to disrupt memory,[23] followed by remacemide HCl injections (20 mg/kg, ip) at 1 hr post ischemia, daily for 3 days, and at 1 hr following 21 daily sessions in the T-maze. The pretreatment, pre-4-VO memory scores between the 2 designated groups of rats (ischemia-saline and ischemia-remacemide HCl) did not differ. The post 4-VO memory scores of the saline-treated rats were, however, significantly lower than their pretreatment scores. Histological evaluations indicated a significant reduction ($p < 0.02$) of CA1 neuronal necrosis in 4-VO rats treated with remacemide HCl compared to those given saline and tested in the T-maze. The data are presented in TABLE 3. In earlier work, doses of remacemide HCl in the range used herein did not influence learning in normal rats.[23]

In the third 4-VO study rats were subjected to 15 min ischemia. At 1 hr after reinstitution of blood flow the animals received either remacemide HCl (20 mg/

TABLE 3. Effects of Remacemide Hydrochloride on Rat Spatial Working Memory Scores in the T-Maze following 30 min 4-VO[a]

| Treatment Group (N) | Correct Responses/Intertrial Memory Delays | | |
|---|---|---|---|
| | 10 Sec Delay | 90 Sec Delay | 180 Sec Delay |
| Pre-ischemia (combined scores) (N = 7) | 11.2 ± 0.4 | 8.9 ± 0.7 | 8.7 ± 1.2 |
| Ischemia-saline (N = 3) | 9.8 ± 1.0 | 7.5 ± 0.9 | 6.9 ± 0.7 |
| Ischemia remacemide HCl (N = 4) | 11.2 ± 0.2 | 9.3 ± 0.5 | 8.2 ± 0.4 |

[a] Values are the mean ± SD correct choices (total correct choices = 12) utilizing 6 separate memory sessions of 12 trials under both preischemia and postischemia conditions. Data are analyzed with an ANOVA followed by Newman Keul's range test. The $p$ value for comparisons between the post-4-VO ischemia-remacemide HCl animals vs ischemia-saline animals was less than 0.01.

kg, ip) or equivalent volume (1 ml/kg) of saline. Injections were maintained daily for 14 days when the brains were removed for histological analyses consisting of gross scoring (CA1/CA3 pyramidal cell evaluation), planimetry (percent volume of damage to the CA1 neuronal sector), and counting of viable neurons in the CA1. Analyses were made comparing 8 sections ($-3.2$ to $-3.8$ bregma) of the left and right sides for each rat. The findings are presented in TABLE 4. All three methods of damage assessment indicated that ischemic rats treated with remacemide HCl had significantly less injury than those receiving saline.[23] This once-a-day dosing regimen did not give the degree of protection observed in experiment 1, suggesting the importance of maintenance of adequate plasma levels of remacemide HCl.

*Global Ischemia: Canine Model*

Beagle dogs were preanesthetized with ketamine, glycopyrrolate and succinylcholine followed by nitrous oxide/halothane general anesthesia. The continued

TABLE 4. Protection of Rat Hippocampal CA1 Neuronal Sector by Remacemide Hydrochloride following 15 Min of 4-VO Ischemia[a]

| Parameter of Stroke Damage Assessment | Saline-Ischemia Score (N = 9) | Remacemide HCl Ischemia Score (N = 10) |
|---|---|---|
| Gross damage scores of CA1/CA3 neurons | 2.82 ± 0.3 | 2.33 ± 0.6 $p < 0.01$ |
| Planimetry (percent volume of CA1 neuronal damage) | 90.8 ± 4.8 | 77.5 ± 15.1 $p = 0.022$ |
| Counting of viable CA1 pyramidal neurons | 25.2 ± 8.0 | 40.7 ± 24.7 $p < 0.05$ |

[a] Values are mean ± SD; remacemide HCl was injected at 20 mg/kg, ip at 1 hr after ischemia and sid for 14 days. Gross scoring: 0 = no damage, 1 = 25% damage, 2 = 50% damage and 3 = 100% damage. Cell counts in sham-operated controls were 254 ± 13.5. Statistics derived from 2 × 2 × 8 ANOVA (2 treatments × left vs right × 8 sections) followed by the Newman Keul's range test.

TABLE 5. Damage Scores of CA1 Pyramidal Neurons from Canine Hippocampus following 8 Min of Global Ischemia[a]

| Treatment Group, N | Gross Damage Septal Area | Gross Damage Middle Area | Cell Counts Middle Area |
|---|---|---|---|
| Sham-control (N = 5) | 0.00 | 0.00 | 96.6 |
| Sham-remacemide (N = 3) | 0.00 | 0.00 | 112.3 |
| Ischemia-saline (N = 7) | 2.35 | 2.28 | 24.6 |
| Ischemia-remacemide (N = 5) | 1.08 | 0.74 | 83.6* |

[a] Remacemide HCl was injected iv (7.5 mg/kg), at 30 min after reflow, 6 hr later, followed by bid for 2 days and sid for 4 days. Mean values are combinations of scores between left and right sides (which were not significantly different from one another). Cell counts are means of the CA1a and CA1c subregions including left vs right sides. Damage scoring as follows: 0 = no damage; 1 = slight (up to 33% cell death); 2 = moderate (34 to 66% cell death); and 3 = severe (67 to 100% cell death). ANOVA treatment effects: ischemia-saline vs ischemia-remacemide, HCl (septal region, $p = 0.009$; middle region, $p = 0.029$).
* Newman Keul's $p = 0.006$ compared to ischemia-saline animals.

presence of an analgesic agent throughout the course of the experiment was required in our approved protocol. Unfortunately morphine administration interfered with the experimental outcome while preanesthetic medication with ketamine did not. We assume that insufficient levels of ketamine (an uncompetitive NMDA receptor antagonist) remained in the brain during postoperative recovery, especially during the time of delayed cell death to the hippocampus. Eight min of ischemia was induced by clamping the ascending aorta followed by reflow. Measurements were monitored before and after surgery of several physiological parameters, including neurological signs. The procedure is that of Michenfelder et al.,[25] as updated by us (Palmer et al., submitted). Remacemide HCl was injected iv at a dose of 7.5 mg/kg at 30 min after reflow, 6 hr later and twice daily for 2 days, then once daily for 4 days. The brains were prepared for histology on day 8 and the CA1 region of the hippocampus examined for neuronal damage. Damage was assessed by either gross scoring of the septal and middle hippocampal regions or counting viable neurons from the CA1a and CA1c subregions from both left and right sides from the middle area. TABLE 5 reveals significant CA1 neuronal protection in the septal and middle regions in the remacemide HCl group. Moreover, on post-op day 4 the neurological scores in the remacemide HCl-treated animals were significantly improved.

## Global Ischemia: Gerbil

The gerbil has been used historically on a routine basis to evaluate compounds for stroke.[17,18] Because of the lack of the posterior communicating arteries, the incomplete circle of Willis allows for testing of compounds in a global model of forebrain ischemia by the simple procedure of clamping the common carotid arteries. A portion of the earlier work may, however, be subject to question as ischemia itself and many compounds produce hypothermia which is highly therapeutic in this species.[17] In our recent study (Dr. D. Corbett, St. Johns, Newfoundland, unpublished) gerbils were subjected to either 3 or 5 min of global forebrain ischemia. Body and head temperature (use of a "Mini Mitter" brain temperature probe) were rigorously maintained at 37°C during occlusion and for several hr thereafter.[17] When evaluated 3 days after ischemia, gerbils displayed an heightened level of open field exploratory activity.[17] Similar testing was completed on postischemia days 7 and 10. At the end of the behavioral experiment the brains were prepared for histological ranking for CA1 neuronal damage in the hippocampus. Neither the acute (40 mg/kg, ip at the end of occlusion and at 4 hr postocclusion) nor subchronic (similar ip dosing schedule, but includes additional oral treatment of 20 mg/kg at 1, 2 and 3 days postischemia) dosing regimens of remacemide HCl were capable of protection in both the behavioral open-field test and CA1 neuronal survival. Drs. D. McCarthy and N. Mahmood (Fisons, unpublished pharmacokinetic study) found that plasma levels of the desglycine metabolite in the gerbil are considerably below the calculated therapeutic level for other species (mouse, cat and rat). Hence the gerbil does not readily convert the parent compound into the desglycine metabolite.

## Focal Ischemia Models

Animal models of focal ischemia consisting of occlusion of the middle cerebral artery at its source or exit from the lateral sulcus are highly amenable to treatment by antagonists of excitatory amino acid receptors.[12,22] We show here that remacemide HCl pretreatment did indeed reduce the volume of cortical infarction in two separate animal models of focal ischemia.

### Focal Ischemia: Wistar and Spontaneously Hypertensive Rats (SHR)

Focal ischemia was produced in anesthetized Wistar or SHR by carotid occlusion (bilateral for Wistar and ipsilateral for SHR) and clamping the right middle cerebral artery for 2 hr.[26] Remacemide HCl was injected ip (20, 10, and 10 mg/kg) at three time points—30 min prior to ischemia plus 4 and 12 hr postischemia. Cerebral blood flow was determined at the onset of occlusion, at the time of recirculation, and before sacrifice at 24 hr, at which time the brains were removed and prepared for histological determination of cerebral infarct volume. In the Wistar rat no effect of remacemide HCl on regional blood flow was detected, although there was a tendency (nonsignificant) for reduction in cortical infarct volume (saline-ischemia animals = $152.6 \pm 20.2$ mm$^3$, remacemide HCl animals = $115.1 \pm 20$ mm$^3$, N = 20). In the SHR, which has poor collateral circulation and greater infarct volume as a consequence of middle cerebral artery occlusion,[26] the protective effect of remacemide HCl was significant (saline-ischemia animals = $204 \pm 10.5$ mm$^3$, remacemide HCl = $146 \pm 25$ mm$^3$, N = 10, $p = 0.04$). Interestingly, in the SHR receiving remacemide HCl there was an unexplained reduction in cortical blood flow to the penumbra area within the first hr after recirculation.[27]

## Focal Ischemia: Feline Model

Recently J. McCulloch, P. Bannan and D. I. Graham (Glasgow, Scotland, unpublished) evaluated the effects of remacemide HCl on ischemia damage after middle cerebral artery occlusion in the cat. Remacemide HCl was infused into anesthetized animals at 278 μg/min for 90 min prior to a 6-hr permanent occlusion of one middle cerebral artery. Controls received a similar volume of saline. Drug infusion was terminated at the time of occlusion. Slices of brain prepared for histology were cut at 200 μm intervals throughout each forebrain and examined by light microscopy. Damage was quantified using a computer-based image analysis system which calculated areas of infarction at different coronal planes using anterior-posterior coordinates.[12] Cardiovascular and respiratory parameters of control and remacemide HCl-treated groups were unremarkable. Remacemide HCl administration led to a significant reduction of ischemic damage by 49% and 57% in the total cerebral hemisphere (includes basal ganglia and thalamus) and cerebral cortex, respectively. Absolute values for volume of ischemic damage are: 1) Cerebral hemisphere: vehicle = 2505 ± 454 mm$^3$, remacemide HCl = 1266 ± 54 mm$^3$; 2) Cerebral cortex: vehicle = 1929 ± 480, remacemide HCl = 822 ± 55 mm$^3$ ($p$ <0.02, N = 6). No protection was observed in the basal ganglia, which receives blood supply via end arteries, obviating any influence from collateral circulation.[12] The amount of tissue salvaged by remacemide HCl stands in comparison with other highly effective NMDA antagonists, namely MK-801 and d-CPPene, that have been evaluated in this model.[12]

### Subarachnoid Hemorrhage Models

Subarachnoid hemorrhage (SAH) is another class of stroke whose most severe problem is the delayed vasospasm that occurs within 48–72 hr following the event. Current therapy is nimodipine which acts to relax the affected vasculature.[28] Two unpublished, preliminary studies by Drs. D. Anderson and M. Zuccarello (Veterans Administration Hospital in Cincinnati) have demonstrated possible efficacy for remacemide HCl. The initial experiment looked at the ability of either remacemide HCl or MK-801 to reduce the subsequent edema in rats resulting from opening the blood-brain barrier by ipsilateral cortical (left side) application of either nonheparinized blood (300 μl) or FeCl$_2$ (50 mM).[29] Animals received remacemide HCl (10 mg/kg, ip), MK-801 (3 mg/kg, ip) or saline at 30 min before SAH and again at 1 hr post-SAH (remacemide HCl now given at 20 mg/kg). Evans blue dye was injected (50 mg/kg) 1 hr after SAH and was cleared from the cerebral vasculature at 3 hr post-SAH by perfusion of the brain. The brains were removed, dried, the Evans blue dye extracted, and determined spectrophotometrically. Both remacemide HCl and MK-801 significantly reduced extravasation of the dye on the left side when compared to saline-treated animals: 1) Blood-induced SAH, remacemide HCl = 70% reduction, MK-801 = 63% reduction; 2) FeCl$_2$ = induced SAH, remacemide HCl = 45% reduction, MK-801 = 43% reduction. In support of these findings, NMDA receptors have been identified on cerebral microvessels and have been shown to mediate trauma-induced breakdown of the blood-brain barrier.[30]

Another recent study by M. Zuccarello (unpublished) involved injection of autologous arterial blood into the cisterna magna of anesthetized rabbits. The resultant vasospasm of the basilar artery was monitored prior to SAH and at 72 hr post-SAH using angiovist 282 coupled to serial digital substraction angiography.[31] Remacemide HCl was injected ip at 15 mg/kg at 30 min after SAH, again at 6 hr and bid for 3 additional days. At 72 hr following SAH, when vasospasm was apparent in untreated rabbits, a second angiogram was obtained and the diameter of the basilar artery measured at 3 separate loci. The percent constriction averaged 35.3 ± 6.8% and was significantly ameliorated by remacemide HCl pretreatment (27.3 ± 5.4%, $p$ <0.001). The degree of reduction in vasospasm was about half that reported for the 21-aminosteroid, U-74006F.[31] The significance of both findings with remacemide HCl on experimental SAH is interesting, albeit preliminary, and will require further verification, especially regarding possible influence of remacemide HCl on cerebrovascular smooth muscle.

*Parkinson's Models*

Excessive stimulation by excitatory amino acid transmitters at critical neuronal connections within the brain has been linked to both Parkinson's and Huntington's disorders. In this regard the diminished dopamine input to the basal ganglia from the substantia nigra has long been regarded as a link and mode of treatment for Parkinson's disease. However, replenishment of dopamine with the precursor levodopa (L-dopa) does not result in consistent alleviation from the sequela of the disorder, and patients may experience troublesome side effects, especially during the later stages of disease progression. More recent information has revealed that neuronal output from the basal ganglia is regulated in part by excitatory inputs from the subthalamic nucleus. In primate models of Parkinson's disease the glutamate projection from the subthalamus to the globus pallidus and substantia nigra becomes overactive and contributes to the expression of the clinical symptoms. There is now information to suggest that glutamate receptor antagonists might reduce the consequences of over activity of the subthalamic nuclei and exert antiparkinson effects in synergy with L-dopa.[32]

Regarding an anti-parkinson role for remacemide HCl, two investigations were carried out by Dr. T. Greenamyre and his colleagues.[33] In the first study rats were made akinetic by injection of 5 mg/kg, ip of reserpine. Twenty-four hr later the rats were treated with varying oral doses of levodopa (methylester form, ip) followed by saline or remacemide HCl (po) 30 min later. After another 30 min had elapsed, behavioral testing commenced which consisted of measuring horizontal motor activity for 30 min in a darkened "Optovarimex-Auto Track" apparatus. Oral doses of remacemide HCl (5–40 mg/kg) did not influence motor activity in normal or reserpinized rats. Rats pretreated for 24 hr with reserpine were akinetic. Motor activity increased gradually in a dose-related manner in response to levodopa alone (100–200 mg/kg), but was elevated to a marked extent when levodopa was given in conjunction with remacemide HCl (10 mg/kg). If a threshold dose of levodopa (75 mg/kg) was administered with varying doses of remacemide HCl, a dose-related increase in horizontal motor activity was again evident. Significant responses occurred with 5 mg/kg of remacemide HCl.

The second experiment evaluated remacemide HCl in aged female rhesus monkeys rendered parkinsonic with MPTP (1-methyl-4-phenyl-1,2,3,6-tetra-hydropyridine). After several weeks recovery behavioral testing was initiated. Both levodopa-carbidopa and remacemide HCl were administered orally. Behavior was remotely monitored for 10–20 min at hourly intervals, for 5 hr. The 3 MPTP monkeys each had a stable parkinsonian syndrome that was dose-dependently alleviated with levodopa-carbidopa. Remacemide HCl (5 mg/kg) plus levodopa-carbidopa gave a better clinical score (42% improvement) than either the vehicle control or vehicle plus levodopa-carbidopa groups. Except for tremor each of the component scores (posture, gait, bradykinesia, balance gross motor and defense) showed significant and substantial improvement with the remacemide HCl levodopa-carbidopa group. Moreover the effect of remacemide HCl was prolonged for over 5 hr and during this time the plasma levels of the desglycine metabolite were nondetectable (Greenamyre, unpublished).

Taken together, the two investigations support the contention of Greenamyre and O'Brien[32] that NMDA receptor antagonists potentiate the action of L-dopa to alleviate symptoms of Parkinson's disease and may in the future allow for better clinical management of the disorder.

### *Overall Preclinical Conclusions*

The studies conducted to date along with others in progress indicate remacemide HCl is a safe, effective compound for epilepsy, whose efficacy in stroke models has been established, and therefore shows promise for clinical trials. Anticonvulsant efficacy most likely results from prevention of seizure initiation via uncompetitive antagonism of NMDA receptors and seizure spread by inhibition of selected states of activity associated with $Na^+$ channel. As a neuroprotective agent, remacemide HCl exhibits efficacy in animal models of global and focal ischemia, subarachnoid hemorrhage, and Parkinson's disease. These findings are likely due to the ability of the compound to limit activity at excitatory amino acid receptors, principally of the NMDA-type. The role of remacemide HCl in conditions of cerebral trauma remain to be investigated. The following discussion will review the protocols for the clinical trials in progress (see also Ref. [34] from this symposium).

### *Clinical Studies to Investigate the Neuroprotective Properties of Remacemide HCl*

Clinical investigations regarding the neuroprotective properties of remacemide HCl are being conducted in three groups of patients, namely, those undergoing coronary artery bypass surgery (CABS), patients with acute ischemic stroke, and patients with Huntington's disease.

Acute, transient neuropsychological deficit has been demonstrated in up to 77% of patients undergoing CABS.[35] Furthermore, long-term follow-up studies have suggested that a proportion of patients have persistent deficits at 6 months.[36,37] The precise origin of these deficits is unknown, but "showers" of microemboli to the brain[38] or cerebral hypoperfusion may be implicated. A pilot safety and tolerability study of remacemide HCl in patients undergoing CABS has been completed and has established that 600 mg/day in divided doses is a safe and well tolerated dose in this patient population. A larger double-blind placebo-controlled efficacy study is ongoing in approximately 150 patients undergoing CABS. Neuropsychological tests are employed as the endpoints and functions such as memory, recall, motor speed, attention, reaction times and visual-spatial skills are assessed pre- and postoperatively.

The safety and tolerability of intravenous remacemide HCl is also currently being assessed in a dose-escalation study in patients who have sustained acute ischemic stroke. A preliminary review of the tolerability suggests that remacemide HCl is well tolerated by patients with acute ischemic stroke.[34]

Preliminary work has also been undertaken in patients with Huntington's disease. In this patient group remacemide HCl has been well tolerated up to 600 mg/day.

In conclusion, preliminary results suggest that the tolerability of the neuroprotective agent remacemide HC1 is good in patients undergoing CABS, in patients with acute stroke, and in patients with Huntington's disease.

## ACKNOWLEDGMENTS

The authors express appreciation to Andrew Howell and Dietgard Kamp for excellent technical assistance related to the unpublished studies reported herein.

## REFERENCES

1. PALMER, G. C., B. CLARK & J. B. HUTCHISON. 1993. Drugs Future **18:** 1021–1042.
2. PALMER, G. C., V. JAMIESON & T. JONES. Remacemide hydrochloride. *In* Epilepsy, a Comprehensive Textbook. J. Engel, Jr. & T. A. Pedley, Eds. Raven Press. New York. In press.
3. WAMIL, A. W., H. CHEUNG, H. HARRIS, & M. J. MCLEAN. Epilepsy Res. In press.
4. CRAMER, C. L., M. L. STAGNITTO, M. A. KNOWLES & G. C. PALMER. 1994. Life Sci. **54:** PL271–PL274.
5. MACDONALD, R. L. 1989. Epilepsia **30**(Suppl. 1): S19–S28.
6. ROGAWSKI, M. A. 1992. Drugs **44:** 279–292.
7. HARRIS, E., M. STAGNITTO, G. GARSKE, E. CREGAN, R. RAY, R. JULIEN, T. WILSON, G. MACHULSKIS, P. BIALOBOK, J. WHITE & G. PALMER. 1992. Neuroprotection in animals by remacemide, a prodrug for noncompetitive NMDA antagonism with a high therapeutic index. *In* Multiple Sigma and PCP Receptor Ligands: Mechanisms for Neuromodulation and Neuroprotection? J-M Kamenka & E. F. Domino, Eds. 643–653. NPP Books. Ann Arbor, MI.
8. SUBRAMANIAM, S., S. D. DONEVAN & M. A. ROGAWSKI. 1993. Soc. Neurosci. **19:** 712.
9. PORTER, H. P. & J. T. GREENAMYRE. 1995. J. Neurochem. **64:** 614–623.
10. OLNEY, J. W. 1989. Drug Dev. Res. **17:** 299–319.
11. PORSCHE-WIEBKING, E. 1989. Drug Dev. Res. **17:** 367–376.
12. MCCULLOCH, J. 1992. Br. J. Clin. Pharmacol. **34:** 106–114.
13. WILLETS, J., R. L. BALSTER & J. D. LEANDER. 1990. TIPS 11: 423–428.
14. WILMOT, C. A. 1989. Drug Dev. Res. **17:** 339–365.
15. PULSINELLI, W. A. & A. BUCHAN. 1990. The NMDA receptor/ion channel: its importance to *in vivo* ischemic injury to selectively vulnerable neurons. *In* Pharmacology

of Cerebral Ischemia. J. Krieglestein & H. Oberpichler, Eds. 169–175. Wissenschaftliche Verlagsgellschaft. Stuttgart.
16. BUCHAN, A. & W. A. PULSINELLI. 1990. J. Neurosci. **10:** 311–316.
17. CORBETT, D., S. EVANS, T. C. WANG & R. A. JONES. 1990. Brain Res. **514:** 300–304.
18. CHAPMAN, A. G., J. H. SWAN, S. PATEL, J. L. GRAHAM & B. S. MELDRUM. 1990. Cerebroprotective and anticonvulsant action of competitive and non-competitive NMDA antagonists. *In* Amino Acids, Chemistry, Biology and Medicine. G. Lubec & G. A. Rosenthal, Eds. 219–232. ESCOM Science Publishers. Amsterdam.
19. SWAN, J. H. & B. S. MELDRUM. 1990. J. Cereb. Blood Flow Metab. **10:** 343–351.
20. LIN, B., W. D. DIETRICH, M. D. GINSBERG, M. Y-T. GLOBUS & R. BUSTO. 1993. J. Cereb. Blood Flow Metab. **13:** 925–932.
21. GROTTA, J. C., C. M. PICONE, P. T. OSTROW, R. A. STRONG, R. M. EARLS, L. P. LAO, H. M. RHOADES & J. R. DEDMAN. 1990. Ann Neurol. **27:** 612–619.
22. PULSINELLI, W., U. DIMAGI, M. JACEWICZ & A. BUCHAN. 1992. Antagonists of excitatory amino acid neurotransmitters: a comparison of their effects on global versus focal ischemia. *In* Alfred Benzon Symposium. A. Schousboe, N. H. Biemer & H. Kofod, Eds. 225–238. Munksgaard. Copenhagen.
23. ORDY, J. M., B. VOLPE, R. MURRAY, G. THOMAS, P. BIALOBOK, T. M. WEGENACK & W. DUNLAP. 1992. Pharmacological effects of remacemide and MK-801 on memory and hippocampal CA1 damage in the rat four-vessel occlusion (4-VO) model of global ischemia. *In* The Role of Neurotransmitters in Brain Injury. M. Globus & W. D. Dietrich, Eds. 83–92. Plenum Press. New York.
24. VOLPE, B. T. & C. K. PETITO. 1985. Neurology **35:** 1793–1797.
25. MICHENFELDER, J. D., W. L. LANIER, B. W. SCHEITHAUER, W. J. PERKINS, G. T. SHEARMAN & J. H. MILDE. 1989. Brain Res. **481:** 228–234.
26. BUCHAN, A. M., D. XUE & A. SLIVKA. A new model of temporary focal neocortical ischemia in the rat. 1992. Stroke **23:** 273–279.
27. XUE, D., Z. G. HUANG & A. M. BUCHAN. 1993. Can. J. Neurol. **20(Suppl. 2):** S75.
28. GROTTA, J. C. 1991. Clin. Neuropharmacol. **14:** 373–390.
29. ZUCCARELLO, M. & D. K. ANDERSON. 1989. Stroke **20:** 367–371.
30. KOENIG, H., J. J. TROUT, A. D. GLADSTONE & C. Y. LU. 1992. Brain Res. **588:** 297–303.
31. ZUCCARELLO, M., J. T. MARSCH, G. SCHMITT, J. WOODWARD & D. K. ANDERSON. 1989. J. Neurosurg. **71:** 98–104.
32. GREENAMYRE, J. T. & C. F. O'BRIEN. 1991. Arch. Neurol. **48:** 977–981.
33. GREENAMYRE, J. T., R. V. ELLER, A. ZHANG, A. OLVADIA, R. KURLAN & D. M. GASH. 1994. Ann. Neurol. **35:** 655–661.
34. MUIR, K. W. & LEES, K. R. 1995. Initial experience with remacemide hydrochloride in patients with acute ischaemic stroke. Ann. N.Y. Acad. Sci. This volume.
35. HARRISON, M. J. G., A. SCHNEIDAU, R. HO, P. L. C. SMITH, S. NEWMAN & T. TREASURE. 1989. Stroke **20:** 235–237.
36. SHAW, P. J., D. BATES, N. E. F. CARTLIGE, J. M. FRENCH, D. HEAVSIDE, D. G. JULIAN & D. A. SHAW. 1987. Q. J. Med. **239:** 259–268.
37. SAVAGEAU, J. A., B. STANTON, C. D. JENKINS & R. W. M. FRASER. 1982. J. Thorac. Cardiovasc. Surg. **84:** 595–600.
38. PUGSLEY, W., L. KLINGER, C. PASCHALIS, S. NEWMAN, M. HARRISON & T. TREASURE. 1990. Vasc. Surg. **24:** 34–43.

# Discussion

ANONYMOUS: Could you speculate on the post-stroke efficacy of remacemide vis-à-vis slow metabolism to active metabolite?

G. C. PALMER (*Fisons Pharmaceuticals, Rochester, NY*): The potential efficacy of remacemide after stroke depends to some extent on the mechanism of action. If the primary preclinical efficacy is due to $N$-methyl-D-aspartate ion-channel block, then the parent drug will have no significant effect, and the rather slow rise of cerebrospinal fluid metabolite concentrations after permanent middle cerebral artery occlusion in cat shown by Prof. James McCulloch in Glasgow is of theoretical concern. However, both parent drug and desglycine metabolite have significant voltage-sensitive sodium channel-blocking properties, which may also contribute to neuroprotective efficacy.

# Safety, Tolerability and Pharmacokinetics of the N-Methyl-D-Aspartate Antagonist Ro-01-6794/706 in Patients with Acute Ischemic Stroke[a,b]

THE DEXTRORPHAN STUDY GROUP[c] AND
HOFFMANN-LA ROCHE[d]

[c] G. W. Albers, Stanford Stroke Center, Stanford University Medical Center, Palo Alto, California; R. Atkinson, Mercy General Hospital, Sacramento, California; R. E. Kelley, University of Miami Medical Center, Miami, Florida; D. M. Rosenbaum and P. Katz, Montefiore Medical Center, New York, New York
[d] L. M. Lesko, K. Paul, J. Rae, M. Modi, K. Yoo, V. Pitman, and L. Lehr, Hoffmann-La-Roche, Nutley, New Jersey; G. Magni, Basel, Switzerland

## INTRODUCTION

Excitatory neurotransmitters (*e.g.*, glutamate and aspartate) may function as neurotoxins and have been implicated in mediating cell injury in the ischemic brain by triggering a complex cascade of chemical events.[1-4] Glutamate antagonists, particularly those active at the *N*-methyl-D-aspartate (NMDA) receptor sites, have been shown to attenuate glutamate-induced neuronal damage *in vitro* and *in vivo*. NMDA-receptor antagonists are potent anticonvulsants[5] and have demonstrated an ability to protect neurons from the degeneration associated with ischemia,[4-6] hypoxia,[7] and hypoglycemia,[8] in both *in vivo* and *in vitro* models.

Dextrorphan HCl (Ro 01-6794/706) is the O-demethylated monohydrochloride derivative of dextromethorphan, a drug that has been used as an over-the-counter antitussive agent for over 30 years.[9] Both dextrorphan and its parent compound, dextromethorphan, are synthetic nonopioid dextrorotatory morphinans which act as noncompetitive antagonists of the NMDA subtype of the glutamate receptor complex in the central nervous system.[10-14] Dextrorphan is a more potent glutamate antagonist than dextromethorphan in both *in vivo* and *in vitro* models of neuronal injury/damage. Both bind to the part of the NMDA receptor complex that is labelled by tritiated phencyclidine or by $^3$H-MK-801.[14-17]

---

[a] Data from this paper were presented in part at: the May 1994 American Academy of Neurology Meeting in Washington, DC, the July 1994 International Symposium on Pharmacology of Cerebral Ischemia in Marburg, Germany, and this conference.

[b] Address correspondence to: Lynna M. Lesko, M.D., Ph.D., Division of General Medicine, Boehringer Ingelheim Pharmaceuticals, Inc., 900 Ridgebury Road, P.O. Box 368, Ridgefield, CT 06877.

In both rabbit and rat models of focal ischemia, dextrorphan reduced the size of infarcted brain tissue when administered before, during, or after ischemic insult in both transient and permanent middle cerebral artery occlusion.[18-23] Dextrorphan freely crosses the blood-brain barrier after systemic administration. Consequently, it is under development as a neuroprotective agent for the treatment of acute ischemic stroke in man.[24] In preparation for an efficacy trial in acute stroke patients, the following study was undertaken to determine the highest tolerated loading dose and maintenance infusion of dextrorphan that could be given safely to patients with an acute ischemic stroke. The clinical pharmacokinetic profile of dextrorphan in this acute stroke patient population was also evaluated.

## METHODS

The study was a multicenter (7 US clinical sites), ascending-dose study in which dextrorphan or placebo was to be administered intravenously to eleven groups of patients as a one-hour loading dose followed by an 11- or 23-hour maintenance infusion. The study design included three parts: 1) a single-blind administration of placebo; 2) a randomized, placebo-controlled, double-blind administration of placebo or dextrorphan in ascending doses of both a one-hour loading dose and an 11- or 23-hour maintenance infusion and 3) an open-label administration of dextrorphan in an ascending one-hour load followed by an 11-hour ascending constant rate maintenance infusion. The total planned cumulative doses were 475 to 1280 mg for the 12-hour administration schema and 945 to 2140 mg for the 24-hour administration schema. Study drug administration was to be accomplished in a monitored clinical environment (*e.g.,* intensive care unit (ICU), Med-ICU, Neuro-ICU or other special care unit) with careful evaluation of electrocardiographic and respiratory function. Patients admitted to the study included those 1) with an acute, supratentorial ischemic stroke within 48 hours before receiving study drug, 2) who had a stable neurological deficit and had no apparent significant medical or psychiatric illness and 3) who were alert and responsive. No minimum neurological deficit was required for study entry. Patients were allowed any concomitant medications other than digoxin, cimetidine, or warfarin. They underwent a head computerized tomography (CT) scan, 12-lead electrocardiogram (ECG), and two to four hours of cardiac telemetry before study drug administration. Vital signs, blood samples for assessment of clinical laboratory parameters/pharmacokinetics were taken at specified times before, during, and after the study drug administration. While this was not a study examining the efficacy of dextrorphan, a NIH Stroke Scale Score[25-27] was obtained at baseline as a measure of neurological impairment, and at least at 12, 24 and 48 hours after study drug administration when feasible. Pharmacologic effects of dextrorphan were monitored and reported as adverse experiences, and their severity and relatedness to study drug were also recorded throughout the study drug administration period for an additional 24-hour period after drug administration and during follow-up visits.

TABLE 1. Baseline Characteristics of Patients Enrolled

| Characteristic | Placebo (N = 16) | | Dextrorphan Loading Infusion (mg/h) | | | | | |
|---|---|---|---|---|---|---|---|---|
| | | | 60–120 (N = 15) | | 145–180 (N = 15) | | 200–260 (N = 21) | |
| | n | (%) | n | (%) | n | (%) | n | (%) |
| Age, mean ± SD | 16 | 68 ± 11 | 15 | 64 ± 13 | 15 | 63 ± 14 | 21 | 66 ± 10 |
| Sex, male | 8 | (50) | 8 | (53) | 9 | (60) | 8 | (38) |
| Race, white | 9 | (56) | 8 | (53) | 8 | (53) | 12 | (57) |
| black | 6 | (38) | 4 | (27) | 4 | (27) | 5 | (24) |
| NIH Stroke Scale (median, range) | 5 | 1–19 | 6 | 2–15 | 8 | 1–14 | 6 | 1–20 |
| Previous stroke | 2 | (12) | 5 | (33) | 7 | (47) | 9 | (43) |
| Renal disease | 0 | (0) | 2 | (13) | 1 | (7) | 1 | (5) |
| Angina | 0 | (0) | 3 | (20) | 1 | (7) | 2 | (10) |

TABLE 2. Distribution of Loading Infusion Doses

| Loading Infusion Doses (mg/h) | Dextrorphan (N = 51) n (%) | Placebo (N = 16) n (%) |
|---|---|---|
| 0 | 0 | 16 (100) |
| 60–120 | 15 (29) | 0 |
| 145–180 | 15 (29) | 0 |
| 200–260 | 21 (42) | 0 |

## RESULTS

### Safety and Tolerability

Fifty-one of 67 patients enrolled in the study received dextrorphan, the remainder received placebo. TABLE 1 summarizes baseline characteristics for the group of patients who were enrolled. The placebo and dextrorphan treatment group had similar demographic characteristics, medical histories and previous medications. Their secondary diagnoses, previous and concomitant medications were considered to be clinically age appropriate and similar to a typical population of patients having an ischemic stroke. TABLES 2 and 3 list the distribution of patients and doses of test drug for both the loading and maintenance infusions. Loading doses

TABLE 3. Distribution of Maintenance Infusion Rates

| Maintenance Infusion Rate (mg/h) | Dextrorphan (N = 51) n (%) | Placebo (N = 16) n (%) |
|---|---|---|
| 0 | 2 (4) | 16 (100) |
| 15–30 | 8 (16) | 0 |
| >30–50 | 19 (37) | 0 |
| >50–70 | 12 (24) | 0 |
| >70–135 | 10 (20) | 0 |

TABLE 4. Number and Percentage of Patients Showing Selected Adverse Events for All Doses

| Selected Adverse Event | Dextrorphan (N = 51) n (%) | Placebo (N = 16) n (%) |
|---|---|---|
| Nystagmus | 43 (84) | 0 |
| Somnolence | 37 (73) | 0 |
| Agitation | 31 (61) | 0 |
| Hallucinations | 28 (55) | 0 |
| Confusion | 27 (53) | 1 (6) |
| Hypertension | 22 (43) | 2 (13) |
| Nausea | 21 (43) | 2 (13) |
| Dizziness | 18 (35) | 3 (19) |
| Stupor | 13 (26) | 1 (6) |
| Vomiting | 13 (26) | 1 (6) |
| Hypotension | 9 (18) | 0 |
| Total patients with one or more adverse events | 51 (100) | 13 (81) |

for dextrorphan were grouped *post hoc* into low (60–120 mg/hr, N = 16), intermediate (145–180 mg/hr, N = 15) and high doses (200–260 mg/hr, N = 21). Total cumulative doses of drug ranged from 120 mg to 3310 mg.

Administration of low, intermediate and high loading doses and maintenance doses of dextrorphan produced no clinically significant abnormalities in laboratory test values. Mean values for blood chemistry, urinalysis and hematology were all within normal ranges when obtained within five days after administration of test drug. There were no clinically significant ECG findings on routine monitoring. No patients died during administration of the drug, though one patient developed a malignant pleural effusion and died from an occult carcinoma one month after drug administration.

TABLE 4 summarizes the common pharmacologic effects/adverse experiences for the dextrorphan and placebo group; the profile differs quite extensively for both groups. One hundred percent of patients who received dextrorphan reported one or more adverse experiences compared to 81% of placebo patients. The most commonly reported pharmacologic effects for the dextrorphan-treated group were those in the peripheral and central nervous system. In general, most pharmacologic effects tended to be mild to moderate, self-limiting and reversible. Many of these common effects/adverse experiences occurred with different frequencies during the load and maintenance infusion periods; these are shown in FIGURES 1 and 2. Nystagmus, somnolence, nausea, vomiting and hypotension were seen with greater frequency during the first 90 minutes of dextrorphan administration, while agitation, confusion, hallucinations and hypertension occurred more frequently during the maintenance infusion period. Patients with agitation and confusion responded well to reassurance, and medication was generally not required. The incidence of the most common adverse experiences in the load and maintenance infusions was lower at the intermediate dose group than at the higher dose group as depicted in FIGURES 3 and 4.

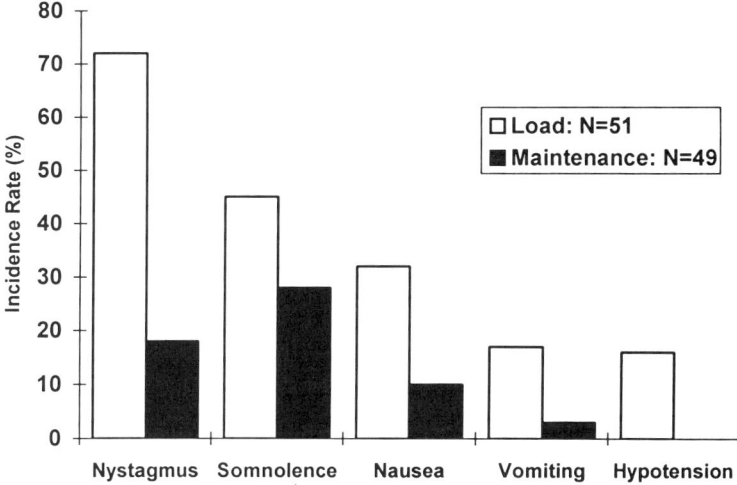

**FIGURE 1.** Incidence of pharmacologic effects associated with the loading infusion, compared to their incidence during the maintenance infusion.

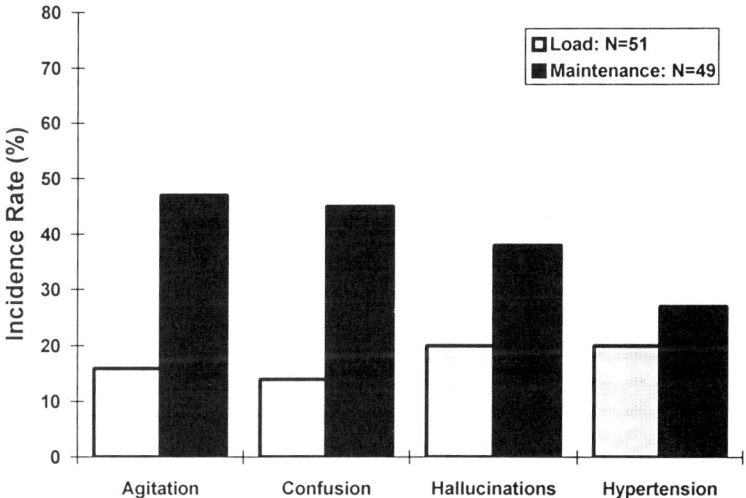

**FIGURE 2.** Incidence of pharmacologic effects associated with the maintenance infusion, compared with their incidence during the loading infusion.

The escalation of the loading dose was terminated after 7 of 21 patients in the highest loading dose group (200–260 mg/hr) developed rapid, symptomatic (*e.g.*, pallor, diaphoresis) drops in systolic blood pressure within 90 minutes after the start of the loading dose administration. A total of 9 patients had hypotension

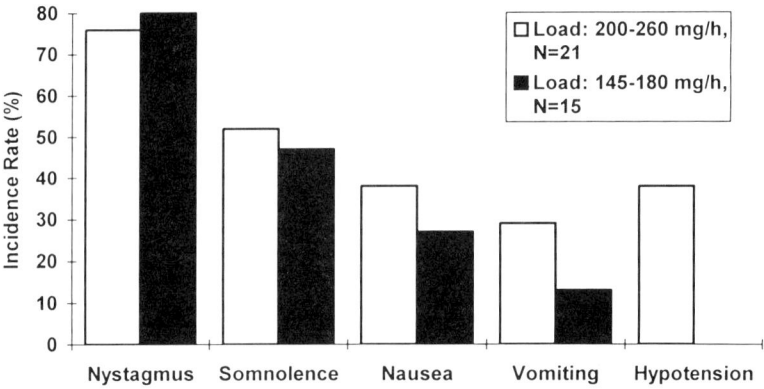

**FIGURE 3.** Lower vs higher loading dose groups: lower dose has decreased incidence of adverse experiences.

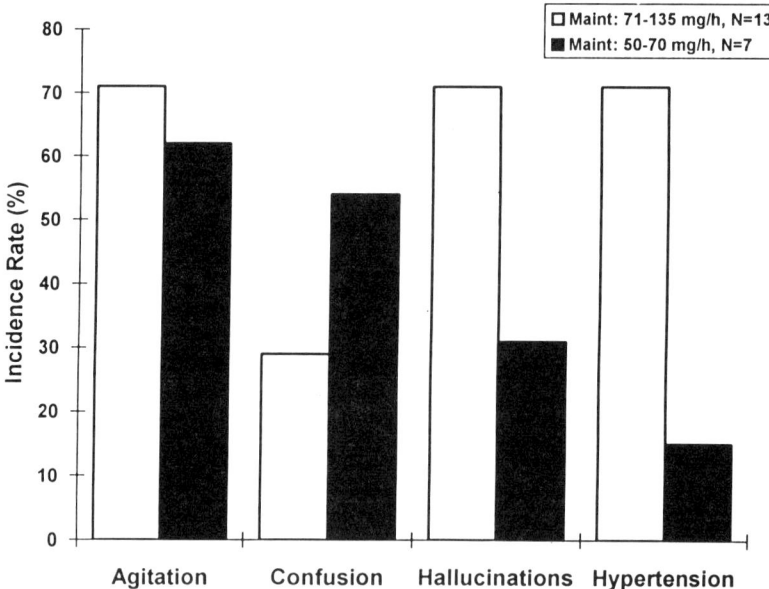

**FIGURE 4.** Lower vs higher maintenance infusion groups: lower infusion rate associated with decreased adverse experience rate.

reported as an adverse experience in the case report form. However, not all events reported as hypotension were clinically significant or similar in presentation, since no specific criteria for reporting "hypotension" were defined before the start of the study. Hypotension was reported in 1 of the 9 patients (loading dose: 60 mg/

TABLE 5. Decreases in Systolic Blood Pressure within 90 Minutes of the Start of Test Drug Administration, by Loading Dose Administered

| Systolic Pressure: Decrease from Baseline (mm Hg) | Loading Infusion Rate (mg/h) | | | |
|---|---|---|---|---|
| | 0 (n = 16) n (%) | 60–120 (n = 15) n (%) | 145–180 (n = 15) n (%) | 200–260 (n = 21) n (%) |
| >20–30 | 2 | 1 | 3 | 2 |
| >30–50 | 3 | 0 | 0 | 2 |
| >50 | 1 | 1 | 0 | 6 |
| Total n (%) | 6 (38) | 2 (13) | 3 (20) | 10 (48) |

hr) after review of the case report form; the blood pressure change was not rapid in onset and the patient was asymptomatic. A second patient had hypotension that occurred 3 hours after the end of the maintenance infusion, after receiving intravenous antihypertensive medication for 24 hours. These latter two cases clearly differed from the other reports of hypotension that resulted in the termination of the loading dose escalation. An additional 8 other dextrorphan-treated patients and 6 placebo-treated patients also had drops in systolic blood pressure ranging from greater than 20 mm Hg to greater than 50 mm Hg during the first 90 minutes after the start of the loading dose infusion (TABLE 5). However, these drops in blood pressure were neither as symptomatic (pallor, diaphoresis) nor as rapid as those that resulted in termination of the loading dose escalation. All symptomatic blood pressure drops were short-lived and reversible by placing patients supine, administering intravenous fluids and in two patients, administering low-dose dopamine; none of these blood pressure drops produced any neurologic physical sequelae. The major factor contributing to the production of hypotension during the loading dose infusion appeared to be the rate of dextrorphan administration. No other common predisposing factors (*e.g.*, concomitant medication, preexisting illness, dextrorphan plasma concentration) could be determined in a *post hoc* analysis of the data. In summary, the physiologic loading period was considered to be 90 minutes, since the limiting/clinically significant hypotensive episodes occurred mostly during the first 90 minutes after the start of dextrorphan administration.

The escalation of the maintenance infusion was stopped only because of the termination of the escalation of the loading infusion. However, at maintenance infusion rates above 90 mg/hr, 3 of 49 patients had their infusion discontinued for reasons of decreased level of consciousness (2/49) and respiratory depression (1/49).

Of note, NIH Stroke Scale scores obtained at 48 hours after test drug administration showed no difference between the placebo and dextrorphan treatment groups as shown in TABLE 6.

### *Clinical Pharmacokinetics*

Preliminary pharmacokinetic results showed that intravenous dextrorphan has a short half-life (range 1.7–5.4 hr). Dextrorphan plasma concentrations increased

TABLE 6. NIH Stroke Scale Scores at Baseline and 48 Hours

| Loading Infusion Dose (mg/h) | Baseline | | 48 Hours | | Mean Change |
|---|---|---|---|---|---|
| | Mean Score | Range | Mean Score | Range | |
| Placebo (n = 16) | 5.9 | 1–19 | 5.5 | 1–19 | −0.6 |
| 60–120 (n = 14) | 6.5 | 2–15 | 5.1 | 0–15 | −1.4 |
| 145–180 (n = 15) | 8.5 | 1–14 | 9.0 | 1–27 | 0.4 |
| 200–260 (n = 21) | 7.4 | 1–20 | 6.4 | 0.19 | −1.0 |

in a dose-proportional manner; the ranges of plasma concentrations after a 160 and 260 mg/hr loading dose in stroke patients were 413–506 and 375–1050 ng/mL, respectively. Higher loading doses were associated with higher dextrorphan plasma concentrations at one hour after the start of the loading lose and greater variability in plasma concentration (FIG. 5). Plasma concentrations decreased relatively rapidly after stopping the infusion in both the 12- and 24-hour treatment groups (FIG. 6). Dextrorphan was rapidly distributed out of the blood when given intravenously and had a large volume of distribution of 250 to 650 L. Clearance of drug was high in stroke patients (range 47–259 L/hr) with considerable variability (greater than 30%). Females greater than 65 yrs of age had the lowest clearance of the stroke patients studied (FIG. 7). Some variability in clearance could be explained by the influence of age and gender.

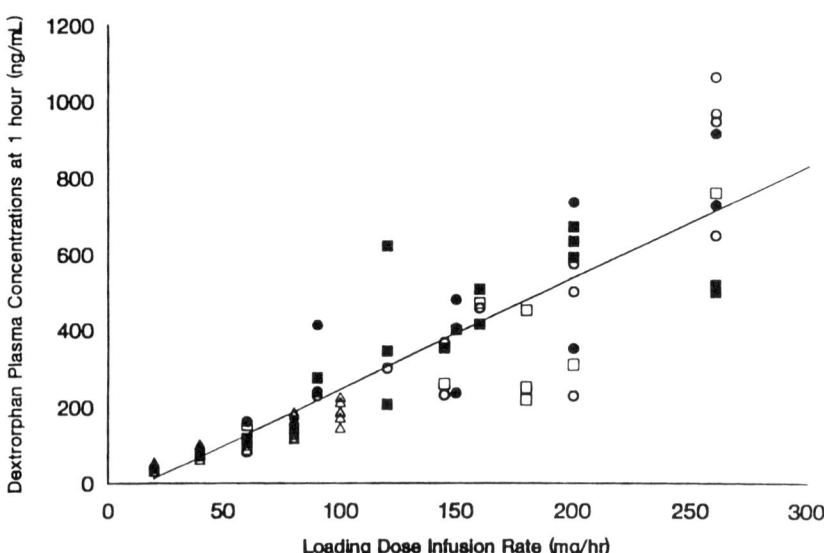

FIGURE 5. The relationship between dextrorphan plasma concentrations at 1 hour and loading dose infusion rate in healthy male subjects (△, N3494C) and stroke patients (□ males <65 yr, ■ males >65 yr, ○ females <65 yr, ● females >65 yr).

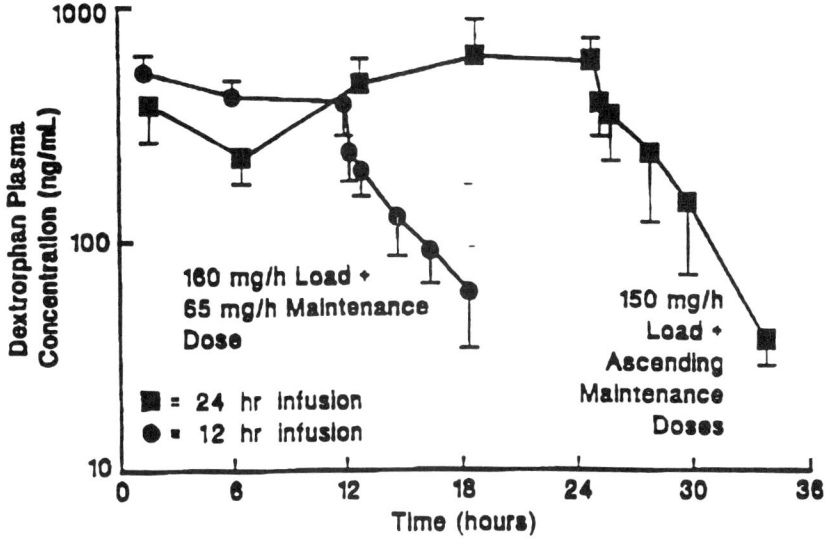

**FIGURE 6.** Mean dextrorphan plasma concentrations: 12- and 24-hour infusions.

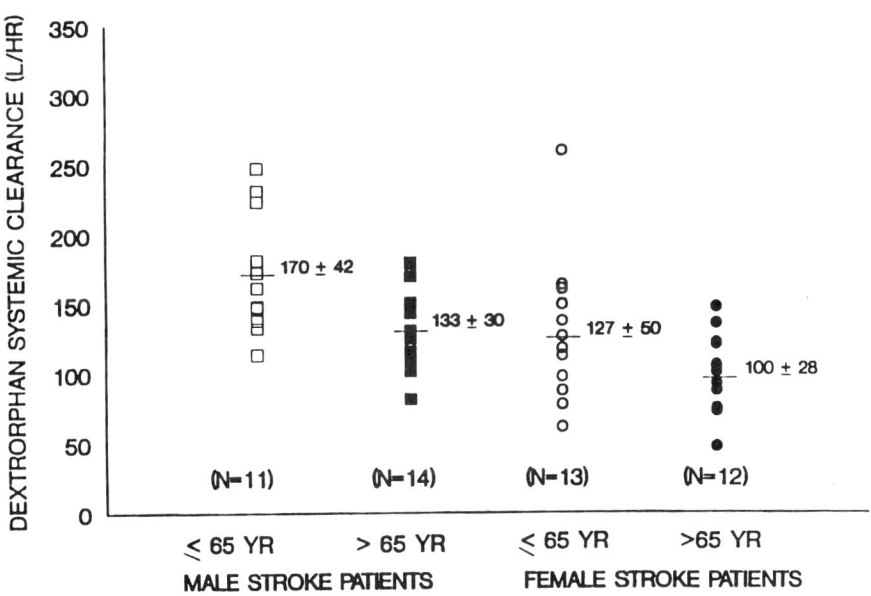

**FIGURE 7.** Dextrorphan systemic clearance (L/h) in male and female stroke patients.

## DISCUSSION

During the last several years in *in vitro* and *in vivo* experiments, it has been recognized that dextrorphan HCl is a noncompetitive antagonist at the NMDA receptor complex and is neuroprotective in various animal models of ischemic stroke. *In vivo* models of ischemic stroke have suggested that the neuroprotective effects of dextrorphan are dose-dependent and increase with higher serum concentrations of drug. With this caveat in mind, several Phase I trials in volunteers and an acute stroke patient population were undertaken to study the safety and pharmacokinetics of escalating doses of dextrorphan. The results of these recent clinical trials indicate that dextrorphan can be safely administered to an elderly population of acute stroke patients while achieving plasma concentrations between 300 and 1000 ng/mL in an extended infusion schema. These plasma concentrations in the acute stroke population are thought to be comparable to those levels found to be neuroprotective in *in vitro* and *in vivo* models of ischemic injury.

In this study, dextrorphan was administered to acute stroke patients within 48 hours after their ischemic stroke to determine the "maximum tolerated" one-hour loading dose and maintenance infusion rate. Dextrorphan administration was associated with a high incidence of pharmacologic effects, predominantly, CNS in nature (*e.g.*, nystagmus, nausea, agitation, hallucinations, confusion and somnolence), which indicated NMDA receptor blockade. Even though 100% of dextrorphan-treated patients experienced pharmacologic effects, most of these effects were mild to moderate in severity, were short-lived, and were fairly well tolerated by elderly patients. The frequency of the most pharmacologic common effects differed between the loading dose and maintenance infusion periods. Nystagmus, nausea, vomiting and somnolence were seen with a greater frequency during the first 90 minutes (loading period); confusion, agitation, hallucinations and hypertension were seen more frequently throughout the maintenance period. The incidence of these pharmacologic effects was generally lower in the low and intermediate dose group (145–180 mg/hr) than in the highest dose group (200–260 mg/hr) in both the loading and maintenance infusion periods. It is encouraging that dextrorphan administration produced no clinically significant alterations in ECG findings or in hematologic, urine, or serum chemistries.

Loading dose escalation was eventually limited by abrupt drops in systolic blood pressure. Dose escalation was terminated after 7 of 21 patients, receiving the highest range loading dose (200–260 mg/hr) developed rapid, symptomatic but reversible drops in systolic blood pressure. These abrupt drops in systolic blood pressure, which occurred without neurologic sequelae, occurred within a very predictable loading window of 90 minutes from onset of drug infusion and at a rate of more than 3 mg/min. After careful evaluation of patient characteristics and pharmacokinetic data, no other common predisposing factors (*e.g.*, dextrorphan plasma concentrations, preexisting illnesses, concomitant medications, weight or lean body mass) were determined. Hypotension appeared to be related to the rate of the loading dose administration and not the plasma concentration. The escalation of the maintenance infusion was terminated secondarily to the termination of the escalation of the loading infusion. Decreased level of consciousness and respiratory depression in three patients was seen at maintenance infusion rates greater than 90 mg/hr and lead to discontinuation of the maintenance infusion. Subsequently, it was felt that the highest safe and tolerable loading dose and maintenance infusion dose were <180 mg/hr and between 50 to 90 mg/hr, respectively. Clinical investigators had a lengthy window of opportunity to enter patients into the trial since its goal was not to evaluate dextrorphan's efficacy. Consequently, it would be unlikely to expect neuroprotective results from treatment with dextrorphan in this study. It is encouraging that even though the dextrorphan-treated patients did not show greater improvement on their NIH Stroke Scale scores at 48 hours than the placebo patients, they did not neurologically worsen even when developing symptomatic hypotension.

Dextrorphan has a 1) relatively short half-life, 2) a large volume of distribution and, 3) a high clearance in acute stroke patients. Plasma concentrations decreased rapidly for six hours after the termination of the infusion in both the 12- and 24-hour treatment groups. This pharmacokinetic profile suggests that the abovementioned pharmcologic effects of the drug would also rapidly clear after the end of the infusion, and patients would return to their poststroke but predrug physical status.

## SUMMARY

Dextrorphan HCl (Ro 01-6794/706) is an NMDA receptor antagonist with clinical potential for administration in an elderly population of acute ischemic stroke patients. *In vivo* experience with such patients demonstrated a consistent pharmcologic effect/adverse experience profile that is typical of an NMDA receptor antagonist (*e.g.,* nystagmus, nausea, vomiting, agitation, somnolence, hallucinations and hypertension). For the most part, these pharmacologic effects were mild to moderate in severity; short-lived; reversible; not life-threatening and subjectively tolerated. The most serious pharmacologic effect produced by dextrorphan administration was hypotension, which occurred within a well-defined window of 90 minutes from the start of the loading dose infusion in patients who received 200 mg/hr or greater loading dose infusions. In all cases it was reversible without neurologic sequelae. Careful review of demographic and pharmacokinetic parameters did not demonstrate any overriding factor(s) to the production of hypotension other than the rate of the loading dose infusion. Severe hypotension, severe decreased levels of consciousness and respiratory depression should not be generally expected at loading doses less than 200 mg/hr. In summary, dextrorphan can be safely given to an elderly population of ischemic stroke patients as a loading dose rate below 200 mg/hr and as a maintenance dose rate between 50–90 mg/hr for 24 hours when patients are monitored carefully for pharmacologic effects.

## REFERENCES

1. ROTHMAN, S. M. & J. W. OLNEY. 1986. Glutamate and the pathophysiology of hypoxic-ischemic brain damage. Ann. Neurol. **19:** 105–111.
2. MCBEAN, G. J. & P. J. ROBERTS. 1984. Chronic infusion of L-glutamate causes neurotoxicity in rat striatum. Brain Res. **290:** 372–375.

3. MANGANO, R. M. & R. SCHWARCZ. 1983. Chronic infusion of endogenous excitatory amino acids into rat striatum and hippocampus. Brain Res. Bull. **10:** 47–51.
4. MCLENNAN, H. 1981. On the nature of the receptors for various excitatory amino acids in the mammalian central nervous system. *In* Glutamate as a Neurotransmitter. G. DiChiara & G. L. Gessa, Eds. 253–262. Raven Press. New York.
5. CROUCHER, M. J., J. F. COLLINS & B. S. MELDRUM. 1982. Anticonvulsant action of excitatory amino acid antagonists. Science **216:** 899–901.
6. SIMON, R. P., J. H. SWAN, T. GRIFFITHS *et al.* 1994. Blockade of $N$-methyl-D-aspartate receptors may protect against ischemic damage in the brain. Science **226:** 850–852.
7. MELDRUM, B. S., T. GRIFFITHS & M. EVANS. 1982. Hypoxia and neuronal hyperexcitability: a clue to mechanisms of brain protection. *In* Protection of Tissues against Hypoxia. 275–286. A. WAQUIER, M. BORGERS & W. K. AMERY, Eds. Elsevier Biomedical Press. Amsterdam.
8. WIELOCH, T. 1985. Hypoglycemia-induced neuronal damage prevented by an $N$-methyl-D-aspartate antagonist. Science **230:** 681–683.
9. ISBELL, H. & H. F. FRASER. 1953. Actions and addiction liabilities of dromoran derivatives in man. J. Pharmacol. Exp. Ther. **107:** 524–530.
10. WONG, B. Y., D. A. COULTER, D. W. CHOI *et al.* 1988. Dextrorphan and dextromethorphan, common antitussives, are antiepileptic and antagonize $N$-methyl-D-aspartate in brain slices. Neurosci. Lett. **85:** 261–266.
11. CHOI, D. W. 1987. Dextrorphan and dextromethorphan attenuate glutamate neurotoxicity. Brain Res. **403:** 333–336.
12. CHOI, D. W., S. PETERS & V. VISEKUL. 1987. Dextrorphan and levorphanol selectively block $N$-methyl-D-aspartate receptor-mediated neurotoxicity on cortical neurons. J. Pharmacol. Exp. Ther. **272:** 713–720.
13. CHURCH, J., D. LODGE & S. C. BERRY. 1985. Differential effects of dextrorphan and levorphanol on excitation of rat spinal neurons by amino acids. Eur. J. Pharmacol. **111:** 185–190.
14. HAMPTON, R. Y., F. MEDZIHRADSKY, J. H. WOODS *et al.* 1982. Stereospecific binding of $^3$H-phencyclidine in brain membranes. Life Sci. **30:** 2147–2154.
15. MURRAY, T. F. & M. E. LEID. 1984. Interaction of dextrorotatory opoids with phencyclidine recognition sites in rat membranes. Life Sci. **34:** 1899–1911.
16. SUN, F-Y., H. ZHU, L-M. ZHANG *et al.* 1987. Dextrorphan: an antagonist for phencyclidine receptors. Life Sci. **40:** 2303–2307.
17. WONG, E. H. F., A. R. KNIGHT & G. N. WOODRUFF. 1988. [$^3$H]MK-801 labels a site of the $N$-methyl-D-aspartate receptor channel complex in rat brain membranes. J. Neurochem. **50:** 274–281.
18. STEINBERG, G. K., J. SALEH & D. KUNIS. 1988. Delayed treatment with dextromethorphan and dextrorphan reduces cerebral damage after transient focal ischemia. Neurosci. Lett. **89:** 193–197.
19. STEINBERG, G. K., J. SALEH, R. DELAPAZ *et al.* 1989. Pretreatment with the NMDA-antagonist, dextrorphan, reduces cerebral damage after transient focal ischemia in rabbits. Brain Res. **497:** 382–386.
20. STEINBERG, G. K., J. SALEH, R. DELAPAZ *et al.* 1989. Protective effect of $N$-methyl-D-aspartate antagonists after transient focal ischemia in rabbits. Stroke **20:** 1247–1252.
21. STEINBERG, G. K., J. SALEH, D. KUNIS & R. DELAPAZ. 1989. Protection against cerebral ischemia by the NMDA antagonist dextrorphan is dose dependent and correlated with plasma and brain levels. Annual Meeting of the Society for Neuroscience. Abstracts 15, No. 1, 45, Abstr. No. 23.23.
22. STEINBERG, G. K., J. SALEH, D. KUNIS & R. DELAPAZ. 1989. Post-ischemic treatment with the NMDA antagonist dextrorphan protects against cerebral injury after focal ischemia: a dose-dependent response. J. Cereb. Blood Flow Metab. **9**(Suppl. 1): S238.
23. GRAHAM, S. H., J. CHEN & R. P. SIMON. 1993. A dose response study of dextrorphan in permanent focal ischemia. Neurosci Lett. **160:** 21–23.
24. MELDRUM, B. S. 1985. Possible therapeutic applications of antagonists of excitatory amino acid neurotransmitters. Clin. Sci. **68:** 113–122.

25. LYDEN, P. D. & G. T. LAU. 1991. A critical appraisal of stroke evaluation and rating scales. Stroke **22:** 1345–1352.
26. BROTT, T., H. P. ADAMS, C. P. OLINGER *et al.* 1989. Measurements of acute cerebral infarction: a clinical examination scale. Stroke **20:** 864–870.
27. GOLDSTEIN, L. B., C. BERTELS & J. N. DAVIS. 1989. Interrater reliability of the NIH Stroke Scale. Arch Neurol. **46:** 660–662.

# The Rationale for Glutamate Antagonists in the Treatment of Traumatic Brain Injury

J. S. MYSEROS AND R. BULLOCK

*Division of Neurosurgery*
*MCV Station*
*Box 980631*
*Richmond, Virginia 23298-0631*

## INTRODUCTION

There is clear evidence from both clinical and neuropathological studies that a substantial proportion (30–40%) of those patients who die after severe head injury have spoken at some stage after the impact.[1] This suggests that secondary processes are responsible for a substantial part of subsequent brain damage. This provides the opportunity for drug treatment prior to these secondary processes, at least in a proportion of head-injured patients.

Converging lines of evidence from several animal studies suggest that excitotoxic damage to neurons and glia may develop as a consequence of excessive release of excitatory amino acids after primary impact injury, ischemic events, and hematoma.[2–7] Therefore, it appears that the potent neuroprotective effects that have been shown for NMDA antagonist drugs in the laboratory can now be translated into clinical benefit for head-injured patients.

### Mechanisms That Cause Brain Damage after Severe Human Head Injury

Our present understanding of the pathophysiological events in human head injury has been developed from several sources: (1) neuropathological studies, (2) monitoring and imaging the head-injured patients during life, and (3) study of animal models. Unfortunately, neuropathological studies are biased toward the poorest outcome in the head injury spectrum, and may, therefore, overestimate the incidence and severity of both ischemic damage and structural axonal shearing in those who survive. Despite recent advances, dynamic imaging and invasive physiological monitoring of the living brain after severe head injury remain relatively poorly developed. Although studies such as magnetic resonance imaging (MRI) scanning have provided important structural insight, our ability to monitor hemodynamically stabilized head injury patients within the intensive care unit has allowed us to detect only the aftereffects of harmful events that occurred within the first minutes or hours after the injury and before the patient has reached the intensive care unit.

It has been the study of animal models that has given us information regarding these important early posttraumatic events. These model studies have given an insight into early dynamic events ranging from the macroanatomical/biomechanical level to the intracellular and extracellular microenvironment. The events concerned with intracellular energy metabolism, maintenance of neuronal membrane potential, and homeostasis at synapses are currently the focus of intense interest.

Postmortem studies of fatally head-injured patients have shown that most ischemic damage is focal, not global. Moreover, NMDA antagonists are more effective in focal ischemia models.[8] This type of ischemic damage is associated with raised intracranial pressure, hypoxic or hypotensive events during life, and intracranial hematomas.

Hippocampal ischemic damage is especially common after severe head injury and occurs in 50% without raised intracranial pressure, hypotension, or hypoxia.[9,10] This suggests that alternative mechanisms may damage the hippocampus, which appears to be preferentially vulnerable in the head-injured patient.

Intra- and extraaxial hematomas may complicate the clinical course of patients with even mild head injury and transform it into a life-threatening event. Present in 25–45% of severely injured patients, they remain an important cause of secondary ischemia due to raised intracranial pressure.[11] Of course, acute subdural hematoma carries the worst prognosis. Paradoxically, 55–70% of patients have been lucid at some time after injury and before demonstration of the hematoma, yet over 60% remain disabled or die after a subdural hematoma is removed, supporting the idea of a secondary insult.[12] In addition, we have found marked reductions in cerebral blood flow focally around cerebral contusions, and beneath acute hematoma.[13]

Previously, diffuse axonal injury was thought to have been an instantaneous event in which widespread physical and functional disruption of axons occurred at the moment of impact.[14] Numerous studies using fluid percussion injury models (FPI) have shown that impact is immediately followed by massive release of neurotransmitter, including catecholamines, acetylcholine, and glutamate.[2,3,7] Studies have also shown, however, that structural axonal disruption only develops later,[15] perhaps by widespread depolarization with ingress of sodium and calcium ions and efflux of potassium into the extracellular space.[16] This may then cause swelling of axoplasm and glia, which may proceed to cause mechanical disruption in some axons, eventually causing the reactive axonal swellings, or retraction balls, as seen on silver stains more than 24 h after impact. Further evidence for this consequential damage comes from clinical studies that have shown that 30% of patients with histological diffuse axonal injury at postmortem examination had spoken at some time after impact and before death.[1]

### Evidence from Animal Models Depicting Human Head Injury

Potent glutamate receptor antagonists, now available for investigation, have made excitotoxicity a focus of intense interest in the field of ischemia and neurotrauma research.[8] There is now evidence from four categories of animal model that demonstrates glutamate-induced brain damage or functional disruption after head injury-related events.

## Middle Cerebral Artery (MCA) Occlusion: Pure Focal Cerebral Ischemia Models

Because of the frequency of focal and global ischemia, models of focal ischemia are highly relevant to human head injury. We have demonstrated up to a 40-fold increase in extracellular glutamate in the striatum after MCA occlusion in the rat.[17] The time course of this increase accords with the increase in glucose utilization demonstrated in the periphery of an MCA occlusion, persisting up to 4 h after the onset of ischemia.[18] This pattern of glucose hypermetabolism in the peri-ischemic zone corresponds both topographically and temporally with the uptake of both $^3$H-MK-801 and $^{123}$I-MK-801 after MCA occlusion.[19] $^3$H-MK-801 is a specific ligand for the agonist gated ion channel. The increased *in vivo* binding is, therefore, indicative of glutamate-induced ion channel activation.

The most powerful evidence in support of glutamate-induced neurotoxicity in focal ischemia comes from many neuroprotection studies, performed with a variety of NMDA and non-NMDA glutamate antagonists, in the majority of which, neuroprotective efficacy has been shown (TABLE 1). NMDA antagonists are most effective when administered before the insult (especially competitive antagonists), but MK-801 and GYKI 52466 have been effective when given up to 2 h after the ischemic event. This consistency and magnitude of neuroprotection exceed that which has been shown for any other category of neuroprotective compound in the past.

Such effects of NMDA antagonists after transient global ischemic insults are much less certain. In addition, a new category of glutamate antagonist has recently been studied, in that they block release of glutamate from the presynaptic vesicle. These (*e.g.*, BW 619) have now shown convincing evidence of neuroprotective efficacy in models of both global and focal ischemia.[20]

## Diffuse Axonal Shearing Injury Models

Several animal models have been devised to attempt to replicate the shearing injury produced in the human brain by high energy acceleration or deceleration. Since only the PENN I and PENN II primate studies closely reproduced the neuropathological findings seen in humans, it has not been possible to use these models to seek evidence of glutamate neurotoxicity.[14] The fluid percussion inury (FPI) models in the cat and rat, although less similar to human head injury, have provided important evidence of EAA-mediated changes.[21] There is now much support for the hypothesis that the structural axonal lesions seen by light microscopy after shear injury may be caused not by a mechanical process, but by failure of ionic homeostasis, perhaps mediated via the glutamate channel. Microdialysis has demonstrated a surge in extracellular fluid (ECF) glutamate to twice basal and six times basal levels following fluid percussion in the rat, respectively, lasting only a few minutes.[3,16] In Katayama's studies, massive efflux of potassium was demonstrated supporting sustained depolarization of both voltage-dependent and EAA-mediated ion channels.

Mild to moderate fluid percussion injury produces a consistent impairment of short-term memory in the rat, such that performance in the radial arm maze or

TABLE 1. NMDA Receptor-Associated Antagonists Following Experimental Fluid-Percussion Injury in Rats

| Investigator | Type of Antagonist | Compound | Findings |
|---|---|---|---|
| McIntosh[33] | noncompetitive NMDA | MK-801 | reduced focal brain edema, restored ion homeostasis, improved metabolic status |
| Shapira[34] | noncompetitive NMDA | MK-801 | reduced focal brain edema, improved neurologic function |
| Smith[42] | noncompetitive NMDA | dextromethorphan | improved neurologic function |
| Smith[43] | noncompetitive NMDA | magnesium | improved cognitive function |
| Smith[43] | noncompetitive NMDA | ketamine | improved cognitive function |
| Hayes[35] | noncompetitive NMDA | PCP | attenuated long-term motor deficits |
| Jenkins[36] | noncompetitive NMDA | PCP | attenuated 2° vulnerability superimposed ischemia and decreased $CA_1$ death |
| McIntosh[37] | noncompetitive NMDA | MK-801 | improved cardiovascular variables, improved motor function |
| Lyeth[39] | noncompetitive NMDA | MK-801 | improved motor function |
| Hamm[40] | noncompetitive NMDA | MK-801 | decreased memory deficits |
| Faden[3] | noncompetitive NMDA | dextrorphan | improved motor function and bioenergetic status |
| McIntosh[38] | noncompetitive NMDA | magnesium | improved neurologic function |
| Faden[3] | competitive NMDA | CPP | improved neurologic function |
| Smith[42] | competitive NMDA | CGS 19755 | no effect when administered |
| Smith[44] | glycine site | indole-2-carboxylic acid | improved posttraumatic cognitive function |
| Katayama[16] | glycine site | kynurenate | decreased $K^+$ efflux |
| Smith[41] | glycine site | kynurenate | reduced regional edema formation, reduced regional total $Ca^{2+}$ increases |
| Smith[41] | glycine site | indol-2-carboxylic acid | reduced regional edema formation, decreased regional total $Ca^{2+}$ and $Na^+$ increases |

the Morris water maze is impaired for periods up to 2 weeks. Treatment with NMDA antagonists, both with MK-801 and the competitive antagonist CGS 19755, before FPI results in a dose-dependent improvement in both mortality (severe FPI) and memory and motor tasks (moderate FPI).[21]

*Excitotoxic Mechanisms following Acute Subdural Hematoma in the Rat*

We have devised a model of acute subdural hematoma in the rat that produces a consistent zone of focal cerebral ischemia (14% of hemisphere volume) beneath the hematoma.[22] Using this model, we have demonstrated a sevenfold increase in glutamate after induction of the hematoma. This hypermetabolic process persisted for between 2 and 4 h, suggesting that this may be the window of opportunity during which glutamate neurotoxicity is occurring in this model. When the experiments were repeated with an inert silicone mass within the subdural space, hippocampal hyperactivation was not seen.[23] Ultrastructural studies have shown vacuolation and cell death in 2–3% of neurons within the CA3 sector of the hippocampus in this model, although blood flow is preserved at levels well above the thresholds for ischemia. Pretreatment with the competitive NMDA antagonist D-CPP-ene abolishes the hypermetabolism and significantly reduces (by 54%) the extent of ischemic damage that occurs under the subdural hematoma.[6,24]

*Double-Insult Models*

Clinical studies have shown secondary events such as ischemia or hypoxia to carry a poor prognosis, in that 100% of patients who sustained both hypotensive and hypoxic insults after severe head injury were dead or severely disabled in one study.[25] Both the ischemic damage and impaired memory performance in rats after FPI were abolished by pretreating with the NMDA antagonist phencyclidine or scopolamine.[26]

Mild ischemia may inactivate or reverse glutamate reuptake mechanisms at the synaptic cleft, particularly in the areas with a high density of glutamatergic synapses, such as the hippocampus. Therefore, the glutamate released by the FPI may reach toxic levels at the synaptic cleft to cause or predispose to cell damage. Such mechanisms may explain some of the phenomena seen in head-injured patients, and they also may explain the phenomenon of delayed neuronal death.[27] However, such speculative hypotheses require rigorous testing.

### *Choosing the Appropriate Glutamate Antagonist for Human Head Injury*

The putative sites of action for selected glutamate antagonists that may have a clinical role in the future are shown in FIGURE 1. Only CGS 19755, D-CPP-ene, and CNS 1102 have completed safety assessments in humans and are in phase II and III clinical trials. CGS 19755 is currently in a phase III trial in human stroke, while MK-801 has been withdrawn from clinical use. A series of "second generation" glutamate antagonists, *e.g.*, ACEA 1021, Pfizer CP 101-606, and BW 619 C81, with putatively less side effects, are now being evaluated in phase II studies.

Magnesium chloride administration has achieved striking neuroprotection in a rat middle cerebral occlusion model.[28] Unfortunately, magnesium is difficult to administer to patients because of its narrow safety margin. All these drugs are of clinical interest because theoretically they may provide the opportunity to pretreat the glutamate-vulnerable injured brain against the effects of secondary ischemia with less side effects.

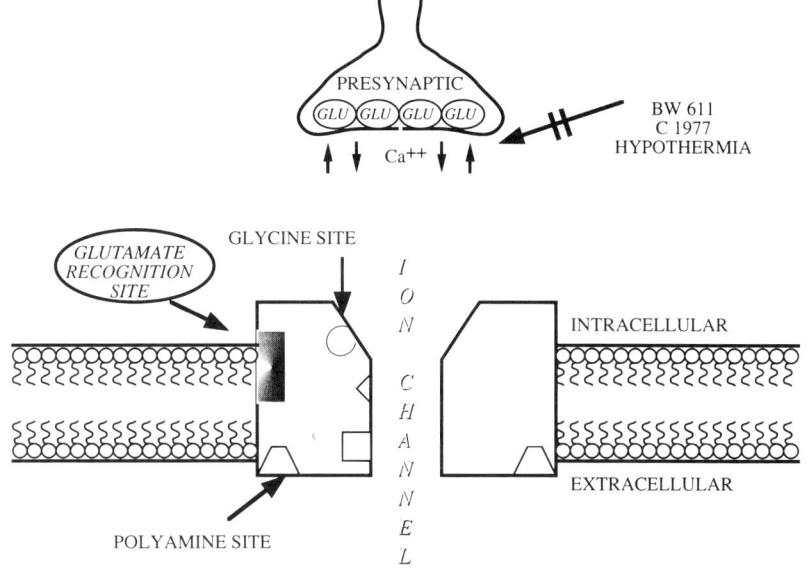
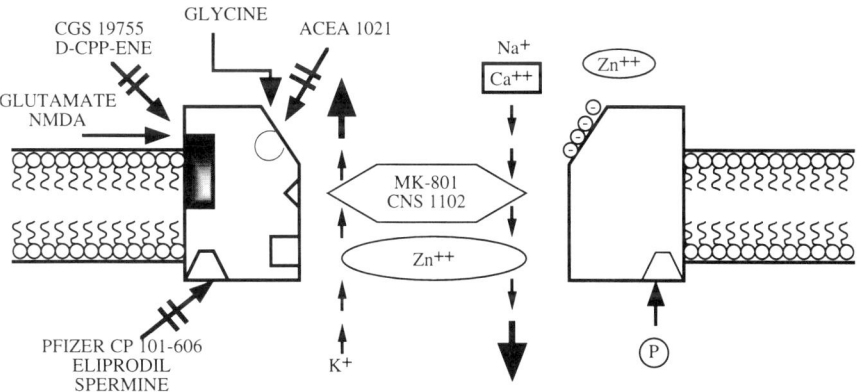

**FIGURE 1.** Putative sites of action for selected glutamate antagonists.

### Other Advantages and Disadvantages of NMDA Antagonist Drugs in Management of Head-Injured Patients

In addition to their neuroprotective properties, both competitive and noncompetitive NMDA antagonists possess other effects that may be beneficial in head injury.

Studies in a variety of normal animals and models of cerebral ischemia have shown that D-CPP-ene, MK-801, and C1977 are powerful sedative agents that possess analgesic properties. Therefore, this could reduce the requirements for neuromuscular paralytics and narcotics during the ventilation and resuscitation of these head-injured patients. Fortunately, neither D-CPP-ene, CGS 19755, or MK-801 demonstrated any adverse influence on intracranial pressure.[29]

Although the neuroprotective effect of glutamate antagonists is primarily independent of their effects on cerebral blood flow (CBF), these agents also increase regional CBF. MK-801 produced significant increases in regional CBF, particularly in limbic structures. This probably reflects intact coupling of flow and metabolism.[30] Similar increases in CBF have been shown with CGS 19755.[31] The CBF effects of NMDA antagonists may be abolished or attenuated by concomitant anesthesia.

The competitive antagonists D-CPP-ene and CGS 19755 are also potent anticonvulsants.[32] In the severely head-injured population, where the incidence of seizures ranges from 14% to 43%, this effect will be of major benefit.

Neurotoxicity, psychotropic effects, retention of $CO_2$, and hypotension have been observed with some NMDA antagonists. As such, these patients should be closely monitored, particularly during the use of these agents.

## THE FUTURE

The clinical dilemmas facing physicians who deal with severely head-injured patients are now becoming clear. Techniques must be developed to detect mechanisms of brain damage in humans such as glutamate-induced neurotoxicity, free radical-induced membrane damage and voltage-dependent calcium-mediated damage. Strategies then must be devised for the optimal administration of appropriate pharmacological agents or physical techniques (hypothermia) to ameliorate these processes. The prospect of achieving a major reduction in head injury-induced morbidity and mortality is at least becoming tangible.

## SUMMARY

The recent development of potent antagonists for the most widespread neurotransmitter in the mammalian brain has opened up possibilities for many forms of therapy. The excitotoxic hypothesis implicates excessive release of excitatory amino acids (EAAs) as an important cause of brain damage, especially in acute ischemia, and chronic neurodegeneration. Focal ischemic damage and diffuse axonal injury are the major causes of brain damage after traumatic human brain injury. Evidence from animal models has shown that excitatory amino acid-induced events maybe responsible for a proportion of the posttraumatic sequelae and that these effects can be blocked by EAA antagonists. This evidence is reviewed, and the implications for human pathophysiology and treatment are discussed.

## REFERENCES

1. BLUMBERG, P. C., N. R. JONES & J. B. NORTH. 1989. Diffuse axonal injury in head trauma. J. Neurol. Neurosurg. Psychiatry **52:** 838–842.
2. BECKER, D. P., Y. KATAYAMA, T. TAMURA, L. GORMAN & M. K. CHEUNG. 1989. Excitotoxic ion fluxes and neuronal dysfunction following traumatic brain injury. J. Cereb. Blood Flow Metab. **9**(Suppl. 1): S302.
3. FADEN, A. I., DEMEDIUK, S. S. PANTER & R. VINK. 1989. The role of excitatory amino acids and NMDA receptors in traumatic brain injury. Science **244:** 798–800.
4. INGLIS, F. M., R. BULLOCK, M-H. CHEN, D. I. GRAHAM, J. D. MILLER, J. MCCULLOCH & G. M. TEASDALE. 1990. Ischemic brain damage associated with tissue hypermetabolism in acute haematoma: reduction by a glutamate antagonist. *In* Proceedings of Eighth International Symposium on Brain Oedema. H. J. Reulen, Ed. 277–280. Springer-Verlag. Bern, Vienna.
5. BULLOCK, R., S. P. BUTCHER, M-H CHEN, L. KENDALL & J. MCCULLOCH. 1991. Correlation of the extracellular glutamate concentration with extent of blood flow reduction after subdural haematoma in the rat. J. Neurosurg. **74:** 794–802.
6. BULLOCK, R., F. M. INGLIS, Y. KURODA, S. BUTCHER, J. MCCULLOCH & W. MAXWELL. 1991. Transient hippocampal hypermetabolism associated with glutamate release after acute subdural haematoma in the rat: a potentially neurotoxic mechanism: Brain '91. XVth International Symposium on Cerebral Blood Flow and Metabolism. Miami, FL, June 1991. J. Cereb. Blood Flow Metab. **11**(Suppl. 2): S109.
7. KAWAMATA, T., Y. KATAYAMA, D. HOVDA, A. YOSHIRO & D. P. BECKER. 1992. Administration of excitatory amino acid antagonists via microdialysis attenuates the increase in glucose use seen following concussive brain injury. J. Cereb. Blood Flow Metab. **12:** 12–24.
8. MELDRUM, B. 1990. Protection against ischemic neuronal damage by drugs acting on excitatory neurotransmission. Cerebrovasc. Brain Metab. Rev. **2:** 27–57.
9. KOTAPKA, M., D. I. GRAHAM, J. H. ADAMS & T. A. GENNARELLI. 1992. Hippocampal pathology in fatal non-missile human head injury. Acta Neuropathol. (Berlin) **83:** 530–534.
10. GRAHAM, D. I., A. LAWRENCE, J. H. ADAMS, D. DOYLE & D. R. MCLENNAN. 1988. Brain damage in fatal non-missile head injury without high intracranial pressure. J. Clin Pathol. **41:** 34–37.
11. BULLOCK, R. & G. M. TEASDALE. 1990. Head injuries—surgical management: traumatic intracranial hematomas. *In* Vinken and Bruyn's Handbook of Clinical Neurology: Head Injury. R. Braakman, Ed. Vol. 24: 249–298. Elsevier Science Publishers. Amsterdam.
12. STONE, J. L., M. H. S. RIFAI, O. SUGAR, R. G. A. LANG, J. B. OLDERSHAW & R. A. MOODY. 1983. Subdural hematomas. Acute subdural hematoma: progress in definition, clinical pathology and therapy. Surg. Neurol. **19:** 216–231.
13. SCHRODER, M. L., J. P. MUIZELAAR & A. J. KUTA. 1994. Documented reversal of global ischemia immediately after removal of an acute subdural hematoma. J. Neurosurg. **80:** 324–327.
14. ADAMS, J. H., D. L. GRAHAM & T. A. GENNARELLI. 1983. Head injury in man and experimental animals: neuropathology. Acta Neurochir. Suppl. **32:** 15–30.
15. ERB, D. I. & J. T. POVLISHOCK. 1988. Axonal damage in severe traumatic brain injury: an experimental study in the cat. Acta Neuropathol. **76:** 347–358.
16. KATAYAMA, Y., D. P. BECKER, T. TAMURA & D. A. HOVDA. 1990. Massive increases in extracellular potassium and the indiscriminate release of glutamate following concussive brain injury. J. Neurosurg. **73:** 889–900.
17. BUTCHER, S. P., R. BULLOCK, D. L. GRAHAM & J. MCCULLOCH. 1990. Correlation between amino acid release and neuropathological outcome in rat striatum and cortex following middle cerebral artery occlusion. Stroke **21:** 1727–1733.
18. SHIRAISHI, K., F. R. SHARP & R. P. SIMON. 1989. Sequential metabolic changes in rat brain following middle cerebral artery occlusion: a 2-deoxyglucose study. J. Cereb. Blood Flow Metab. **9:** 765–773.

19. WALLACE, M. C., G. M. TEASDALE & J. MCCULLOCH. 1992. Autoradiographic analysis of $^3$H-MK801 *in vivo* uptake, and *in vitro* binding, after focal cerebral ischemia in the rat. J. Neurosurg. **76:** 127–134.
20. MELDRUM, B., J. H. SWAN, M. MILLAN, M. J. LEACH, G. RYDER & R. P. SIMON. 1992. A pyrimidine derivative, Wellcome BW 1003 C 87, decreases glutamate release and protects against ischemic damage. *In* Proceedings of an Official Satellite Symposium of BRAIN-91: the Role of Neurotransmitters in Brain Injury. M. Y. Globus & W. D. Dietrich, Eds. 15–20. Plenum Press. New York.
21. HAYES, R., L. W. JENKINS & B. G. LYETH. 1992. Neurotransmitter mediated mechanisms of traumatic brain injury: acetylcholine and excitatory amino acids. J. Neurotrauma **9**(Suppl 1): S173.
22. MILLER, J. D., R. BULLOCK, D. I. GRAHAM, M-H CHEN & G. M. TEASDALE. 1990. Ischemic brain damage in a model of acute subdural hematoma. Neurosurgery **27:** 433–439.
23. KURODA, Y., F. M. INGLIS, J. D. MILLER, J. MCCULLOCH, D. I. GRAHAM & R. BULLOCK. 1992. Transient glucose hypermetabolism after acute subdural hematoma in the rat. J. Neurosurg. **76:** 944–950.
24. CHEN, M-H., R. BULLOCK, D. L. GRAHAM, J. D. MILLER & J. MCCULLOCH. 1991. Ischemic neuronal damage after acute subdural hematoma in the rat: effects of pretreatment with a glutamate antagonist. J. Neurosurg. **74:** 944–950.
25. GENTLEMAN, D. & B. JENNETT. 1981. Hazards of interhospital transfer of comatose head injured patients. Lancet **2:** 853–855.
26. JENKINS, L. W., K. MOSZYNSKI, B. G. LYETH *et al.* 1989. Increased vulnerability of the mildly injured rat brain to cerebral ischemia: the use of controlled secondary ischemia as a research tool to identify common or different mechanisms contributing to mechanical and ischemic brain injury. Brain Res. **477:** 211–224.
27. KIRINO, T., A. TAMURA & K. SANO. 1984. Delayed neuronal death in the rat hippocampus following transient forebrain ischaemia. Acta Neuropathol. (Berlin) **64:** 139–147.
28. PINARD, E., Y. IZUMI, S. ROUSEL & J. SEYLAG. 1992. Comparative effects of magnesium chloride and MK 801 on the infarct volume after MCA occlusion in Fischer 344 rats. *In* Proceedings of an Official Satellite Symposium of BRAIN-91: the Role of Neurotransmitters in Brain Injury. M. Y. Globus & W. D. Dietrich, Eds. 93–98. Plenum Press. New York.
29. KURODA Y., H. FUJISAWA, S. STREBEL, D. I. GRAHAM & R. BULLOCK. 1994. Effect of neuroprotective *N*-methyl-D-aspartate antagonists on increased intracranial pressure: studies in the rat acute subdural hematoma model. Neurosurgery **35:** 106–112.
30. NEHLS, D. G., C. K. PARK, A. G. MCCORMACK & J. MCCULLOCH. 1990. The effects of *N*-methyl-D-aspartate receptor blockade with MK 801 upon the relationship between cerebral blood flow and glucose use. Brain Res. **511:** 271–279.
31. TAKIZAWA, S., M. HOGAN & A. M. HAKIM. 1991. The effects of a competitive NMDA receptor antagonist (CGS 19755) on cerebral blood flow and pH in focal ischemia. J. Cereb. Blood Flow Metab. **11:** 786–793.
32. CHAPMAN, A. 1990. Excitatory amino acid antagonists and therapy of epilepsy. *In* Excitatory Amino Acid Antagonists. B. Meldrum, Ed. 265–285. Blackwell Scientific. London.
33. MCINTOSH, T. K., R. VINK, H. SOARES, R. HAYES & R. SIMON. 1990. Effect of noncompetitive blockade of *N*-methyl-D-aspartate receptors on the neurochemical sequelae of experimental brain injury. J. Neurochem. **55:** 1170–1179.
34. SHAPIRA Y., G. YADID, S. COTEV, A. NISKA & E. SHOHAMI. 1990. Protective effect of MK801 in experimental brain injury. J. Neurotrauma **7:** 131–139.
35. HAYES, R. L., L. W. JENKINS, B. G. LYETH, R. L. BALSTER, S. E. ROBINSON, G. L. CLIFTON, J. F. STUBBINS & H. F. YOUNG. 1988. Pretreatment with phencyclidine, an *N*-methyl-D-aspartate antagonist, attenuates long-term behavioral deficits in the rat produced by traumatic brain injury. J. Neurotrauma **5:** 259–274.
36. JENKINS, L. W., B. G. LYETH, W. LEWELT, K. MOSZYNSKI, D. S. DEWITT, R. L. BALSTER, L. P. MILLER, G. L. CLIFTON, H. F. YOUNG & R. L. HAYES. 1988. Com-

bined pretrauma scopolamine and phencyclidine attenuates posttraumatic increased sensitivity to delayed secondary ischemia. J. Neurotrauma **5:** 275–287.
37. McIntosh, T. K., R. Vink, H. Soares, R. Hayes & R. Simon. 1989. Effects of the $N$-methyl-D-aspartate receptor blocker MK-801 on neurologic function after experimental brain injury. J. Neurotrauma **6:** 247–259.
38. McIntosh, T. K., R. Vink, I. Yamakami & A. I. Faden. Magnesium protects against neurological deficit after brain injury. Brain Res. **482:** 252–260.
39. Lyeth, B. G., L. W. Jenkins, R. J. Hamm, L. L. Phillips, C. E. Dixon, H. F. Young, J. F. Stubbins, G. L. Clifton & R. L. Hayes. 1989. Pretreatment with MK-801 reduces behavioral deficits following traumatic brain injury (TBI) in rats. Soc. Neurosci. Abstr. **15:** 1113.
40. Hamm, R. J., D. M. O'Dell, B. R. Pike & B. G. Lyeth. 1993. Cognitive impairment following traumatic brain injury: the effect of pre- and postinjury administration of scopolamine and MK-801. J. Cognit. Brain Res. **1:** 223–226, 1993.
41. Smith, D. H., K. Okiyama, M. Thomas, B. Nolan & T. K. McIntosh. 1991. The effects of two novel NMDA antagonists on regional cation concentration and edema formation following experimental brain injury. J. Cereb. Blood Flow Metab. 11(Suppl. 2): S 300.
42. Smith, D. H., M. Thomas, H. Soares & T. K. McIntosh. 1990. Differential effects of competitive and non-competitive $N$-methyl-D-aspartate (NMDA) receptor antagonists in experimental brain injury. FASEB J. **4:** 773.
43. Smith, D. H., K. Okiyama & T. K. McIntosh. 1991. Ketamine and magnesium attenuate memory loss after experimental brain injury. Soc. Neurosci. Abstr. **17:** 167.
44. Smith, D. H., K. Okiyama, M. Thomas & T. K. McIntosh. 1990. An NMDA receptor-associated glycine site antagonist attenuates memory loss after experimental brain injury. Soc. Neurosci. Abstr. **2:** 779.

# Strategies for Neuroprotection with Glutamate Antagonists

## Extrapolating from Evidence Taken from the First Stroke and Head Injury Studies

R. BULLOCK

*Division of Neurosurgery*
*School of Medicine*
*Medical College of Virginia*
*MCV Station, Box 980631*
*Richmond, Virginia 23298-0631*

### INTRODUCTION

The pharmaceutical industry has produced at least nine glutamate antagonists which have completed or are currently completing normal human volunteer studies and which are now involved in clinical trials, chiefly of the Phase II type although for some of these compounds, Phase III efficacy studies have been commenced (TABLE 1).[1-8] Clinical data regarding the safety, tolerability and pharmacokinetics of these compounds is only now becoming public knowledge. For this new category of neuroprotective compounds as a whole, one of the most difficult problems has been the identification of a tolerated dose which is likely to have neuroprotective effects.[10] Many of these compounds have been shown to produce disturbances of higher mental function consistent with their effect upon the limbic system and hippocampus in particular, because of the high density of $N$-methyl-D-aspartate (NMDA) receptors in these structures.

The aim of this report is, therefore, to draw generalized conclusions regarding neuroprotective efficacy, tolerated dose, side effects and pharmacokinetics, particularly from data which was recently presented concerning the first studies with the competitive NMDA antagonist CGS 19755 in both neurotrauma and stroke patients. We will compare this data with information reported in this volume and elsewhere regarding the other agents which are listed in TABLE 1.

### PATIENTS, PHARMACEUTICAL AGENTS, AND METHODS

CGS 19755 has now been given to over 100 stroke patients, and over 50 severe neurotrauma patients.[1,2] For stroke, a double and single dose escalation study was performed in moderate stroke patients with the aim of identifying the optimal tolerated dose for this population. For head trauma, a similar dose escalation regime was performed, using three or four intravenous doses, each 24 hours apart. For stroke, hematologic, hemodynamic, and behavioral safety data were col-

TABLE 1. Glutamate Antagonists and Clinical Trial Indications (as of August, 1994)

| Company | Agent | Category | Trial Indications |
|---|---|---|---|
| Ciba Geigy | CGS 19755 (selfotel) | Competitive glutamate site NMDA antagonist | stroke, brain trauma, high risk neurosurgical prophylaxis |
| Sandoz | D-CPP-ene (EAA494) | competitive glutamate site NMDA antagonist | seizures, brain trauma |
| Cambridge Neuroscience | CNS 1102 (cenestat) | noncompetitive NMDA gated ion channel blocker | stroke, brain trauma |
| Synthelabo | SL 82 (eliprodil) | polyamine site NMDA glutamate antagonist | stroke, brain trauma |
| Burroughs-Wellcome | BW 619C89 | presynaptic glutamate release blocker | stroke, brain trauma |
| Pfizer | CP 101606 | polyamine site NMDA glutamate antagonist | brain trauma, neurodegeneration, stroke |
| ACEA | ACEA 1021 | glycine site NMDA glutamate antagonist | stroke, brain trauma |
| Hoffmann-La Roche | Ro-01-6794/706 (dextromethophan derivative) | noncompetitive NMDA channel blocker (moderate affinity) | stroke |
| Fisons | remacemide | noncompetitive NMDA channel blocker (moderate affinity) | seizures, stroke, coronary bypass |
| Parke-Davis | CI 977 enadoline | Kappa opiate agonist, with glutamate release inhibition | analgesia, brain trauma |

lected, and efficacy was determined by assessing outcome using the NIH and Barthell stroke scales. For the head injury study, outcome was assessed using the Glasgow outcome scale, at 1 and 3 months. Cerebral hemodynamic perameters such as intracranial pressure, cerebral perfusion pressure, middle cerebral artery flow velocity, and cerebral oxygen consumption were also determined in this patient population, who was subjected to uniform intensive care unit (ICU) care.

The noncompetitive NMDA channel blocker CNS 1102, which has much more rapid brain penetration and clearance ($^1/2 \pm 4$ hours) than the competitive agents CGS 19755 and D-CPP-ene, has now been administered to many stroke and head-injured patients, using a trial design broadly similar to the CGS 19755 study.[8-10] Similarly, D-CPP-ene has now been administered to over 30 severe neurotrauma patients in a dose escalation paradigm, as is also the case for the Synthelabo compound, eliprodil.

*Seizure Studies*

The low-affinity noncompetitive NMDA channel blocker remacemide has been administered to a large number of seizure patients[6] and the high affinity competi-

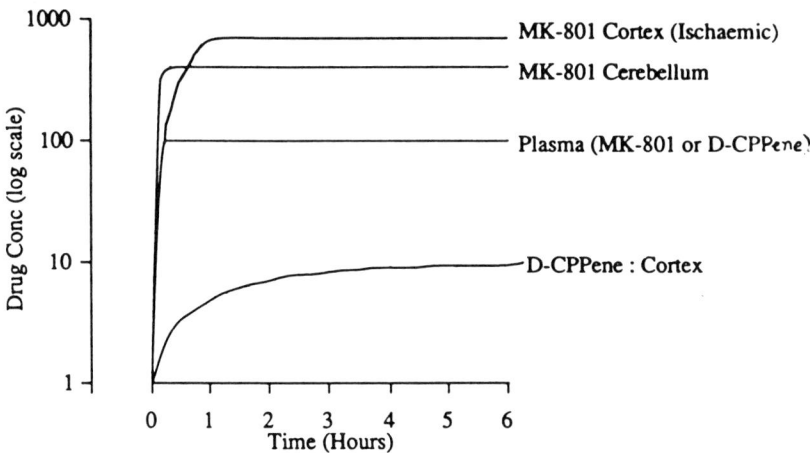

**FIGURE 1.** Theoretical modeling to depict brain penetration, and plasma pharmacokinetics for different classes of NMDA antagonists. The use-dependent receptor binding of noncompetitive agents may theoretically facilitate uptake of drug by ischemic tissue.

tive agent D-CPP-ene has also been given to severe epileptic patients in an "add-on study" design.[11]

## RESULTS AND DISCUSSION

### How to Determine the Optimal Neuroprotective Dose for Glutamate Antagonists?

The diverse pharmacokinetic characteristics, particularly brain penetration, which are seen in the different glutamate antagonists listed in TABLE 1, mean that determining the optimal dose which will balance neuroprotective efficacy against unwanted effects may be difficult, and will clearly vary from compound to compound.[9] FIGURE 1 depicts theoretical modeling of brain uptake for the use-dependent noncompetitive channel blockers, such as MK-801 and dextrometorphan, and for competitive NMDA antagonists, such as D-CPP-ene and selfotel. Since "neuroprotective" plasma concentrations are known from animal studies, and Phase I human volunteer studies yield pharmacokinetic data, and since the concentration of drug which is necessary to inhibit the receptor is known from Scatchard analysis, it is possible to arrive at theoretical dose predictions (TABLE 2).

Neuroprotection studies in gyrencelphalic species such as cats and primates

TABLE 2. Dose-Finding Studies with Glutamate Antagonists Published to Date

| Compound | Indication | Dose | *Estimated* Human "Neuroprotective" Dose | Reported Side Effects and Benefits |
|---|---|---|---|---|
| CGS 19755 (selfotel) | Stroke | 1.75–2 mg/Kg | 4–5 mg/Kg | agitation, paranoia, confusion, delirium outcome (% improvement on MH scale) 7% vs 36% |
| | severe head injury | 1–6 mg/Kg | | ICP lowered by 16 ± 10 mmHg at 5 mg/Kg no adverse effects—patients in coma |
| CNS 1102 (cerestat) | normal volunteers | 3–100 μgm/Kg + infusion | 25 nmol. plasma level | disinhibition, depression, nystagmus (dose-dependent) independent of rate of administration |
| | severe head injury | up to 268 μg/Kg | | no adverse effects—patients in coma |
| Ro-01-764-706 (Dextrometorphan) | acute stroke | 200–260 mg/hr | ? | agitation, confusion, hallucination, somnolence, hypertension in 30–50% of drug patients outcome data awaited |
| BW 619-C89 | healthy volunteers | 0.125–1 mg/Kg | 1–2 mg/Kg | mild dizziness, EEG changes |
| | acute stroke | 1–1.25 mg/Kg | | vomiting, visual hallucinations in 3/7 patients at 1.25 mg/Kg outcome data awaited |
| Remacemide | stroke | 200–300 mg, BD, iv | ? | agitation in 1/28 patients outcome data awaited |
| D-CPP-ene | epilepsy | 250 mg, BD, oral 500 mg, BD, oral | 1–2 mg/Kg iv | sedation, disorientation, confusion, ataxia, amnesia seizures not improved |
| | severe head injury | | | data awaited |

have yielded solid data to show the doses which are needed for neuroprotection. For example, for D-CPP-ene, the lowest effective neuroprotective dose in the cat is 4.5 mg per kilogram, while the comparable dose in the rat is 15 mg per kg.

Many authors have speculated that a four- to fivefold interspecies difference exists between the cat and man, so that a theoretical neuroprotective dose for CGS 19755 would be 5–6 mg/kg and for D-CPP-ene, 1–2 mg/kg.

### *Surrogate Evidence of Brain Penetration in Man*

While direct sampling and analysis of brain concentration in man may be possible under certain rare circumstances, *e.g.*, if the drug is given prior to resectional cerebral surgery, this is not often easy. The onset of psychometric effects (see below) and electroencephalogram (EEG) changes have been considered to be surrogate markers of brain penetration with these compounds, although these effects may begin at doses somewhat lower than those required for neuroprotection.[4] The intracranial pressure (ICP) effect, seen for CGS 19755 in head trauma, may also be evidence of brain penetration.[2]

### Unwanted Effects of Glutamate Antagonists

Although there is relatively little published information available regarding unwanted effects of these agents, it appears that psychomotor and behavioral effects have been seen with all these compounds in different dose paradigms and indications (TABLE 2), especially in normal volunteers and stroke. These side effects are summarized in TABLE 2. For all the compounds, however, the effects have been mild, self limiting and controllable with concomitant sedation such as haloperidol or benzodiazepines.[1,3-7] Hemodynamic side effects are of far more importance. Hypotension could be highly deleterious in unstable stroke or neurotrauma patients, particularly when ICP is high. Although hypotension has been seen with MK-801 in animal models, it has thus far not proved to be a problem with the glutamate antagonists so far tested in humans.

### Experience with Selfotel in Human Stroke

In a seven-center double-blind ascending dose study to assess safety and tolerability, CGS 19755 was administered within twelve hours of hemispheric occlusive stroke to over 100 acute stroke patients, as two doses twelve hours apart or as a single dose, in an ascending dose design.[1] Side effects such as agitation, hallucinations, confusion, paranoia, and delirium occurred in all six patients treated with 2 mg/kg, and in four of six patients treated with 1.75 mg/kg. However, this is also seen in placebo patients in similar studies.

Surprisingly, these side effects began up to 22 hours after treatment and lasted for two to sixty hours (mean 24 hours). None of these side effects was severe. Importantly, the percentage improvement in the NIH stroke scale was 71% for the drug-treated patients, versus 36% for the placebo patients. On the Barthel scale, the percentage of patients with a score of greater than 70 was 95% in the drug-treated group versus 29% in the placebo group. Thus, it does appear that even at the low doses used, outcome was better, although behavioral side effects were the major limiting factor for dosing.[1] Experience with BW 619 and the weak noncompetitive NMDA antagonist Ro-1-764-706 have shown a very similar profile of psychomotor changes, although these effects were not seen with the weak NMDA antagonist remacemide[5,6] (TABLE 2).

### Glutamate Antagonists in Severe Head Injury

Initial experience with selfotel and severe head injury in over 50 patients at 3–5 mg/kg has shown only minimal evidence of psychomotor effect.[2] This is because the compound has been administered to patients who were initially in coma, or concomitantly sedated with morphine or benzodiazepines. Two patients who were interviewed months after their injuries, however, recalled formed visual hallucinations, which they likened to vivid dreams. Selfotel also reduced intracranial pressure at the 5-mg/kg dose. Similarly, initial experience with CNS 1102 in severe head injury (seristat) revealed no evidence of adverse effects.[8] Preliminary data is also available to show that the Sandoz compound D-CPP-ene is likewise well tolerated at neuroprotective doses in head-injured patients. Therefore, in order to achieve the full neuroprotective effect and maximize the benefit of agents in this category, it is likely that conscious or alert but confused patients will need to be concomitantly sedated, based upon the evidence in TABLE 2.

The early evidence of apparent efficacy which is seen with selfotel in treatment for acute stroke, even at doses which may be below the optimal range for neuroprotection, is a strong indication of the likely efficacy of these compounds in future studies.

## *Epilepsy*

Side effects for the weak NMDA antagonist remacemide have been much less significant, and this compound is being primarily investigated for the epilepsy indication. In contrast, the high-affinity competitive NMDA antagonist D-CPP-ene could not be tolerated by epileptic patients because of psychomotor effect.[11] The majority of effective antiseizure medications are weak ion channel blockers with comparatively low receptor affinity, thus *allowing* normal brain receptor interactions to take place. For *neuroprotective* efficacy, by contrast, much higher receptor affinity is probably necessary to prevent the supraphysiological concentrations of glutamate from binding to receptors so that successful neuroprotection may thus only be possible with compounds having sufficient receptor affinity, and sufficient brain concentration to influence these pathological processes.

## SUMMARY

Over fifty patients with severe head injury, and one hundred with stroke, have now been treated with the competitive NMDA antagonist CGS 19755 (selfotel). Preliminary analysis has shown possible evidence of benefit for both these clinical indications, and several other glutamate antagonists are now being evaluated for these indications in Phase II trials.

The optimal dose of CGS 19755 (selfotel) for efficacy for severe head trauma has not yet been identified, but may be >3 mg/kg, as at this dose there was evidence of an ICP lowering effect and improved CPP. For stroke, however, the maximal tolerated dose was 1.5 mg/kg, because these conscious patients developed hallucinations and agitation. There were no other significant drug-associated adverse events in either of these studies. It is difficult to determine the "neuroprotective" dose for this compound in humans. By extrapolating from animal studies the "best estimate" would be around 5 mg/kg in patients with severe head trauma.

For stroke, behavioral side effects were the major limiting factor for dosing.

Although several NMDA antagonists, including CGS 19755 (selfotel), are currently entering efficacy trials for stroke, based upon their tremendous potency in animal models, the problem of psychomimetic effects may necessitate the use of additional management strategies, *e.g.*, more intensive monitoring and concomitant medications.

## REFERENCES

1. GROTTA, J. *et al.* 1994. Safety and tolerability of the glutamate antagonist CGS 19755 in acute stroke patients. Stroke **25(1):** 12.
2. STEWART, L., R. BULLOCK, M. JONES, A. KOTAKE & G. M. TEASDALE. 1993. The cerebral hemodynamic and metabolic effects of the competitive NMDA antagonist, CGS19755, in humans with severe head injury. J. Neurotrauma **10**(Suppl. 1): S104.
3. MUIR, K. W., R. LEES, S. HAMILTON, C. GEORGE, S. HOBBIGER & M. W. LUNNON. 1995. A randomized double-blind placebo controlled ascending dose tolerance study of BW619C89 in acute stroke. This volume.
4. MERCER, A. J., R. LAMB, S. HOBBIGER & J. POSNER. 1995. The tolerability, pharmacokinetics and pharmacodynamics of increasing intravenous doses of BW619C89, a novel compound for the acute treatment of stroke in healthy volunteers. This volume.
5. LESCO, L. M. 1995. Safety, tolerability and pharmacokinetics of the $N$-methyl-D-aspartate antagonist Ro-01-6794/706 in patients with acute ischemic stroke. This volume.
6. MUIR, K. W. & K. R. LEES. 1995. Initial experience with remacemide hydrochloride in patients with acute ischemic strokes. This volume.
7. MUIR, K. W., D. G. GROSSETT & K. R. LEES. 1995. Clinical pharmacology of CNS 1102 in man. This volume.
8. WAGSTAFF, A., G. M. TEASDALE, G. CLIFTON & L. STEWART. 1995. The cerebral hemodynamic and metabolic effects of the noncompetitive NMDA antagonist CNS 1102 in humans with severe head injury. This volume.
9. CHEN, M. H., R. BULLOCK, D. I. GRAHAM, D. FRAY, D. LOWE & J. MCCULLOCH. 1991. Evaluation of a competitive NMDA antagonist (DCPPN) in feline focal cerebral ischemia. Neural **30:** 62–70.
10. MCCULLOCH, J., R. BULLOCK & G. M. TEASDALE. 1991. Excitatory amino acid antagonists: opportunities for the treatment of ischemic brain damage. *In* Excitatory Amino Acid Antagonists. B. Meldrum, Ed. 287–326. Blackwell Scientific. Oxford.
11. SVEINBJORNSDOTTIR, S., J. SANDER, D. UPTON, P. J. THOMPSON, P. PATSALOS, D. HINT, M. EMRE, D. LOWE & J. DUNCAN. 1993. The excitatory amino acid antagonist D-CPP-ene (SDZEAA-494) in patients with epilepsy. Epilepsy Res. **16:** 165–174.

# Clinical Pharmacology of CNS 1102 in Volunteers

KEITH W. MUIR,[a] DONALD G. GROSSET, AND
KENNEDY R. LEES

*University Department of Medicine and Therapeutics*
*Gardiner Institute*
*Western Infirmary*
*Glasgow G11 6NT,*
*Scotland*

## INTRODUCTION

Excitotoxic injury to neurones following focal cerebral ischemia is mediated by the glutametergic $N$-methyl-D-aspartate (NMDA) receptor, a ligand-gated ion channel which increases postsynaptic membrane sodium and calcium conductance. Excessive release of glutamate from depolarised presynaptic neurones, together with failure of glial and neuronal reuptake mechanisms causes large increases in synaptic glutamate concentrations and pathological stimulation of NMDA receptors. Drugs which block the NMDA receptor have been found consistently to reduce the volume of cerebral infarction in models of focal ischemia,[1] and are being developed for potential use in man.

CNS-1102 (*Cerestat*$^{TM}$, *aptiganel hydrochloride*, $N$-(1-naphthyl)$N'$-(3-ethyl phenyl)-$N'$methyl guanidine hydrochloride, Cambridge NeuroScience Inc., Cambridge, MA.) is a selective ligand for the NMDA ion-channel modulatory site to which dizocilpine (MK-801) and ketamine bind. In rat *focal cerebral ischemia* models, CNS 1102 reduced the extent of cerebral infarction by 66% when given prior to ischemia,[2] and by 40% when administered up to 30 minutes after permanent middle cerebral artery occlusion.[3]

We describe a series of three studies performed to investigate the safety, tolerability, and clinical pharmacology of CNS 1102 in humans.

## METHODS

All studies were conducted in the Clinical Investigation and Research Unit of the University Department of Medicine and Therapeutics. Ethical approval for each study protocol was granted by the West Ethical Committee of Greater Glasgow Health Board and written informed consent was obtained from all volunteers.

---

[a] Correspondence to Dr. Muir.

## Study One[4]

Healthy male volunteers aged 18–32 years were randomized in groups of 4 subjects each to CNS 1102 or placebo (3 active drug: 1 placebo) in a double-blind ascending dose tolerability and safety study. CNS 1102 was administered as an intravenous (iv) infusion over 15 minutes. Dosing commenced at 3 µg/kg, and increased to 10, 30, and 100 µg/kg. Notable clinical symptoms were encountered at 100 µg/kg, and intermediate doses of 45 and 60 µg/kg were tested. One further group of 4 received 45 µg/kg over 30 minutes.

## Study Two[5]

Further healthy male volunteers aged 18–35 years were randomized in groups of 4 subjects to CNS 1102 or placebo in a 3 : 1 active:placebo ratio in a double-blind study. CNS 1102 was administered as an iv loading dose over 15 minutes, followed by a continuous infusion over 4 hours. Four dose groups were tested:

10 µg/kg loading, 1.25 µg/kg/h for 4 hours (total dose 15 µg/kg) n = 4
20 µg/kg loading, 3 µg/kg/h for 4 hours (total dose 32 µg/kg) n = 8
30 µg/kg loading, 5 µg/kg/h for 4 hours (total dose 50 µg/kg) n = 4
45 µg/kg loading, 7 µg/kg/h for 4 hours (total dose 73 µg/kg) n = 4

In addition to cardiovascular and symptom monitoring, plasma levels of catecholamines, angiotensin II and renin activity were determined. Computerized testing of reaction times was undertaken using a well-validated system,[6] which obtained motor and recognition reaction times.

## Study Three[7]

This study was undertaken to ascertain the need for weight-adjustment of drug doses, to assess the cerebrovascular effects of CNS 1102, and to clarify cardiovascular effects. Eight further healthy male volunteers received placebo, CNS 1102 2 mg as iv bolus, and CNS 1102 2 mg as 15 minute iv infusion in random order in a single-blind crossover study, with a minimum of one week between study phases. Subjects were deliberately recruited to be heavy (80–120 kg) or light (65 kg or less). Cerebral blood flow was determined by color flow Doppler ultrasound of common, internal and external carotid arteries with a computerized ultrasonic wall tracker device to determine vessel diameter, and middle cerebral artery flow velocity was measured by transcranial Doppler (TCD) ultrasound.

### *Phamacokinetics*

Blood samples for plasma drug level determination were collected from indwelling iv cannulae at predetermined intervals in all studies. Samples were analyzed by a high-performance liquid chromatography (HPLC) assay, as previously described in detail.[4] The lower limit of detection was 1.25 µg/l, and the intraassay coefficient of variation was 0.69–2.68%.

Area under the curve (AUC) for concentration-time profiles was calculated by the trapezoidal rule and expressed in hours x ng/ml. Clearance was calculated from AUC and dose (Cl = Dose/AUC) and expressed in litres/hour. The slope of the final four detectable concentrations during the elimination phase on a semilogarithmic plot was calculated by linear regression. Where the variability appeared excessive, the final five concentrations were used. Terminal half-life was taken to be $ln(2)$ / slope, expressed in hours.

The volume of the central compartment ($V_1$) was obtained by model-dependent methods. A 2-compartment open model with zero order input and first order elimination from the central (plasma) compartment was chosen. The biomedical statistics package BMD-PAR was used to model the data, using weighted least squares nonlinear regression analysis. Weighting was set to be the reciprocal of the measured concentration and undetectable values were regarded as missing. The volume of distribution at steady state (VDss) was taken to be $V_1 \cdot (1 + k_{12}/k_{21})$. Volumes are expressed in litres.

### Statistics

Inferential statistical analysis was not undertaken for cardiovascular data in Study One. Analysis of covariance for blood pressure, with dose group as the covariate, was performed for Study Two. MAP for Study Three was analyzed by repeated measures analysis of variance with Bonferroni multiple pairwise comparisons. Reaction time-dose group correlations were analyzed by Pearson product moment correlation coefficient. All coefficients of determination were determined by simple linear regression.

## RESULTS

Twenty-seven subjects received CNS (n = 20) or placebo (n = 7) in Study One; one subject was excluded from study due to a finding of chemical hematuria immediately prior to drug administration. Twenty subjects participated in Study Two (CNS 1102 n = 15, placebo n = 5), and eight in Study Three.

### Tolerability

No clinically significant laboratory abnormalities were identified during the studies.

Symptoms and signs are detailed in TABLE 1. These were classified as general effects, CNS effects, and cardiovascular effects. Perioral and peripheral paresthesia have been considered to be CNS symptoms, but may represent a cardiovascular manifestation.

Symptoms and signs appear to be related principally to the total dose of CNS 1102 administered regardless of duration of administration. Symptoms of light-

TABLE 1. Symptoms and Signs Associated with CNS 1102 Administration.

| Total Dose (ug/kg) | Placebo | Placebo | Placebo | 3 | 10 | 15 | 30 | 32 | 2 mg* | 2 mg* | 45 | 45 | 50 | 60 | 73 | 100 |
|---|---|---|---|---|---|---|---|---|---|---|---|---|---|---|---|---|
| Infusion Duration (mins) | 15 | 255 | — | 15 | 15 | 255 | 15 | 255 | 2 | 15 | 15 | 30 | 255 | 15 | 255 | 15 |
| Number of Subjects | 7 | 5 | 8 | 3 | 3 | 3 | 3 | 6 | 8 | 8 | 3 | 3 | 3 | 2 | 3** | 3 |
| **Symptoms** | | | | | | | | | | | | | | | | |
| *General* | | | | | | | | | | | | | | | | |
| Nausea | | | | | | | | 1 | 2 | | 2 | 2 | | | 2 | 2 |
| Vomiting | | | | | | | | | 1 | | | | | 1 | 2 | 2 |
| Dry mouth | | | | | | 1 | | 4 | | | | 2 | 1 | 2 | 1 | 1 |
| Sweating | | | | | | | 1 | 2 | | | 1 | | 2 | 1 | 2 | |
| Flushing | | | | | | | 1 | 3 | 1 | 3 | 1 | 1 | 3 | 1 | 1 | 1 |
| Headache | 1 | | | 1 | 1 | 1 | | | 2 | 1 | | 2 | | 1 | | 1 |
| Tiredness | | 1 | | | 1 | | 1 | 3 | 2 | 2 | 4 | | 2 | | 1 | |
| Cold extremities | 1 | | | | | | | 2 | | | 1 | 1 | 2 | 2 | 2 | 3 |
| Labored respiration | | | | | | | | | | | | | 1 | | | 1 |
| *Central nervous system* | | | | | | | | | | | | | | | | |
| *Paresthesia* | | | | | | | | | | | | | | | | |
| General | | | | | | 1 | | 2 | 2 | 2 | 5 | 2 | 2 | 1 | 2 | 1 | 3 |
| Perioral | | | | | | 1 | | 6 | 6 | 5 | | | 3 | | 3 | |
| Extremities | | | 1 | | 1 | | | 6 | | | | | 2 | | 2 | |
| Nystagmus | | | | | | | | | | | | 3 | | 2 | 1 | 3 |
| Blurred vision | | | | | | | | 2 | | | 1 | 3 | 1 | 2 | 1 | 1 |
| Diplopia | | | | | | | | | | | 1 | 2 | 2 | 1 | 1 | |
| Lightheadedness | | 1 | | | | | 2 | 2 | 3 | 5 | 3 | 2 | 3 | 2 | 2 | 3 | 3 |
| Disorientation | | 1 | | | | | | 2 | | | | | 2 | 1 | 1 | 2 |
| Sedation | 2 | | | | | 1 | | 2 | 2 | | | 1 | 2 | 1 | 3 | 3 |
| Dysarthria | | | | | | | 1 | 1 | 2 | | | | 2 | 1 | 2 | 1 |
| Disinhibition | | | | | | | | | | | 1 | 1 | | | | |
| Dulled senses | | | | | | | | | | 1 | 1 | 1 | | | | |
| Heightened senses | | | | | | | | | | | 1 | 2 | 1 | | | |
| Hallucinations | | | | | | | | | | | | | | | 1 | |
| Vivid memories | | | | | | | | | | | | | | 1 | | |
| Paranoia, anxiety | | | | | | | | | | 1 | | 1 | | | 1 | |
| Choreiform movements | | | | | | | | | | | | | | | | 1 |
| Catatonia | | | | | | | | | | | | | | 2 | | 2 |

\* Fixed dose of 2 mg (Study Three).
\*\* Infusion discontinued in one subject after total dose of 66 ug/kg administered.

headedness, detachment and paresthesia were evident at doses of 30 μg/kg or 2 mg; these progressed to disinhibition, euphoria, gait ataxia, nystagmus, flushing and sweating, with some individuals expressing nonspecific anxiety and restlessness at doses of 45–50 μg/kg. One individual experienced olfactory and visual hallucinations, and one other experienced intense and vivid recollection of memories (both in Study Two). At doses of 60–100 μg/kg, paranoia, marked detachment from reality, severe psychomotor retardation (catatonia in four instances in Study One), nausea and vomiting were manifested. Symptoms appeared within minutes after bolus drug infusion (or during infusion at doses of 60 μg/kg and higher), and persisted for 1–4 hours. After the acute phase of symptoms, subjects who received 60 μg/kg and over were sedated for several hours further, and appeared amnesic for the symptomatic period.

No symptom persisted for longer than 24 hours after drug administration, and all symptoms resolved without sequelae.

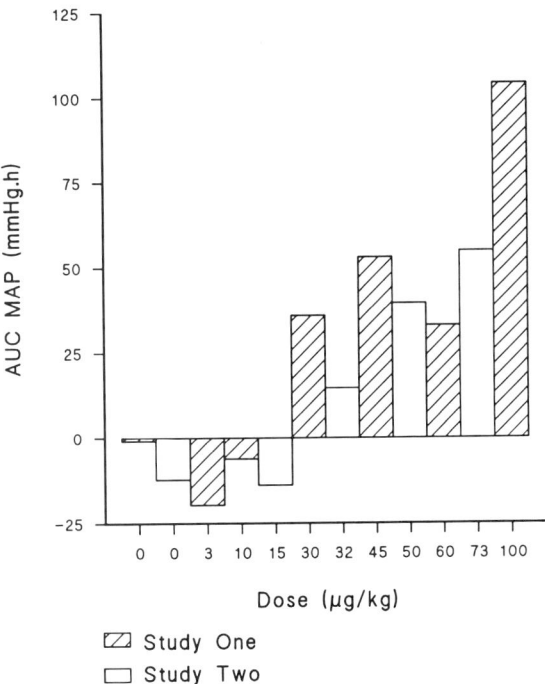

**FIGURE 1.** Area under the mean arterial pressure-time curve by dose group, Studies One and Two.

## Cardiovascular Effects

No electrocardiogram (ECG) abnormality was observed during the course of any of the studies.

Systolic, diastolic and mean arterial pressure (MAP) demonstrated dose-dependent increases during infusion in Studies One and Two (FIG. 1). Doses up to a total of 15 μg/kg did not appear different from placebo. The maximum mean rise in blood pressure was 33/24 mmHg in Study One (100 μg/kg group), and 27/21 mmHg in Study Two (73 μg/kg group). Blood pressure elevation occurred within a few minutes of drug administration, reaching a peak within 15–30 minutes, and remaining elevated for 2–4 hours. The most accurate blood pressure data were obtained from Study Three (FIG. 2), where both 2-mg bolus and 15-minute infusion significantly raised MAP above placebo from 45–120 minutes, with no difference between methods of drug administration.

While Studies One and Two suggested an increased pulse rate during the study period, data were inconsistent and fluctuated greatly. No significant difference between CNS 1102 and placebo was found in Study Three.

Changes in adrenaline, noradrenaline, angiotensin II or plasma renin activity

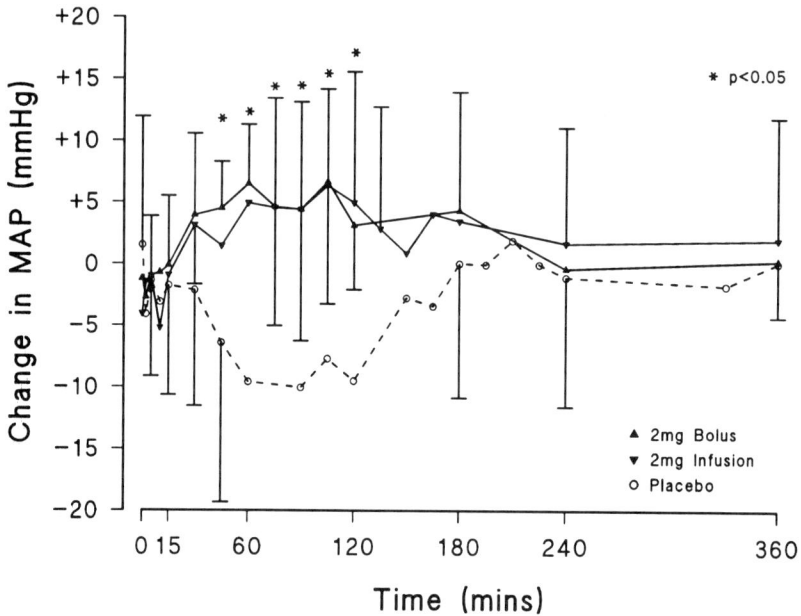

**FIGURE 2.** Mean arterial pressure changes from baseline following 2-mg bolus or 2-mg infusion of CNS 1102 over 15 minutes, or placebo.

from pre- to postdose did not differ between placebo and active groups in Study Two.

Global cerebral blood flow was unaltered by CNS 1102. Flow velocity increased significantly in both middle cerebral arteries following CNS 1102 administration, and was accompanied by an 11% reduction in pulsatility index.

### Reaction Time

Motor reaction time (MRT) was prolonged in a dose-dependent fashion in Study Two, with significant correlation of the area under the MRT-time curve with both dose group and maximal plasma concentration of CNS 1102 ($r^2 = 0.21$, $p = 0.04$; and $r^2 = 0.48$, $p = 0.0004$, respectively). Recognition reaction time (RRT) was not related to dose group, $C_{max}$ or total dose administered ($r^2 = 0.03$, $p > 0.40$ for all) (FIG. 3).

### Pharmacokinetics

Combined pharmacokinetic parameters from Studies One and Two are given in TABLE 2.

The observed $C_{max}$ occurred at, or shortly after, the end of the bolus, as ex-

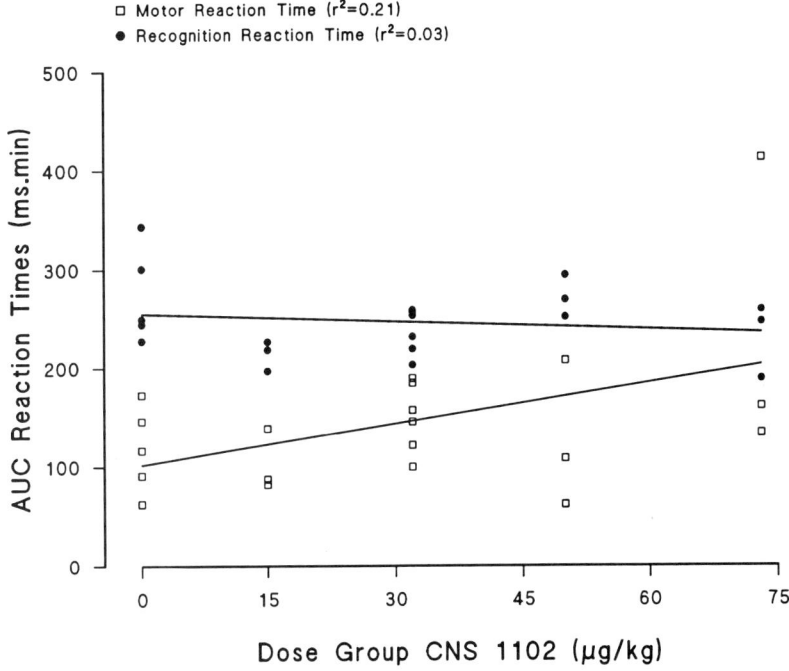

**FIGURE 3.** Motor reaction time (MRT) and recognition reaction time (RRT) versus dose group in Study Two. $r^2$ is the coefficient of determination.

TABLE 2. Pharmacokinetics of CNS-1102 in Normal Volunteers

| | | | | | | | | | | | | | | Mean | SD | n |
|---|---|---|---|---|---|---|---|---|---|---|---|---|---|---|---|---|
| Dose/kg μg/kg | 3 | 10 | 15 | 30 | 32 | 32 | 45 | 45 | 50 | 60 | 67 | 100 | | | | |
| Dose μg | 196 | 757 | 1200 | 2190 | 2240 | 2443 | 3480 | 3390 | 3617 | 5940 | 4787 | 7800 | | | | |
| Infusion Duration min | 15 | 15 | 255 | 15 | 255 | 255 | 15 | 30 | 255 | 15 | 255 | 15 | | | | |
| Weight kg | 65 | 76 | 80 | 73 | 70 | 76 | 77 | 75 | 72 | 99 | 71 | 78 | | 76 | 10 | 32 |
| Height cm | 175 | 174 | 179 | 177 | 171 | 175 | 178 | 171 | 181 | 178 | 177 | 180 | | 176 | 6 | 32 |
| AUC h.ng/ml | | 8.0 | 6.3 | 36.1 | 23.1 | 17.7 | 38.6 | 39.1 | 48.7 | 77.9 | 52.5 | 108.1 | | | | |
| $C_{max}$ ng/ml | 2.6 | 4.7 | 4.2 | 16.1 | 6.1 | 8.4 | 18.5 | 16.8 | 9.1 | 41.4 | 21.1 | 40.4 | | | | |
| Clearance l/h | | 232 | 198 | 61 | 105 | 145 | 94 | 90 | 82 | 77 | 97 | 73 | | 115 | 77 | 32 |
| VDss l/kg | | 3.1 | 7.9 | 4.8 | 8.1 | 5.7 | 6.9 | 5.0 | 8.2 | 4.7 | 6.4 | 6.8 | | 6.2 | 1.9 | 32 |
| T-half h | | 1.2 | 5.8 | 4.2 | 7.0 | 2.1 | 3.8 | 3.0 | 5.6 | 6.1 | 2.6 | 4.5 | | 4.1 | 2.5 | 32 |

pected (FIG. 4). $C_{max}$ increased with dose and no unexpected accumulation occurred. The use of doses adjusted according to body weight did not reduce variability in AUC and $C_{max}$.

Clearance was 115 ± 77 l/h (mean ± SD, n = 32), and terminal half-life was 4.1 ± 2.5 hours (mean ± SD, n = 32). VDss was 6.2 ± 1.9 l/kg (mean ± SD, n = 32).

No relation was demonstrated between body weight and VDss ($r^2$ = 0.9%) or body weight and clearance ($r^2$ = 1.6%).

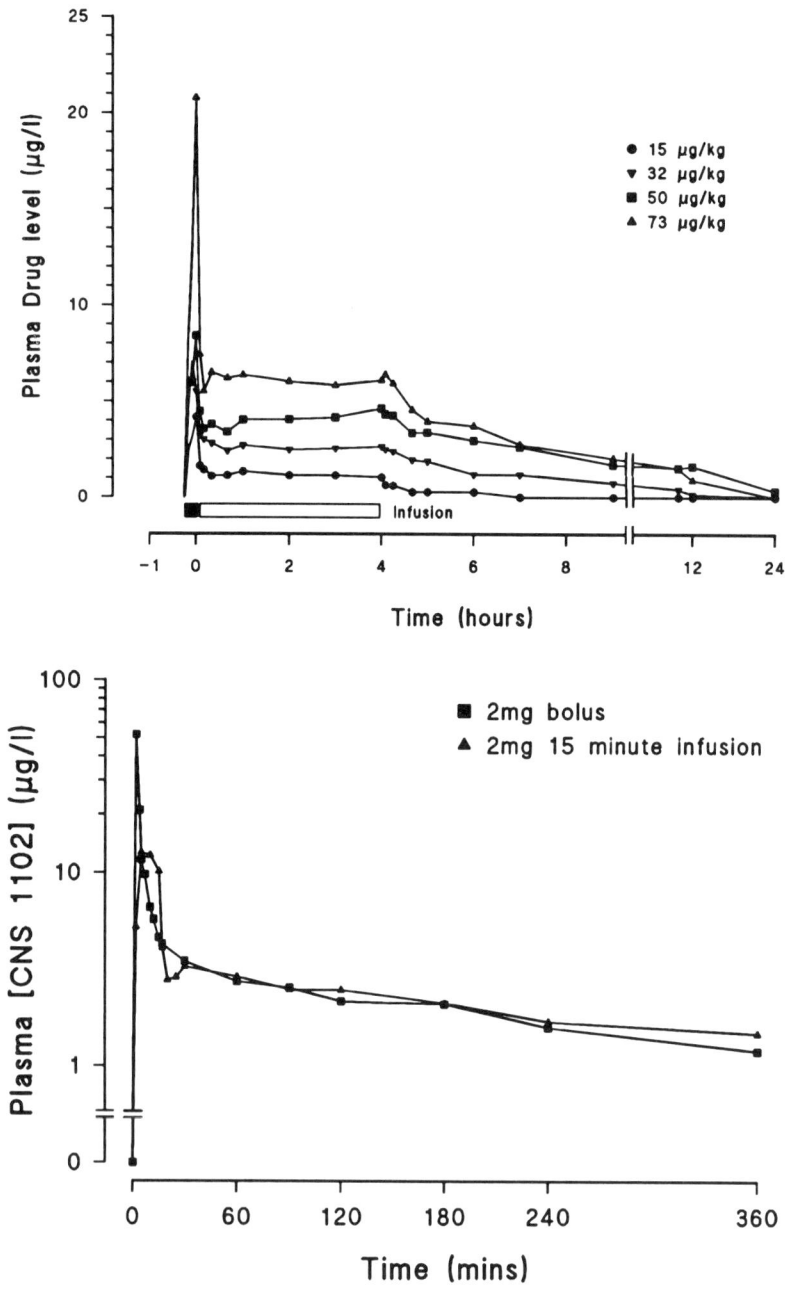

**FIGURE 4.** Plasma levels of CNS 1102 for Study Two (*above*) and Study Three (*below*).

There was 31% variability in VDss and 65% variability in clearance amongst these normal subjects.

## DISCUSSION

The results of these studies define the clinical pharmacology of CNS 1102 in healthy volunteers. Clinical experience has subsequently shown that the effects in normal volunteers may not necessarily extrapolate to patients after stroke or traumatic brain injury. Whether the observed differences are due predominantly to pharmacokinetic or to pharmacodynamic factors remains to be determined.

CNS 1102 is a high-affinity noncompetitive antagonist of the NMDA receptor ion channel. There are notable similarities between the effects of CNS 1102 and those of other drugs known to block the NMDA receptor ion channel, such as the anesthetic agent ketamine,[8] a low-affinity blocker. Ketamine administration is associated with light-headedness, disorientation, hallucinations, sedation, euphoria, and analgesia, accompanied by a state of catatonia at high doses. Dose-dependent elevation of blood pressure[9] is also seen.

CNS 1102 produces a dose-dependent hierarchy of symptoms and signs similar to those of ketamine in normal volunteers, as outlined above. There are some notable differences. The paresthesiae which were a prominent early finding in all three studies with CNS 1102 were not recorded with ketamine. Psychotomimetic emergence phenomena, which are predominant after ketamine anesthesia,[10] have not been seen with CNS 1102: even in subjects who experienced paranoid ideation or hallucinations, these effects were transient, lasting at most 2 hours, and resolved with no sequelae. This was confirmed by follow-up to 6–8 weeks. These differences may be important for future clinical applications.

The cardiovascular and cerebrovascular effects of CNS 1102 are also similar to those reported for ketamine. It has been demonstrated by the Intravenous Nimodipine West European Stroke Trial (INWEST)[11] that pharmacological lowering of blood pressure after acute stroke is detrimental to outcome. Both the rise in blood pressure, and the demonstration of unaltered global cerebral blood flow after CNS 1102, even at the point of maximal elevation of blood pressure, are thus reassuring for further clinical development. In studies with ketamine, the rise in blood pressure appears to result from central sympathetic nervous system stimulation,[12] with secondary changes in the renin-angiotensin system[13] and circulating catecholamine levels.[12] Increased middle cerebral artery blood flow velocities have also been shown with TCD in patients given ketamine.[9] The observed changes may either result from primary change in vascular tone—vasoconstriction of arterioles distal to the middle cerebral artery as a result of general sympathetic stimulation—or may be a secondary vascular change reflecting increased metabolic demand in certain brain regions induced by noncompetitive NMDA antagonists.

The large volume of distribution is compatible with a highly lipid soluble compound predominantly distributed to tissues. Rapid onset of CNS symptoms indicates that drug rapidly enters the brain. There is considerable intersubject variability in CNS 1102 volume of distribution and clearance. The low values of coefficients of determination for VDss and clearance versus weight suggested that weight adjustment of doses was not likely to offer any advantages over a fixed dose of CNS 1102, and Study Three confirmed this impression. Both light and heavy weight subjects showed variable clinical symptoms, signs and blood pressure response to a fixed 2-mg dose. Pharmacokinetic variability was not adversely affected by fixed rather than weight-adjusted doses. The opportunity to administer a single fixed dose of drug is advantageous for simplicity of future clinical trials.

As noted above, phase II studies of CNS 1102 in stroke and traumatic brain injury have administered doses considerably higher than those tolerated by volunteers without replication of the associated symptoms and signs. Stroke patients have received up to 150 μg/kg over 4 hours[14] without either elevation of blood pressure or consistent side effects, and doses of over 250 μg/kg have been well tolerated in traumatic brain injury patients[15] who are paralyzed and ventilated. Although no differences in pharmacokinetics between young healthy individuals and the more elderly stroke population have been observed so far, direct comparisons of pharmacokinetics and pharmacodynamics in contrasting age groups or disease states have not been undertaken.

## SUMMARY

The high affinity noncompetitive $N$-methyl-D-aspartate receptor antagonist CNS 1102 (aptiganel hydrochloride, Cambridge NeuroScience, Cambridge, MA.) is neuroprotective in preclinical models of stroke when administered as pretreatment or up to 60 minutes postischemia, and has potential for treatment of acute stroke or traumatic brain injury in man. A total of 55 healthy male subjects have participated in three separate studies to determine the clinical pharmacology of CNS 1102, 43 of whom have received CNS 1102 in doses of up to 100 μg/kg. Administration of CNS 1102 has been studied as a 15-minute intravenous infusion, as a 15-minute loading intravenous infusion followed by a 4-hour maintenance infusion, or as a fixed-dose intravenous bolus over 90 seconds.

CNS 1102 in normal volunteers is well tolerated in total doses up to 32 μg/kg whether as a bolus injection, 15-minute infusion or 4-hour infusion. Central nervous system affects are evident within minutes of administration, implying rapid drug penetration. CNS 1102 has a large and variable volume of distribution (mean ± standard deviation, 6.2 ± 1.9 l/kg), variable clearance (115 ± 77 l/h), and plasma half-life of approximately 4.5 hours. Adjustment of doses by subject weight does not improve variability of these parameters, and fixed doses may thus be administered. CNS 1102 causes dose-dependent elevation of blood pressure, accompanied by clinical evidence of vasoconstriction. Global cerebral blood flow is maintained, whilst middle cerebral artery flow velocity increases. Symptoms of light-headedness, disorientation and paresthesia progress through euphoria, disinhibition, and hallucinations to psychomotor retardation, paranoia and catatonia as total administered dose increases.

## ACKNOWLEDGMENTS

We wish to thank Cambridge NeuroScience Inc. for drug supplies and support; Wendy Fallon for drug preparation and randomisation; Jean Fenton and the staff of the Clinical Investigation and Research Unit; Dr. Peter Meredith and Charles McNeill for CNS 1102 assays; and Dr. Martin Brodie and Elizabeth Colquhoun for help with reaction time testing.

## REFERENCES

1. McCulloch, J. 1992. Excitatory amino acid antagonists and their potential for the treatment of ischaemic brain damage in man. Br. J. Clin. Pharmacol. **34:** 106–114.
2. Minematsu, K., M. Fisher, L. Li, M. A. Davis, A. G. Knapp, R. E. Cotter, R. N. McBurney & C. H. Sotak. 1993. Effects of a novel NMDA antagonist on experimental stroke rapidly and quantitatively assessed by diffusion-weighted MRI. Neurology **43:** 397–403.
3. Meadows, M-E., M. Fisher & K. Minematsu. 1994. Delayed treatment with a noncompetitive NMDA antagonist, CNS 1102, reduces infarct size in rats. Cerebrovasc. Dis. **4:** 26–31.
4. Muir, K. W., D. G. Grosset, E. Gamzu & K. R. Lees. 1994. Pharmacological effects of the non-competitive NMDA antagonist CNS 1102 in normal volunteers. Br. J. Clin. Pharmacol. **38:** 33–38.
5. Muir, K. W. et al. Submitted for publication.
6. Hindmarch, I. 1980. Psychomotor function and psychoactive drugs. Br. J. Clin. Pharmacol. **10:** 189–209.
7. Grosset, D. G., K. W. Muir & K. R. Lees. 1995. Systemic and cerebral hemodynamic responses to the non-competitive $N$-methyl-D-aspartate (NMDA) antagonist, CNS 1102. J. Cardiovasc. Pharmacol. **25:** 705–709.
8. White, P. F., W. L. Way & A. J. Trevor. 1982. Ketamine—its pharmacology and therapeutic uses. Anesthesiology **56:** 119–136.
9. Kochs, E., C. Werner, W. E. Hoffman, O. Mollenberg & J. Schulte 1991. Concurrent increases in brain electrical activity and intracranial blood flow velocity during low-dose ketamine anaesthesia. Can. J. Anaesth. **38:** 826–830.
10. Albin, M. S., L. Bunegin & C. Garcia. 1990. Ketamine and postanesthetic emergence reactions. In Status of Ketamine in Anesthesiology. E. F. Domino, Ed. 17–25. NPP Books. Ann Arbor.
11. Wahlgren, N. G., D. G. MacMahon, J. Dekeyser, B. Indredavik & T. Ryman. 1994. Intravenous Nimodipine West European Stroke Trial (INWEST) of nimodipine in the treatment of acute ischaemic stroke. Cerebrovasc. Dis. **4:** 204–210.
12. Appel, E., R. Dudziak, D. Palm & A. Wnuk. 1979. Sympathoneuronal and sympathoadrenal activation during ketamine anesthesia. Eur. J. Clin. Pharmacol. **16:** 91–95.
13. Pipkin, F. B. & B. A. Waldron. 1983. Ketamine hypertension and the renin-angiotensin system. Clin. Exp. Hypertens. Part A Theory Pract. **5:** 875–883.
14. Fisher, M. 1994. Cerestat (CNS 1102), a non-competitive NMDA antagonist, in ischemic stroke patients: dose-escalating safety study. Cerebrovasc. Dis. **4:** 245.
15. Wagstaff, A., G. M. Teasdale, G. Clifton & L. Stewart. 1994. The cerebral haemodynamic and metabolic effects of the non-competitive NMDA antagonist CNS 1102 in humans with severe head injury. Proceedings of the Second International Conference on Neuroprotective Therapy (Abstract).

# Evidence for Prolonged Release of Excitatory Amino Acids in Severe Human Head Trauma

## Relationship to Clinical Events

R. BULLOCK,[a] A. ZAUNER, J. S. MYSEROS, A. MARMAROU,
J. J. WOODWARD,[b] AND H. F. YOUNG

*Division of Neurosurgery
and
[b] Department of Pharmacology and Toxicology
School of Medicine
Medical College of Virginia
Richmond, Virginia 23298-0631*

## INTRODUCTION

Many neuroprotective agents which block the putatively excitotoxic effects of glutamate are now available, and several of these are well advanced in clinical trials.[1,2] Some agents, however, have side effect profiles which could preclude their use for categories of conscious or confused head-injured patients.[3] We have, therefore, sought evidence of excitatory amino acid (EAA) release in a spectrum of patients with severe head trauma.

The aim of these studies was as follows: 1) to determine the relationship of EAA release to the clinical type of head trauma, 2) to determine the time course of EAA release in order to determine the "therapeutic window", and 3) to determine any relationship between EAA release, intracranial pressure (ICP), cerebral perfusion pressure (CPP), and ionic changes.

## METHODS

### Patients

The characteristics of the seventeen patients in this report are shown in TABLE 1. In seven patients, excitatory amino acids were measured within the hemisphere underlying an acute subdural hematoma, and in one patient, under an epidural hematoma. In four, microdialysis monitoring was established in edematous cortical tissue, adjacent to a focal cerebral contusion, which had been previously surgically resected. In the remaining five patients, the microdialysis probe was inserted

---

[a] To whom correspondence should be addressed: Division of Neurosurgery, MCV Station, Box 980631, Richmond, VA 23298-0631.

TABLE 1. The Characteristics and Glutamate and Aspartate Levels of the 17 Patients in This Study[a]

| Injury Category | N | GCS Range | Outcome | | | | Mean Glutamate ($\mu$mol ± SD) | ($\mu$ mol ± SD) |
|---|---|---|---|---|---|---|---|---|
| | | | Death | Veget | SD | GR/MD | | |
| Diffuse injury | 5 | 3–6 | 1 | | 2 | 1 | 1.8 ± 1.7 | 0.6 ± 0.3 |
| Subdural hematoma | 2 | 7 | 1 | | | 1 | 2.0 ± 0.6 | 0.6 ± 0.2 |
| Epidural hematoma | 1 | 6 | | | | 1 | 0.6 | 0.2 |
| Focal contusion | 4 | 3–10 | | | 1 | 3 | 28.5 ± 26.2 | 9.2 ± 8.2 |
| 2° ischemia or hypoxia | 5 | 3 | 2 | | 2 | 1 | 28.1 ± 33.0 | 9.4 ± 14.9 |

[a] N = number of patients in each group, Veget = vegetative, SD = severe disability, GR = good recovery, and MD = moderate disability.

via a twist drill ventriculostomy opening. In these patients with diffuse injuries who did not undergo craniotomy, the probe was angled at 45 degrees away from the ventriculostomy, and a guide cannula was used to achieve placement of the membrane in cortex not traumatized by the ventriculostomy itself.

### Microdialysis

A 10-mm flexible probe with external diameter of 0.75 mm was used after ethylene oxide sterilization. The active portion of the probe was inserted into cortex, and it was perfused at 2 microliters per minute with sterile 0.9% saline. 60 microliter ($\mu$l) dialysate aliquots were collected every 30 minutes into sealed glass tubes using a CMA 170 refrigerated collector system (4°C). After collection, samples were frozen at $-20°C$ until analyzed. Clinical events which took place during microdialysis were logged into a VAX mainframe computer, along with ICP and mean arterial pressure (MABP).

### Measurement of Extracellular Fluid (ECF) Sodium and Potassium

Sodium ($Na^+$) and potassium $K^+$) were measured by flame photometry using 12-$\mu$l aliquots from every second sample, thus giving hourly measurements. These were entered into the VAX computer for comparison with other parameters.

### Probe Calibration and Standardization of Measurement Techniques

After use, each probe was calibrated *in vitro* by immersion in a bath solution of known glutamate, aspartate, sodium, and potassium concentrations. The probes were perfused with 0.9% saline solution, and recovery rates were calculated for the amino acids and ions. For each probe, six estimations were made. Recovery rates were as follows:

Excitatory amino acids     43 ± 5%
Sodium     63 ± 4%

| | |
|---|---|
| Potassium | 72 ± 5% |

The flame photometry ionic measurement system was also calibrated against known standards, warranted pure by the manufacturer over a wide range of ion concentrations.

### Measurement of Neurochemicals

Aliquots of dialysate were derivatized with an $O$-pthalaldehyde/thiol reagent and injected into a BAS200 high performance liquid chromatography using a BioRad AS-100 autosampler. Derivatized amino acids were separated by reverse-phase C18 column chromatography and peaks were detected using electrochemical detection. Peaks were compared to known standards for identification and quantitation using the Rainin Method Manager running on a Macintosh SE30 microcomputer.[4]

### ICP and CPP Monitoring

In all patients, a frontal ventriculostomy was used to measure intracranial pressure. Continuous data from an arterial line was used to measure MABP. These physiologic parameters were continuously acquired by a VAX mainframe computer system, and the data were smoothed to yield graphs for each parameter for 12-hour epochs, against which neurochemical changes were compared.

## RESULTS

### Patterns of EAA Release and Intracranial Pathology (TABLE 1)

In general, levels of glutamate and aspartate fluctuated together. In patients with *focal cerebral contusion,* EAA release was 6–20 times above the normal level (1–2 μM) observed by other investigators.[4-6] In these patients, EAA levels in extracellular fluid remained elevated and constant, though slowly declining over the entire monitored period (FIG. 1A). In the patients with *diffuse cerebral injuries,* without prior ischemic events or reduced CPP (n = 5), the pattern of EAA release was remarkably constant (FIG. 1B). In these patients, EAA levels were initially 3–4 times above the normal level, but declined over about six hours to within the normal range. The highest levels of EAA release were seen in patients with severe diffuse injuries and *prior ischemic events* (n = 3/5). One patient underwent a prolonged hypotensive period greater than one hour at the scene of a motor vehicle accident due to visceral injuries. In the other two patients, low cerebral blood flow (6 ml/100 g/min and 20 ml/100 g/min) with subsequent transtentorial herniation, and bilateral fixed pupils, plus hypotension for more than 30 minutes was observed. In these three patients, EAA release ranged from 20 to 50 times above normal. In all but one of the nonischemic patients, the EAA trend was of progressive decline. In one patient, however, EAAs rose from 10 times above the normal

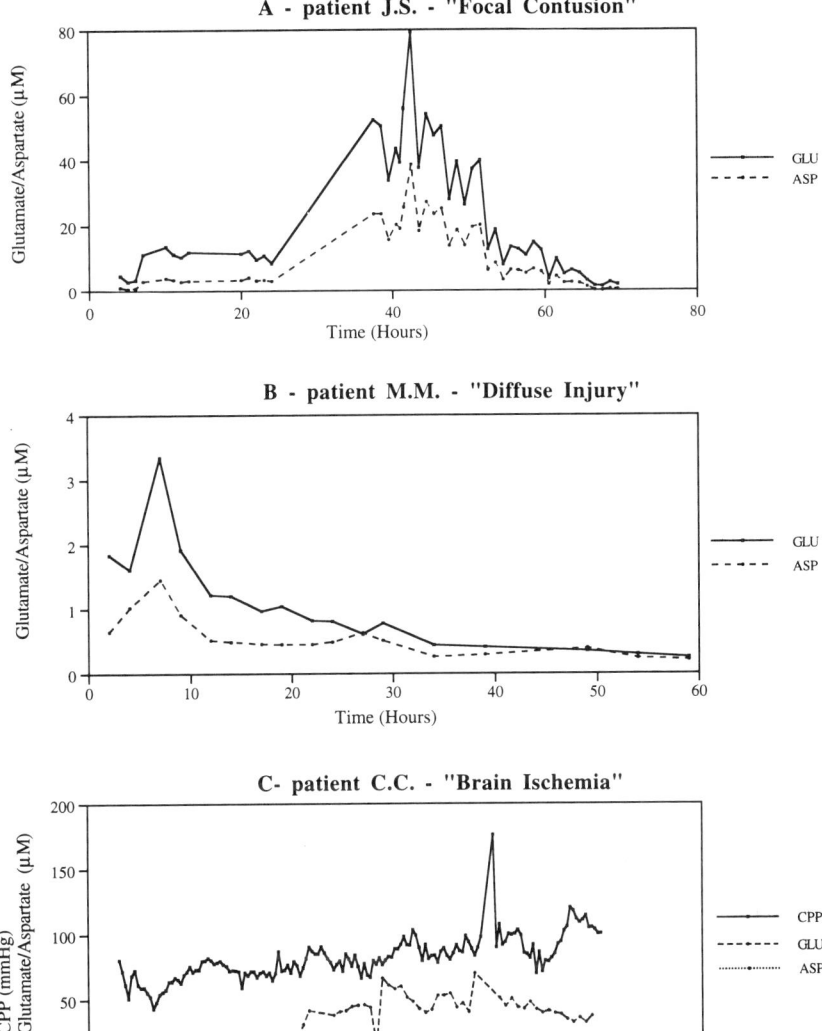

**FIGURE 1.** Glutamate and aspartate levels over time for three different types of patients: (**A**) focal contusion, (**B**) diffuse injury, and (**C**) ischemic or hypoxic event. (C) also shows the cerebral perfusion pressure (CPP).

level to 60 times normal, without any measured change in CPP (FIG. 1C). The factors leading to this rise in this patient remain unknown.

*Time Course*

When EAAs were elevated greater than five times normal, as seen in the patients with contusions and those with secondary ischemic injury, they remained high for the entire monitoring period (up to four days) in most cases.

*Relationship Between ICP, CPP, and EAA Release*

During 1,712 hours of microdialysis in 17 patients, only two patients demonstrated sustained elevations of ICP for greater than 30 minutes. EAA levels in these patients, who both died, increased steadily upward to levels greater than 50 times normal (patient C.C., FIG. 1C). In six patients, 18 brief episodes (less than 5 minutes) of ICP above 40 mmHg were noted. However, none of these episodes was associated with increases in EAA levels greater than 100% over baseline.

## Ionic Changes

The changes in ions in ECF for two patients are shown in FIGURE 2.

*Potassium*

In three patients, $K^+$ increased fivefold or more. In each of these three, EAAs were greater than 50-fold higher than normal. In all three of these patients, however, the $K^+$ increases were transient (~12 hours), while the EAA increases were sustained (2–4 days). In the remaining patients, $K^+$ remained below 2.5–5 mEq in ECF.

*Sodium*

The perfusate for dialysis (0.9% saline) contained 154 ± 3 mEq of $Na^+$, so that changes in the efflux dialysate must be interpreted with care. Striking changes in hour-to-hour $Na^+$ concentrations were seen (FIG. 2). In general, a tendency to reciprocal changes in $Na^+$ were seen, with respect to $K^+$. Patients with the most marked hour-to-hour $Na^+$ fluctuations tended to have high EAAs, but this was not constant. In some patients, $Na^+$ was momentarily below the level in the perfusate, implying ECF levels which were lower still.

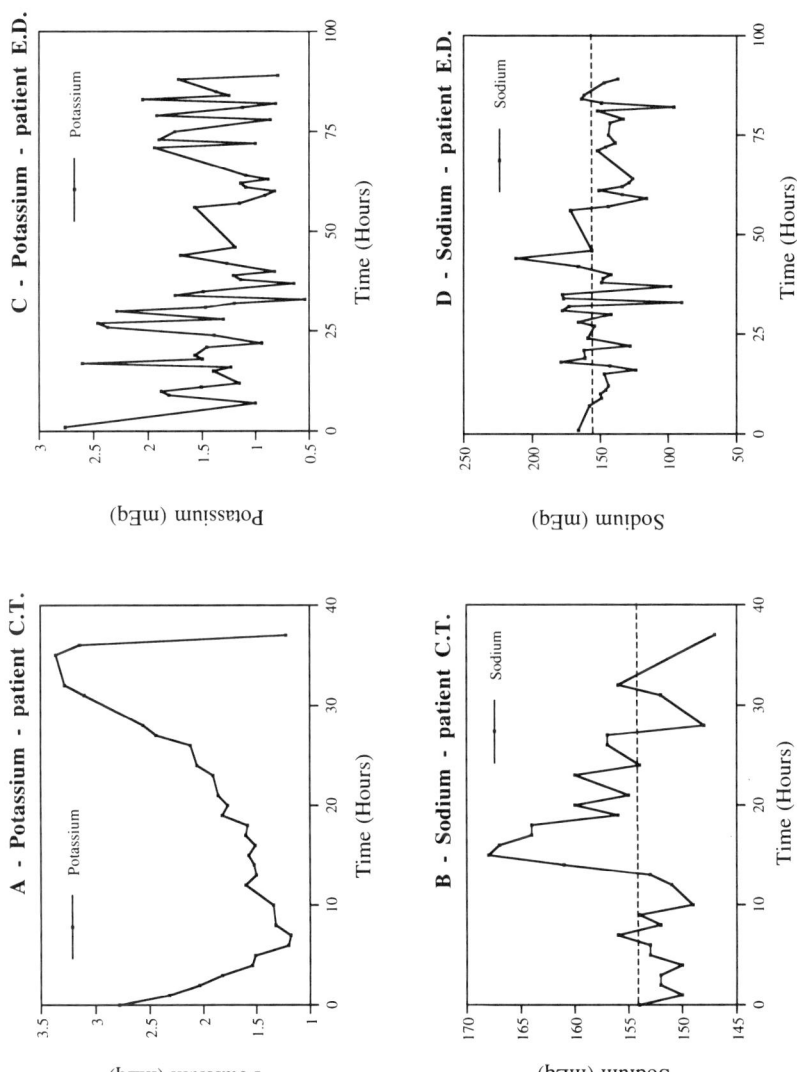

FIGURE 2. Changes in sodium and potassium in two patients, both of whom suffered ischemic injuries. Note the tremendous flux of ions and the apparent reciprocity of changes between sodium and potassium.

## DISCUSSION

The purpose of these studies was to document the patterns and time course of EAA levels in human patients following severe head injury. Overall, 11 of the 17 patients (65%) manifested sustained high glutamate levels in ECF (6–50-fold increase over normal) which generally persisted for the duration of monitoring. Although these studies are primarily descriptive in nature, the following conclusions can be made. First, in patients *without secondary ischemic complications,* increases in EAA levels appeared to be a transient phenomenon, as in animal models, but in some cases these increases persisted for up to about 12 hours following injury. Second, in those patients with no ischemic events and *focal contusions,* causing 'low density' on computerized tomography (CT), EAA levels were increased 6–50-fold and persisted for at least four days. Finally, in those patients *with secondary ischemic events,* EAA levels were very high (20–50 times normal) and persisted for four days or more.

Thus, it appears that the latter two groups would be good candidates for prolonged therapy with EAA antagonist drugs, while patients without contusions or secondary insults may only require treatment during the first 12 hours following injury. For the longer acting competitive antagonists, such as D-CPP-ene or CGS 19755, one dose may be appropriate although more data is needed to validate this conclusion. Our recent animal studies are consistent with the view that secondary ischemic insults cause substantial and sustained increases in EAA release.[7] This agrees with the findings of a study by Persson *et al.* which attempted to validate the apparent relationship between EAA release and ICP.[8,9] Our data suggests that ICP only becomes a significant factor with respect to elevated EAA levels when it is sustained over 40 mmHg, with concomitant CPP reduction (<40 mmHg) for long periods. Brief CPP and ICP fluctuations (<5 minutes) do not seem to significantly affect EAA levels. We therefore hypothesize that severe traumatic shear damage to the brain or major ischemic events occurring shortly after traumatic brain injury (TBI) cause massive EAA release. When this occurs focally, ischemic neuronal necrosis and astrocyte swelling (due to $K^+$ buffering) may result. Brain swelling and high ICP may follow these events when this process is widespread ultimately leading to reduced CPP and brain death. Although our single-site microdialysis monitoring means that only a small region of the brain is being sampled, our data suggest that elevated levels of EAAs may potentiate harmful events after human TBI.

The ionic changes measured in this study generally support these interpretations. The increases in ECF $K^+$ only occurred in the patients with the highest levels of EAAs, which implies a close linkage between ion flux and EAA levels. We speculate that the relatively steady levels of $K^+$ observed in the present microdialysis studies are due to astrocyte buffering which prevents the large, prolonged accumulations of ECF $K^+$ (40–50 mEq) often seen with ion-sensitive microelectrodes in traumatic brain injury models of head trauma.[9,10]

The fluctuations in sodium measured in the present study are more difficult to interpret due to the use of a dialysate fluid (saline) with high levels (154 mEq) of $Na^+$. Any change in ECF $Na^+$ under these conditions would thus be difficult to observe. Further studies are needed to address these issues.

Overall, these findings reinforce the view that significant and prolonged increases in EAA release may occur after trauma and lead to widespread brain damage. These data also suggest that early treatment with EAA antagonists may be beneficial, and phase III trials were recently developed to test this hypothesis.

## ACKNOWLEDGMENTS

The authors would like to thank A. Stout, T. Blevins and J. Harms for their excellent technical assistance during this study.

## REFERENCES

1. BULLOCK, R. & H. FUJISAWA. 1992. The role of glutamate antagonists for the treatment of CNS injury. J. Neurotrauma **9:** 5443–5461.
2. BULLOCK, R. 1993. Opportunities for neuroprotective drugs in clinical management of head injury. J. Emerg. Med. **11:** 23–30.
3. GROTTA, J. et al. 1994. Safety and tolerability of the glutamate antagonist CGS 19755 in acute stroke patients. Stroke **25**(1): 12.
4. PERSSON, L. & L. HILLERED. 1992. Chemical monitoring of neurosurgical intensive care patients using intracerebral microdialysis. J. Neurosurg. **76:** 72–80.
5. DURING, M. J. & D. D. SPENCER. 1993. Extracellular hippocampal glutamate and spontaneous seizure in the conscious human brain. Lancet **341:** 1607–1610.
6. RONNE-ENGSTROM, L. & L. HILLERED. 1992. Intracerebral microdialysis of extracellular amino acids in the human epileptic focus. J. Cereb. Blood Flow Metab. **12:** 873–876.
7. TSUJI, O., A. MARMAROU & R. BULLOCK. 1994. Microdialysis detection of electrolytes and amino acid changes following head impact acceleration, coupled with secondary insult. In 9th International Symposium on Intracranial Pressure. H. Nagai, K. Kamiya & S. Ishii, Eds. 136–138. Springer-Verlag. Tokyo.
8. BULLOCK, R., A. STOUT, J. J. WOODWARD, O. TSUJI, A. MARMAROU & H. F. YOUNG. 1994. EAA release in severe human head trauma: the role of intracranial pressure and cerebral perfusion changes. In 9th International Symposium on Intracranial Pressure. H. Nagai, K. Kamiya & S. Ishii, Eds. 264–267. Springer-Verlag. Tokyo.
9. NILSSON, P., L. HILLERED, Y. OLSSON, M. J. SHEIARDOWN & A. J. HANSON. 1993. Regional changes in interstitial potassium and calcium levels following cortical compression contusion trauma in rats. J. Cereb. Blood Flow Metab. **13:** 183–192.
10. KATAYAMA, Y., D. P. BECKER, T. TAMURA & D. A. HOVDA. 1990. Massive increases in extracellular potassium and the indiscriminate release of glutamate following concussive brain injury. J. Neurosurg. **73:** 899–900.

# Discussion

G. C. PALMER (*Fisons Pharmaceuticals, Rochester, NY*): Have any N-methyl-D-aspartate or glutamate compounds been effective regarding suppression of subsequent seizures that develop in a certain number of head trauma patients?

R. BULLOCK (*Medical College of Virginia*): With CGS 19755 there are over 50 patients under long-term evaluation, but the code has not been broken.

C. WILLIAMS (*University of Aukland, New Zealand*): What endpoints can be used to set a therapeutic window for treatment of hypoxic-ischemic injury?

K. W. MUIR (*Western Infirmary, Glasgow*): A useful endpoint that may help set the outer boundaries of a therapeutic 'window' is the time course of DNA degradation. Following a mild hypoxic-ischemic injury, DNA degradation starts at about 1 day after injury, whereas, after a severe hypoxic-ischemic injury in the developing rat brain, the DNA degradation has started by about 6 h post injury.

# The Neuroprotective Effect of Calcitonin Gene-Related Peptide following Subarachnoid Hemorrhage

B. ANTHONY BELL, FOR THE EUROPEAN CGRP IN
SUBARACHNOID HAEMORRHAGE STUDY GROUP

*Division of Clinical Neuroscience*
*St. George's Hospital Medical School*
*Atkinson Morley Neuroscience Centre*
*Wimbledon, London SW20 0NE, United Kingdom*

More than 5,000 patients a year bleed from cerebral aneurysms in Britain, and cerebral ischemia limits recovery in up to a third. Over 100 drugs have been tried as neuroprotective agents in subarachnoid hemorrhage (SAH),[1] and only nimodipine has been shown to reduce ischemic morbidity from 33.3% to 21.9%, although death and severe disability still supervene in 19.8% of nimodipine-treated patients.[2]

Endogenous calcitonin gene-related peptide (CGRP) is a powerful vasodilator, and in normal volunteers synthetic human alpha CGRP increases cardiac output and internal carotid blood flow, and produces facial flushing. CGRP can improve cerebral blood flow in focal ischemia,[3] and is released in patients who suffer cerebral vasoconstriction following subarachnoid hemorrhage.[4] Early clinical results in vasospasm following subarachnoid hemorrhage have been encouraging,[5] so a randomized multicenter open comparison of CGRP against standard management has been conducted in patients undergoing intracranial aneurysm surgery.

Patients who developed focal neurological deficits or had a reduced Glasgow coma score (GCS) after surgery, were studied after a computerized tomography (CT) scan had excluded nonischemic causes for the deficit. An intravenous infusion of 0.6 µg/min of CGRP for a minimum of four hours up to a maximum of 10 days was given to 62 patients, and 55 patients received standard management. Outcome was measured at three months on the Glasgow outcome scale by an independent investigator blind to their treatment. Of the 117 patients randomized, 99 met the full inclusion criteria of the study protocol. A good outcome was achieved in 66% of patients treated with CGRP and in 59% of patients receiving standard management, but the difference was not significant. Hypotension was a common side effect of the CGRP infusion, and suggests that intravascular administration of CGRP is not the ideal route. Subarachnoid instillation is an attractive route, as the peptide is normally found on the adventitial rather than the endothelial side of the cerebral vessel wall.

A clinically useful benefit has not been excluded by this study, and a subsequent trial of instillation of CGRP into the subarachnoid space at the time of surgery for a cerebral aneurysm has now started and may show a more marked protective effect against cerebral ischemia with a reduced incidence of systemic hypotension.

If CGRP can protect the brain from cerebral ischemia after early intracranial aneurysm surgery, it has the potential to make early surgery safer in a high proportion of SAH patients. This would remove the need to delay surgery, prevent death from rebleeding, and markedly reduce the overall management morbidity and mortality of aneurysmal SAH.

## REFERENCES

1. WILKINS, R. H. 1986. Attempts at prevention or treatment of intracranial arterial spasm: an update. Neurosurgery 18: 808–825.
2. PICKARD, J. D., J. D. MURRAY, R. ILLINGWORTH, M. D. M. SHAW, G. M. TEASDALE, P. M. FOY, P. R. D. HUMPHREY, D. A. LANG, R. NELSON, P. RICHARDS, J. SINAR, S. BAILEY & A. SKENE. 1989. Effect of oral nimodipine on cerebral infarction and outcome after subarachnoid haemorrhage: British Aneurysm Nimodipine Trial. Br. Med. J. 298: 636–642.
3. TAYLOR, W. A. S., S. G. C. SYDSERFF & B. A. BELL. 1992. Focal ischaemic cerebral blood flow can be increased by CGRP. Neuropeptides 22: 65.
4. JUUL, R., L. EDVINSSON, S. E. GISVOLD, R. EKMAN, A. O. BRUBAKK & T. A. FREDRIKSEN. 1990. Calcitonin gene-related peptide-LI in subarachnoid haemorrhage in man. Signs of activation of the trigemino-cerebrovascular system? Br. J. Neurosurg. 4: 171–180.
5. JOHNSTON, F. G., B. A. BELL, I. J. A. ROBERTSON, J. D. MILLER, C. HALIBURN, D. O'SHAUGHNESSY, A. J. RIDDEL & S. A. O'LAOIRE. 1990. Effect of calcitonin-gene-related peptide on postoperative neurological deficits after subarachnoid haemorrhage. Lancet 335: 869–872.

# A Small Animal Model of Focal Cerebral Ischemia for Studying Neuroprotective Agents

JEREMY P. HOLLAND AND B. ANTHONY BELL

*Division of Clinical Neuroscience*
*St. George's Hospital Medical School*
*Atkinson Morley Neuroscience Centre*
*Wimbledon, London SW20 0NE, United Kingdom*

Neuronal damage after focal cerebral ischemia in the middle cerebral artery (MCA) territory has many clinical correlates, and a number of laboratories have evolved animal models of clinical stroke or subarachnoid hemorrhage for the preclinical testing of neuroprotective agents. Early work on primates and cats has produced much useful data, but there is a need for a reproducible model that can accurately quantify the extent of neuronal damage in smaller animals such as the rat.

We have evolved a rat model of MCA occlusion using an endovascular suture.[1] The rats are anesthetized and paralyzed and ventilated via a tracheostomy, and body temperature is maintained at 37 ± 1°C. A femoral artery is cannulated to monitor blood pressure and heart rate and allow sampling for blood gas estimations, and a 3-0 monofilament nylon suture is introduced into the internal carotid artery via an arteriotomy in the isolated external carotid artery to lodge in the narrow proximal segment of the anterior cerebral artery and occlude the origin of the MCA. Regional cerebral blood flow (CBF) is measured using hydrogen clearance.[2]

After 4 hours of MCA occlusion the brain is perfusion-fixed with formalin and cut into blocks to be processed through a series of formalin/alcohol/chloroform solutions and embedded in polyester wax. Coronal sections 7 microns thick are cut on a microtome, mounted on albumin-coated glass slides and baked for 12 hours prior to staining with hematoxylin and eosin. In 8 sections from each brain the extent of cerebral ischemia is determined with light microscopy and marked onto a corresponding section from a stereotactic atlas.[3] The ischemic neurones are shrunken, angulated and densely stained, and readily differentiated from healthy neurones, allowing the quantification of ischemic territory prior to the development of infarction. The marked ischemic area is cut out and weighed for each section and the volume of cerebral ischemia calculated by integration.

The extrapolation of results from animal models to the clinical setting is fraught with difficulty, but the endovascular suture technique of MCA occlusion produces a reproducible volume of ischemic neuronal injury (233.3 ± 19.4 mm$^3$, mean ± SD, comprising 191.4 ± 12.7 mm$^3$ cortex and 41.9 ± 9.8 mm$^3$ basal ganglia). The endovascular technique is minimally invasive, producing an occlusion at the origin of the MCA which can be confirmed by observing the hydrogen clearance CBF curve. It avoids the problems of a craniectomy, with loss of cerebrospinal fluid

(CSF) and alteration of intracranial fluid dynamics. Hydrogen clearance allows the simultaneous determination of quantitative local CBF at multiple sites repeatedly during an experiment, and will detect effects of the neuroprotective agent on CBF.

Histological assessment of neuronal injury by light microscopy after 4 hours ischemia accurately reflects the ultimate volume of cerebral infarction,[4] and provides an ideal parameter for assessing the degree of protection offered by the agent under test.

## REFERENCES

1. LONGA, E. Z., P. R. WEINSTEIN, S. CARLSON & R. CUMMINS. 1989. Reversible middle cerebral artery occlusion without craniectomy in rats. Stroke **20:** 84–91.
2. AUKLAND, K., B. F. BOWER, R. W. BERLINER *et al.* 1987. Measurement of local blood flow with hydrogen gas. Circ. Res. **14:** 164–187.
3. PAXINOS, G. & C. WATSON. 1982. The Rat Brain in Stereotactic Coordinates. Academic Press. New York.
4. BROWN, A. W. & J. B. BRIERLEY. 1968. The nature, distribution and earliest stages of anoxic-ischaemic nerve cell damage in the rat brain as defined by the optical microscope. Br. J. Exp. Pathol. **159:** 87–106.

# Quantitative Histological Evaluation of Neurotoxic Hippocampal Damage

ANDREW C. SCALLET

*Experimental Neuropathology Laboratory*
*Division of Neurotoxicology*
*National Center for Toxicological Research, FDA*
*Jefferson, Arkansas 72079*

Histological evaluation of neurodegenerative changes is vital to neurotoxicology, since it allows interpreting neurochemical or behavioral effects in the light of correlated structural observations. The hippocampus is of particular interest as a target, since it is damaged by a number of compounds with little structural similarity, such as trimethyltin (TMT), domoic and kainic acids, and methionine sulfoxamine. It is also a major target for hypoxia/ischemia. Protection from irreversible damage to neurons may well be the endpoint of greatest relevance to studies seeking to validate the effectiveness of neuroprotective drugs or procedures. However, routine use of histological methods to evaluate protection has been relatively limited, perhaps due to the difficulty of obtaining numerical results. Several quantitative histochemical methods (including Golgi measurement of dendrites, electron microscopic estimation of synaptic density, immunohistochemistry, and silver degeneration-sensitive stains) have been used to evaluate the effects of various neurotoxicants on the hippocampi of rats and monkeys. The measurements of dendrite length and synaptic density were both sensitive to manipulations as subtle as chronic differences in access to operant test chambers on a daily basis. Although quantitative Golgi and synaptic density methods are sensitive to both acute as well as chronic and persistent neurodegenerative changes, they are quite expensive and time-consuming. Immunohistochemical markers such as c-fos and heat shock proteins readily indicate cells that are responding to neurotoxicant stress, but are not invariant markers of cell death. Glial fibrillary acidic protein can act as a marker of reactive gliosis in response to adjacent neuronal damage, but it is only an indirect indication. However, TMT-induced increases in the density of silver grains in the CA1 hippocampal subregion can be measured by densitometry of digitized microscopic images from sections selectively stained for argyrophilic neurodegeneration. Such measured histological increases in grain counts follow a comparable dose-response relationship as do TMT effects on passive avoidance behavior. A silver degeneration-selective method for measuring the number of grains per unit area has also been used to evaluate the quantitative neurotoxicity of domoic acid in monkey and rat brains. The silver degeneration methods are sensitive to both acute axon terminal as well as perikaryal damage, but the argyrophilia of damaged neuronal structures eventually disappears, rendering the methods insensitive to chronic effects. If acute effects (or their reversal) are of primary interest, the silver degeneration-sensitive stains lend themselves well to quantitative analysis and preclinical screening.

# Perinatal Brain Injury
## Pathophysiology and Therapeutic Intervention

CHRIS WILLIAMS, CARINA MALLARD, WILLIAM TAN,
BARBARA JOHNSTON, ALISTAIR GUNN, KYLA MARKS, AND
PETER GLUCKMAN

*Research Centre for Developmental Medicine and Biology*
*University of Auckland*
*Auckland, New Zealand*

It is generally accepted that hypoxic-ischemic insults in the fetus or newborn are an important cause of neurologic morbidity. However, there are difficulties in identifying those who are likely to benefit from therapeutic intervention and deciding exactly when and how to treat. Recent evidence suggests that asphyxic brain injury is associated with evidence of cardiovascular compromise such as hypotension but not hypoxia alone. The data described here were obtained from descriptive studies and therapeutic studies of chronically instrumented late gestation fetal sheep that undergo 30 minutes of forebrain ischemia. Near infrared spectroscopy (NIRS), quantitative electroencephalogram (EEG) analysis, cortical impedance measurements and microdialysis techniques were used. During the ischemia there is cytotoxic swelling that largely, but not completely, resolves within 30 minutes of reperfusion indicating some acute damage. The extracellular concentration of gamma-aminobutyric acid (GABA) increased markedly by 4,400 ± 500%, whereas glutamate increased by 92 ± 20% and glycine by 250 ± 50% during the ischemia. Pretreatment with flunarizine (30 mg/kg but not 45 mg/kg iv) is moderately protective but causes hypotension. Ganglioside $GM_1$ 30 mg/kg/day iv is similarly protective but does not cause hypotension.

Repetitive insults are likely to occur in the severely compromised fetus or neonate. If injuries are repeated before electrophysiologic recovery (1 h intervals) the ability to recover membrane function is impaired. Both ischemic and asphyxic insults markedly sensitized the striatum causing particular loss of the GABAergic projection neurons (striatal-pallidal and striatal-nigral). This distribution cell loss is similar to that occurring in choreoathetoid cerebral palsy. Given that there was cumulative membrane damage with each insult we treated with $GM_1$ (30 mg/kg) part way through a series of ischemic insults. This was markedly protective. Thus $GM_1$ or compounds with similar actions may be useful for protecting the compromised fetus or neonate at risk of further hypoxic-ischemic injuries.

Following reperfusion after 30 min of forebrain ischemia, there is a distinctive pathophysiologic cascade culminating in laminar necrosis of the parasagittal parietal cortex. Electrical activity is depressed for about several hours then becomes hyperexcitable (seizures) as the secondary cytotoxic edema develops. A previous study by us suggests that this seizure activity causes some further damage distal to the primary infarct. Recently we measured the time course of the cerebrovascular responses, concentrations of amino acid neuromodulators, glucose and lactate with NIRS and microdialysis, respectively. There was a mild increase in blood volume during the early reperfusion period, then a more marked increase preceding the onset of the secondary cytotoxic swelling. Citrulline levels were increased during this period suggesting increased nitric oxide (NO) synthesis. There was some loss of oxidized cytochrome aa3 during the primary insult and early reperfusion period, then a further progressive loss. Lactate concentrations increased in the cortex before the secondary cytotoxic swelling. Thus mitochondrial dysfunction may be an important component of the cascade leading to delayed cortical necrosis.

Infusion of 1 µg recombinant human insulin-like growth factor 1 (rhIGF-1) but not 10 µg IGF-1 (n = 8) into the lateral ventricle, during the phase of postischemic depression (2 h post), reduced neuronal loss compared to vehicle treated controls ($p < 0.01$) to an extent comparable to the pretreatment with $G_{M1}$. The IGF-1 treatment did not suppress the seizures but reduced the systemic increase in lactate and delayed the onset of the secondary cytotoxic swelling from $7 \pm 1$ h to $19 \pm 2$ h. The effective dose was lower than that which we observe in adult rats. This difference may be due to the greater homology of sheep IGF-1 to human IGF-1 and/or developmental differences.

In summary, hypoxic-ischemic injury in the developing brain can trigger a distinctive cascade of pathophysiologic processes that can be monitored by cerebral impedance, quantitative EEG and NIRS measurements. Some of these techniques may prove useful for guiding the application of neuronal rescue therapies.

# The Role of the Growth Factors IGF-1 and TGFβ$_1$ after Hypoxic-Ischemic Brain Injury

CHRIS WILLIAMS, JIAN GUAN, ODETTE MILLER,
ERICA BEILHARZ, HEATHER MCNEILL, ERNEST SIRIMANNE,
AND PETER GLUCKMAN

*Research Centre for Developmental Medicine and Biology*
*University of Auckland*
*Auckland, New Zealand*

The immature brain produces neurotrophic factors following injury. These may serve to restrict the extent of neuronal loss and/or to facilitate functional recovery. Therefore, we have examined the time course of cell death and expression of growth factors following moderate (15-minute) and severe (60-minute) unilateral hypoxic-ischemic injuries in the infant (21-day) rat. Following the moderate injury the neurons developed an apoptotic morphology, acidophilia and DNA laddering by 3 days after the initial injury. These changes were preceded by prolonged expression of the immediate early gene *c-jun* in the dying neurons. The apoptotic changes closely correlated temporally and spatially both with the microglial reaction and sites of transforming growth factor β$_1$ (TGFβ$_1$) mRNA expression. After the severe injury the apoptotic changes were accelerated particularly within the striatum where some DNA and mitochondria (triphenyltetrazolium chloride monohydrate (TTC) staining) remained intact and cells basophilic until after 10 h. Widespread necrosis with random DNA degradation developed by 24 h. The results indicate that there are two pathways to delayed cell death; selective neuronal loss which was apoptotic, and closely coupled with a microglial reaction and *c-jun* expression. In contrast delayed necrosis occurred independently from these processes.

Insulin-like growth factor 1 (IGF-1), which is well known for its anabolic effects, is a potent trophic factor for most types of neurons. We have extensively studied the time course of changes in the IGF axis following these injuries. IGF-1 was induced in astrocytes from 3 days after the severe injury. Its binding proteins BP2 and 3 were also induced at this time; subsequently BP5 was induced at 5 days and IGF-2 in severely damaged regions from 7 days. These BPs are thought to modulate the targeting and activity of the IGFs. We studied the effects of rhIGF-1 (20 μg), rhIGF-2 (20 μg), insulin (20 μg), given 2 h into the lateral ventricle after 10-minute unilateral hypoxic-ischemic injury in adult rats. Only the IGF-1 improved outcome. This dose did not modify cortical temperature after injury. Peripheral administration treatment studies and tracer studies suggested that peripheral administration is unlikely to be effective due to low penetration of IGF-1 across the blood-brain barrier. Together these observations were compatible with the hypothesis that IGF-1 was acting centrally via type 1 receptors.

Vicki Sara postulated that in the central nervous system IGF-1 is a prohormone and is cleaved near the site of action to form des(1-3) IGF-1 and the tripeptide GPE (glycine-proline-glutamate). Des IGF-1 has a much lower affinity for binding proteins but a similar affinity for the type 1 IGF-1 receptor and can have more potent anabolic effects than full-length IGF-1. Therefore, we compared the effects of treatment with 2 and 20 μg of des(1-3)IGF-1 with vehicle and there was not a significant effect. GPE can stimulate acetylcholine release. Therefore, we compared the effect of 3 μg of GPE vs vehicle-treated controls (n = 20) in the same paradigm and there was a significant improvement in outcome. Thus the neuronal rescue effect of IGF-1 is likely to be, in part, mediated by GPE.

$TGF\beta_1$ is an important regulator of injury responses and modulates macrophage/microglial reactions and the expression of other growth factors. *In vitro* $rhTGF\beta_1$ can rescue neurons from excitotoxic injury. When $rhTGF\beta_1$ is given into the lateral ventricle 2 h after a 10-min hypoxic-ischemic injury in adult rats, 10 but not 50 ng reduces the incidence of cortical infarction and extent of neuronal loss. In subsequent studies we observed that 10 ng reduced the deficit in water maze learning ability and the asymmetry in somatosensory function during the first 10 days after injury. Thus endogenous IGF-1 and $TGF\beta_1$ are involved during recovery from injury, and treatment studies in animals by ourselves and other groups indicate that these growth factors show promise as neuronal rescue therapies.

# Oxidative Brain Damage in Aged Mice
## Protection by Caloric Reduction

[a]HARBANS LAL, MICHAEL J. FORSTER, AND RAJ S. SOHAL

*Department of Pharmacology*
*University of North Texas Health Science Center at Fort Worth*
*Fort Worth, Texas 76107*
*and*
*Department of Biological Science*
*Southern Methodist University*
*Dallas, Texas 75275.*

Our experiments were undertaken to determine if oxidative brain damage[1] mediates age-associated deterioration reported in brain functions of C57BL/6NNia mice.[2] The aged mice exhibit deficits in sensory, motor and learning/memory capacity. Mice maintained on a caloric intake 40% less (DR) than an ad libitum fed group (AL) exhibited a 43% extension in life span and a 31% prolongation in mortality rate doubling time. Further, there was a significant retardation in the onset of the brain function deterioration in DR mice. There was a significant increase in the protein carbonyl content in brain, heart and kidney of AL and DR groups aged 9, 17, or 23 months suggesting an increase in the oxidative damage with age. Nearly all brain areas showed an increase in protein carbonyl content, with relatively larger increases in striatum and hippocampus of the aging mice. The loss of membrane protein sulfhydral groups also increased with age in all brain regions except hippocampus. The caloric restriction significantly retarded the age-associated increase in carbonyl protein. This reduction was most pronounced in cortex, whereas only a modest reduction was evident in the hippocampus. An investigation of the mechanisms underlying the neuroprotection showed that the mitochondrial state 4 respiratory rate in brain tissue was increased with age in the AL, but not the DR group. Thus, one protective effect in DR mice occurred at a site of oxygen free-radical generation. The rates of mitochondrial superoxide and hydrogen peroxide generation increased with age and were higher in the AL than DR mice in all the three organs at each age. In contrast, there was no clear-cut pattern of age- or diet-related changes in antioxidant defenses provided by superoxide dismutase, catalase, and glutathione peroxidase. These data suggest that increased oxidative stress/damage may be an important mechanism of brain aging and the associated brain dysfunctions. Both of these effects can be modulated significantly via caloric optimization.

### REFERENCES

1. SOHAL, R. S. *et al.* 1994. Mech. Ageing Dev. **74:** 121.
2. FORSTER, M. J. & H. LAL. 1992. Behav. Pharmacol. **3:** 337.

[a] Supported by NIH-NIA Grants AG07657 and AG07695.

# The Role of Hyperthermia in Amphetamine's Interactions with NMDA Receptors, Nitric Oxide, and Age to Produce Neurotoxicity

JOHN F. BOWYER

*Division of Neurotoxicology*
*National Center for Toxicological Research, FDA*
*Jefferson, Arkansas 72079-9502*

Amphetamine (AMPH) and methamphetamine (METH) exposure produces damage, probably confined to nerve terminals and possibly glia, resulting in prominent decreases in striatal dopamine (DA) levels in laboratory animals. Many similarities exist in the mechanisms involved in AMPH/METH neurotoxicity and the cytotoxicity produced by hypoxia/ischemia and excitatory amino acids. Similar factors appearing to affect both AMPH/METH and hypoxia/ischemia neurotoxicity are 1) age, 2) excitatory amino acids levels, 3) nitric oxide (NO) production, 4) acidosis and 5) hyperthermia/hypothermia.

Interactions of these factors to produce AMPH/METH neurotoxicity are complex. Research at NCTR has focused on the hyperthermia produced by AMPH/METH and its interactions with the other factors. Increased environmental temperature greatly potentiates the neurotoxicity and lethality of the amphetamines thus far tested. Changing the environmental temperature from 20°C to 24.5°C can increase lethality and neurotoxicity over 10-fold. This potentiation of toxicity is primarily due to an increased incidence of hyperthermia during AMPH/METH exposure. Furthermore, reductions in body temperature produced by a (10°C) environmental temperature increases the dose necessary to produce lethality and neurotoxicity over 4-fold. To date we have not been able to produce neurotoxicity in rats administered METH or AMPH that do not become hyperthermic. However, hyperthermia generated by 37°C environmental temperatures or by other compounds cannot mimic AMPH/METH neurotoxicity.

Many laboratories, including ours followed the lead of Sonsalla and collaborators that glutamate NMDA receptors may be involved in METH neurotoxicity. As determined in microdialysis, striatal extracellular glutamate levels increase significantly during exposures to AMPH/METH that damage DA terminals and subsequently downregulate the NMDA-mediated DA release for several days. However, these increases are not sufficient to produce cytotoxicity. Furthermore, the blockade of METH neurotoxicity by MK-801 and haloperidol can be reversed if environmental temperatures are elevated so that hyperthermia occurs. What is left to be determined is if hyperthermia alone can either "open" or interfere with MK-801 blockade of NMDA channels because temperature alters membrane fluidity as much as any other factor.

Activation of NMDA receptors has been noted by many prominent laboratories to result in NO generation. We have observed that NO antagonists nitro-L-arginine (NOARG) and nitro-L-arginine methyl ester (L-NAME) but not D-NAME greatly inhibit DA release in the striatum. However, it is not certain whether release inhibition results from NO synthase inhibition and/or if AMPH/METH neurotoxicity is blocked by NOARG and L-NAME. Studies are necessary to determine if NO generation is affected by hyperthermia alone.

The neurotoxicity of both METH and AMPH is significantly increased as laboratory animals age. In older animals both higher striatal extracellular AMPH levels and body temperature are attained during AMPH administration. The appearance of extreme hyperthermia >41°C during AMPH exposure rapidly elevates striatal extracellular AMPH levels and may induce acidosis. Young animals <40 days old are resistant to long-term AMPH/METH neurotoxicity, but it is not certain whether this is due to their resistance to the hyperthermia produced by AMPH/METH or that the levels of cell-line-derived neurotrophic factor (GDNF) are sufficiently elevated at these ages to allow the rapid regeneration of DA terminals. The research conducted thus far shows that many mechanisms involved in AMPH/METH neurotoxicity at DA terminals are similar to those of hypoxia/ischemia cytotoxicity.

# Lack of Mitigation of Methamphetamine-Induced Neurotoxicity by Ganglioside $GM_1$ or Vitamin E

SYED F. ALI

*Neurochemistry Laboratory*
*Division of Neurotoxicology*
*National Center for Toxicological Research/FDA*
*Jefferson, Arkansas 72079*

Recently, it was reported that the ganglioside $GM_1$ protects against 1-methyl-4-phenyl-1,2,3,6-tetrahydropyridine (MPTP)-induced neurotoxicity. $GM_1$ is a monosialoganglioside known to have neurotropic effects on the damaged dopamine system. Vitamin E, an antioxidant, is known to protect against cellular damage produced by oxidative stress. MPTP and methamphetamine (METH) have some parallel effects on dopaminergic neurons, although they may have different underlying mechanisms of action. We have found that both agents are able to effect the release of dopamine. Because dopamine is readily oxidized with concurrent formation of free radicals, excessive formation of reactive oxygen species (ROS) may result. Therefore, the present study was designed to evaluate whether ganglioside $GM_1$ or vitamin E can protect against METH-induced neurotoxicity.

Adult C57BL/6 mice were dosed with either 10 mg/kg, ip $GM_1$ or 50 mg/kg vitamin E, ip for five days (Monday through Friday). On Wednesday animals were also dosed with $4 \times 20$ mg/kg METH, ip. A separate group of animals was also treated with saline or $4 \times 20$ mg/kg METH, ip. Animals were sacrificed three days post METH administration. Brains were rapidly removed and striata were dissected to measure dopamine (DA), serotonin (5-HT) and their metabolites dihydroxyphenylacetic acid (DOPAC), homovanillic acid (HVA), and hydroxyindoleacetic acid (HIAA) by high-performance liquid chromatography combined with electrochemical detection (HPLC/EC). ROS were measured with the use of a fluorescent probe, 2,7-dichloroflurescein diacetate. METH alone produced significant depletion of DA and its metabolites in striatum. Depletion of DA, however, could not be prevented by the several days of pre- and posttreatment with either $GM_1$ or vitamin E. Levels of 5-HT and its metabolite 5-HIAA and rate of formation of ROS were unchanged by the METH treatment. These data indicate that METH-induced neurotoxicity as measured by the depletion of DA is not mediated by mechanisms involving free radicals or oxidative stress.

# Structural-Functional Correlates of Neuroprotection in the Aging Rabbit by a Calcium Channel Blocker

## Nimodipine Reverses Neocortical Dendritic Atrophy and Improves Memory Retention[a]

RONALD F. MERVIS,[b] N. KUNTZ,[b] D. BURTON,[b] R. DVORAK,[b]
R. TANDON,[b] L. HOOVER,[b] M. S. WOOD,[c] AND P. R. SOLOMON[c]

[b]NeuroMetrix Research, Inc.
794 Northwest Boulevard
Columbus, Ohio 43212
[c]Department of Psychology
and
Program in Neuroscience
Williams College
Williamstown, Massachusetts 01267

## INTRODUCTION

In the aging brain loss of calcium homeostasis is believed to be a key factor underlying neuronal damage associated with dendritic atrophy and, ultimately, cell death. The loss of dendritic branching would disrupt brain circuitry and, hence, would be the anatomical basis for cognitive dysfunction. It was reasoned that chronic nimodipine treatment in aging subjects might be able to diminish or restore the calcium homeostatic imbalance with commensurate neuroprotective effects on neuronal morphology and related behavioral measures. The present study was designed to determine: (1) if chronic nimodipine could facilitate long-term memory of a classically conditioned eye-blink (EB) response in aging animals, and (2) using Golgi stained tissue, whether there were relevant neuroanatomical correlates underlying the behavioral effects of the nimodipine treatment.

### Behavioral Studies

Subjects were 30 New Zealand Albino rabbits. Aged (36–42 months). Subjects underwent acquisition training of the EB response. Following acquisition, rabbits received daily injections of nimodipine at either a low dosage (7.5 mg/kg) or a high dosage (15 mg/kg) for 90 consecutive days. At the end of 30 and 90 days, subjects underwent retention testing. In comparison to the aging controls, low-dose nimodipine had no effect. However, aging *rabbits that received the high*

---

[a] Supported by Miles Pharmaceuticals.

*dose nimodipine treatment showed significantly better retention of the conditioned eye-blink response.* The behavioral results, therefore, demonstrated that there was a dose-dependent beneficial effect of nimodipine on memory facilitation over a relatively long period.

### Golgi Studies

A young control rabbit group (4–6 months) was added. Formalin-fixed coronal sections of parietal cortex were stained and coded slides prepared: 103 layer V pyramids from 15 subjects were randomly selected for morphometric analysis; camera lucida drawings of the basilar tree were evaluated. Morphometric analysis showed that with normal aging there was a significant decrease in total dendritic length and atrophy of the dendritic arbor. Low-dose nimodipine had no effect on dendritic branch atrophy. However, *chronic high-dose nimodipine treatment completely reversed age-related atrophic changes: both total dendritic length and distribution of dendritic material of the aging rabbits were the same as in young controls.* The high-dose nimodipine treatment also reversed age-related atrophy of the soma.

## CONCLUSIONS

Treatment with high-dose (but not low-dose) nimodipine facilitated retention of an age-related memory impairment (a classically conditioned eye-blink response) for a protracted period. Treatment also reversed a neuroanatomical correlate of behavioral decline: age-related atrophy of cortical dendritic branching. These results suggest that this calcium channel blocker is effective in restoring calcium homeostasis in the aging brain. Such homeostasis appears to be critical in exerting both neuroprotective and neuroplastic influences on the aging brain. The results suggest that nimodipine treatment may be an appropriate prophylactic or therapeutic strategy to minimize age-related dendritic atrophy and, hence, the synaptic loss underlying cognitive impairment.

# Neuroprotective Activity of HU-211, a Novel Nonpsychotropic Synthetic Cannabinoid

A. BIEGON

*Pharmos Ltd.*
*Rehovot, Israel*

HU-211 is a synthetic cannabinoid with negligible affinity to cannabinoid receptors and no psychotropic effects in animals. This profile is most probably due to the fact that HU-211, unlike psychoactive cannabinoids, is a (+) enantiomer.[1] The compound shows neuroprotective activity in a number of experimental models in culture and *in vivo*.

In primary neuronal cultures exposed to 1 mM *N*-methyl-D-aspartate (NMDA), HU-211 protects the neurons in a dose-dependent manner with complete reversal of toxicity at concentrations below 10 $\mu$M. A similar dose-response relationship was seen in a hypoxia/hypoglycemia paradigm in culture. Micromolar concentrations of HU-211 also rescue neurons from sodium nitroprusside toxicity. Unlike the former two models, this activity is not shared by the selective NMDA antagonist MK-801.

*In vivo*, HU-211 has been shown to reduce neuroclinical signs, brain edema and calcium influx in a rat model of closed head injury, when given up to 5 hours after injury. A single iv injection of HU-211 (4 mg/kg) 30 or 60 minutes after the insult also conferred significant protection on hippocampal CA1 neurons following severe transient forebrain ischemia in gerbils (10 minutes of bilateral common carotid artery occlusion) and rats (20 minutes of 4 vessel occlusion). A two-week, two-species toxicological study of HU-211 revealed no adverse effects at doses up to 8 mg/kg.

*In vitro* studies have demonstrated that HU-211 is a functional noncompetitive antagonist at the NMDA receptor, binding with $\mu$M affinity at a site linked to the well characterized MK-801 open channel site. In addition, HU-211 has a redox potential close to that of several known antioxidants and is a free radical scavenger, as demonstrated in peroxy and hydroxy radical generating systems. This activity, too, occurs at $\mu$M concentrations of the compound.

It is suggested that HU-211 is a promising neuroprotective agent with a dual (NMDA blockade and free radical scavenging) mechanism of action which does not involve cannabinoid activity.

## REFERENCES

1. HOWLETT, A. C. *et al.* 1990. Neuropharmacology **29**: 161.

# A Randomized, Double-Blind, Placebo-Controlled Pilot Trial of Intravenous Magnesium Sulfate in Acute Stroke

KEITH W. MUIR AND KENNEDY R. LEES

*Acute Stroke Unit*
*University Department of Medicine and Therapeutics*
*Gardiner Institute*
*Western Infirmary*
*Glasgow G11 6NT, Scotland*

## INTRODUCTION

Intracellular calcium (Ca) overload due to unregulated entry via voltage-gated channels or the $N$-methyl-D-aspartate (NMDA) receptor ion channel initiates metabolic events which cause cell death. Magnesium (Mg) is a physiological antagonist of Ca which regulates vascular tone and cell membrane function. Mg acts as a voltage-dependent blocker of the NMDA receptor ion channel and behaves pharmacologically as a noncompetitive NMDA antagonist. Parenteral Mg decreases mortality when given early following acute myocardial infarction, probably due to protection against reperfusion injury. Mg decreases the volume of cerebral infarction after middle cerebral artery (MCA) occlusion by up to 20% and is effective against NMDA-mediated brain injury. It has improved functional recovery and decreased infarct volume after focal traumatic ischemia. In healthy subjects, intravenous (iv) Mg causes vasodilatation with a minor fall in blood pressure.

## METHODS

Patients presenting within 12 hours of acute MCA stroke were randomized in a double-blind study to receive iv Mg sulfate, 8 mmol over 15 minutes + 65 mmol infusion over 24 hours, or equal volume of saline as placebo. Patients who were pregnant, had severe intercurrent illness, or renal impairment were excluded. Cardiovascular monitoring was undertaken and routine laboratory information was collected. Outcome was assessed by the Barthel score at 3 months. The study was not powered to detect small outcome differences.

## RESULTS

Sixty patients of 260 admitted over a 6-month period were eligible and were randomized: 30 received Mg and 30 placebo. Baseline characteristics of the two groups were not significantly different. Blood pressure and pulse rate did not differ between the two groups over 48 hours. There were no differences in laboratory indices. Outcome was better in the Mg-treated group (30% dead or disabled compared with 40% in placebo, chi-squared test, $p = 0.42$). There was a trend towards lower early mortality in the Mg group (log-rank test, $p = 0.07$).

## CONCLUSIONS

Intravenous Mg sulfate is safe after acute stroke. In particular, there is no evidence of hypotension. Although not significant due to the small numbers studied, the better outcome in the Mg-treated group is encouraging for further trials.

# Efficacy and Tolerability of Lifarizine in Acute Ischemic Stroke

## A Pilot Study

I. B. SQUIRE,[a,e] K. R. LEES,[a] W. PRYSE-PHILLIPS,[b] A. KERTESZ,[c] AND J. BAMFORD,[d] FOR THE LIFARIZINE STUDY GROUP

[a]*Acute Stroke Unit*
*University Department of Medicine and Therapeutics*
*Gardiner Institute*
*Western Infirmary*
*Glasgow G11 6NT, Scotland*
[b]*Memorial University of Newfoundland*
*Health Sciences Centre*
*300 Prince Philip Drive*
*St. John's, Newfoundland, Canada A1B 3V6.*
[c]*Department of Clinical Neurological Sciences*
*St. Joseph's Hospital*
*268 Grosvenor Street*
*London, Ontario, Canada N6A 4V2.*
[d]*St. James's University Hospital*
*Beckett Street*
*Leeds LS9 7TF, United Kingdom*

Lifarizine (1-[(2-(4-methylphenyl)-5-methyl)-1H-imidazol-4y1-diphenyl-methyl]-piperazine, RS-87476, Syntex) is a novel, lipophilic basic compound with sodium and calcium channel modulation properties. It is neuroprotective in experimental global and focal ischemia, at doses which have minimal systemic vascular effects. Lifarizine binds to dopamine DA2 receptors, the functional correlate of which may be increased prolactin levels. We describe the results of a double-blind, randomized, parallel group, pilot study in human stroke which was conducted in 16 UK and Canadian centers.

Subjects with symptoms and signs of first ever ischemic stroke were randomized in blocks within each center to receive lifarizine (250 $\mu$g/kg iv *stat* plus 60 mg *bd* orally for 5 days) or matching placebo, after stratification for age (21–74 or $\geq$75 years) and for time since stroke onset (<6 or 6–12 hours). Primary endpoints were safety of lifarizine and functional outcome at 3 months, using the modified Barthel score and Rankin scale. Secondary measures included the NIH and Canadian Neurological scales.

Of 147 patients recruited, 30 were ineligible after the computerized tomography (CT) scan results or discovery of preexisting disease, leaving 117 evaluable for

---

[e] Correspondence to Dr. Squire.

efficacy analysis. Treatment groups were well matched. Lifarizine was well tolerated; a single serious adverse event (a seizure) was attributed to active treatment. Minor adverse events were similar with lifarizine and placebo. Biochemical and hematological indices, and serum prolactin levels were unchanged by lifarizine therapy. There was a fall in systolic and diastolic blood pressure over the study period with both active and placebo therapies, although there was a trend towards a greater fall in the lifarizine group. Unplanned subgroup analyses suggested hypotheses for further study of the pharmacokinetics of lifarizine in elderly females and the blood pressure response in stroke patients. Mortality during the 3-month study was 12/75 (16%) for lifarizine and 17/72 (24%) for placebo; amongst evaluable patients, mortality was 9/63 (14%) for lifarizine and 13/54 (24%) for placebo. At 3 months there was a trend towards an increase in the proportion of functionally independent patients in the lifarizine group *versus* the placebo group (16% greater by Rankin scale, $p = 0.52$; and 11% greater by Barthel score, $p = 0.55$).

Lifarizine was well tolerated in this elderly population at the dose used. Both mortality and functional assessment data showed favorable trends with active treatment. Further large scale studies are justified to examine the efficacy of lifarizine in acute stroke.

# Considerations in the Design of Preclinical Safety Evaluation Programs for Novel Therapeutics Used in Neurologic Diseases

J. A. CAVAGNARO AND S. LIU

*Department of Pharmacology and Toxicology*
*Office of Therapeutics Research and Review*
*Center for Biologics Evaluation and Research*
*Federal Drug Administration*
*1401 Rockville Pike*
*Rockville, Maryland 20892*

The introduction of novel therapeutics into the clinic often requires the application of novel strategies to assess their safety. Many newer biological products proposed for use in neurologic diseases have presented unique safety-related issues which have required specific protocol considerations. A diversity of product classes will be discussed including recombinant-derived human proteins, enzymes, monoclonal antibodies and cellular and gene therapies. The impact of route of administration, including the use of delivery devices, will also be considered. In some cases the use of animal models of disease have been important to assess not only the activity of the product (and thereby rationale) but to assess safety as well. Lack of historical precedence in assessing novel products, *i.e.*, the departure from databases accumulated through traditional testing guidelines or approaches, affords academic, industrial and government scientists the opportunity to be creative in designing preclinical studies. It is expected that in the future the continued adherence to a flexible, science-based approach to preclinical safety evaluation will continue to facilitate the introduction of novel products into the clinic for use in a variety of neurological diseases.

# Sensitization and Desensitization of the NMDA Receptor Complex

## Implications for Therapy

LINDA H. FOSSOM AND PHIL SKOLNICK

*Laboratory of Neuroscience*
*NIDDK/NIH*
*Bethesda, Maryland 20892*

Because excessive activation of the N-methyl-D-aspartate (NMDA)-subset of glutamate receptors appears to be responsible for much of the neuronal damage resulting from ischemic events, the use of drugs that specifically block NMDA receptors has been proposed as a means of minimizing ischemia-induced neuronal death and its sequelae. The NMDA receptor is a multi-subunit cation channel, which is gated coordinately by glutamate and glycine, with at least three sites for potential blockade: the glycine site (*e.g.*, by 7-chlorokynurenic acid), the glutamate site (*e.g.*, by 2-amino-5-phosphonopentanoate [APV]) and the channel itself (*e.g.*, by dizocilopine [MK-801]). Specific, use-dependent channel blockers such as MK-801 have received considerable attention as effective antagonists of glutamate-induced neurotoxicity both *in vivo* and in cell culture. Specific, high-affinity glutamate- or glycine-site antagonists are also available, but poor bioavailability (*i.e.*, limited penetration into the CNS) and side effect profile may limit their therapeutic usefulness. On the other hand, several glycine-site partial agonists readily cross the blood-brain barrier and may provide effective NMDA receptor blockade *in vivo* without unwanted side effects. Glycinergic ligands are available that span the spectrum from full agonists (such as glycine itself and D-serine) through partial agonists with varying efficacies (1-aminocyclopropanecarboxylic acid [ACPC], D-cycloserine and ( +/ − )-3-amino-1-hydroxy-2-pyrrolidone [HA-966]) to antagonists (7-chlorokynurenic acid). Our studies have focused on the high affinity, glycine-site partial agonist ACPC, using granule cells cultured from neonatal rat cerebellum to assess the effectiveness of this and other glycinergic ligands to protect against glutamate-induced neurotoxicity and NMDA-induced increases in cyclic guanosine monophosphate (cGMP) levels. Glycinergic partial agonists like ACPC and HA-966 block glutamate-induced neurotoxicity in a concentration-dependent, glycine-reversible manner. However, Boje and co-workers (1993) reported that 24-hr treatment of granule cells with ACPC, or any of several other glycinergic ligands (including glycine, D-cycloserine and HA-966), attenuated the neuroprotective effect of subsequent application of ACPC and other glycinergic partial agonists or antagonists. Boje and co-workers called this phenomenon "desensitization" of the NMDA receptor complex. Our recent data indicates that this phenomenon may not be "desensitization" to glycinergic protection, but may rather be an increased sensitivity to glutamatergic ligands. Thus, following pretreatment with ACPC, the $EC_{50}$ for glutamate-induced neurotoxicity was decreased 2-fold. Moreover, the concentration-response curves for NMDA-induced increases in cGMP levels (at submaximal glycine concentrations) were similarly left-shifted in ACPC-pretreated granule cells. Furthermore, this increased sensitivity to glutamate was accompanied by an altered pattern of NMDA receptor subunit expression. The implications of these phenomena for the clinical use of glycinergic ligands will be discussed.

# Initial Experience with Remacemide Hydrochloride in Patients with Acute Ischemic Stroke

KEITH W. MUIR AND KENNEDY R. LEES

*Acute Stroke Unit*
*University Department of Medicine and Therapeutics*
*Gardiner Institute*
*Western Infirmary*
*Glasgow G11 6NT, Scotland*

## BACKGROUND

Remacemide hydrochloride (Fisons, UK) is in advanced clinical development for epilepsy, where it has a good safety profile during chronic oral administration. It produces an active desglycinated metabolite which has moderate-affinity noncompetitive $N$-methyl-D-aspartate (NMDA) antagonist properties. Remacemide hydrochloride has been shown to be neuroprotective in global and focal models of cerebral ischemia in a number of species, and particularly in a permanent middle cerebral artery (MCA) occlusion model in the cat. We describe preliminary experience with iv administration in a Phase II tolerability and safety acute stroke study. The chosen doses of remacemide hydrochloride are predicted to produce plasma concentrations in patients approximating to neuroprotective concentrations from experimental studies.

## METHODS

Twenty-nine patients (mean age 66, range 41–84; 9 females) presenting within 12 hours of onset (mean 8.6 h, range 3–12) of an acute MCA territory stroke were randomized (3:1) to receive remacemide hydrochloride or placebo. Dose groups (A–C) were 100 mg bd (A, n = 16), 200 mg bd (B, n = 8) or 300 mg bd (C, n = 5). In group A, treatment was iv for 2 doses then oral for 6 days; in groups B and C, treatment was iv for 72 hours. Primary endpoints are safety and tolerability; outcome is also assessed by Canadian Neurological Scale and Barthel Index at 1 month. Patients with nonischemic lesions on computerized tomography (CT) scan are replaced but included in the safety analysis.

## RESULTS

In view of continuing follow-up, we remain blinded to treatment allocation; only safety information is available to date. The use of oral administration was abandoned after group A in view of the high incidence of stroke-related dysphagia. No treatment-related major adverse events have occurred in any group. Eight deaths have occurred, none considered related to treatment. One patient (group A) developed transiently increased liver enzymes, possibly related to test treatment, 2 weeks after dosing. One instance of agitation was seen after the initial dose (B) which was possibly treatment related; 2 patients (B) developed venous irritation (probably related to treatment) and one patient withdrew after 4 doses because of this. In group C, treatment has been well tolerated, with only minor venous irritation in 3/5 subjects.

## CONCLUSIONS

Remacemide hydrochloride has been well tolerated by the small number of patients with acute stroke who have been studied thus far. The study continues with planned dose escalation up to 400 mg bd. The results will guide dose selection for future efficacy trials.

# The Tolerability, Pharmacokinetics and Pharmacodynamics of Increasing Intravenous Doses of 619C89, a Novel Compound for the Acute Treatment of Stroke, in Healthy Volunteers

A. J. MERCER,[a] R. J. LAMB, Z. HUSSEIN, S. HOBBIGER
AND J. POSNER

*Department of Clinical Pharmacology*
*Wellcome Research Laboratories*
*Beckenham, Kent BR3 3BS, United Kingdom*

619C89, 4-amino-2-[4-methyl-1-piperazinyl]-5-[2,3,5-trichlorophenyl]pyrimidine, is an inhibitor of neuronal sodium ion channels and glutamate release in development for the acute treatment of stroke. In animal models of stroke 619C89 provides significant neuroprotection of ischemic tissue.[1] This study examined the pharmacokinetics and effects on vital signs, electrocardiogram (ECG) and electroencephalogram (EEG) of increasing intravenous doses of 619C89.

Twelve healthy male volunteers took part in a double-blind, randomized, placebo-controlled dose-escalation study. 619C89 or matched placebo was given as an intravenous infusion over 0.5 h. Doses administered were 0.125, 0.25, 0.5, 0.75 and 1 mg/kg$^{-1}$. At each dose level 8 volunteers received 619C89 and 4 received placebo. Supine and erect systolic and diastolic blood pressure and heart rate, ECG variables, adverse experiences (AEs) and blood samples were collected at regular intervals during the study day and EEG was recorded 0, 0.5, 2 and 6 h after dosing. Data were analyzed by analysis of variance (ANOVA) and 95% confidence intervals.

The infusion of 619C89 to healthy volunteers was well tolerated, and no significant changes in heart rate, supine or erect systolic or diastolic blood pressure, respiration rate, ECG morphology or intervals were observed at any dose. Transient (<5 min) mild dizziness was reported at the time of maximum plasma concentrations and was dose-related and reported by 4 of 8 volunteers at 1 mg/kg$^{-1}$ of 619C89. These AEs were not accompanied by cardiovascular or neurological signs. Full blood counts and plasma biochemistry were normal throughout the study. The alpha power of the EEG was decreased in a dose-related fashion (FIG. 1) with significant differences from placebo ($p < 0.05$) observed at a dose of 0.5 mg/kg$^{-1}$ of 619C89 or greater. The AUC$_{0-\infty}$ and C$_{max}$ of 619C89 were linearly related to dose (FIG. 2), with mean ($\pm$ SD) C$_{max}$ of 123 (52.7) ng/mL$^{-1}$, AUC$_{0-\infty}$

---

[a] Corresponding author.

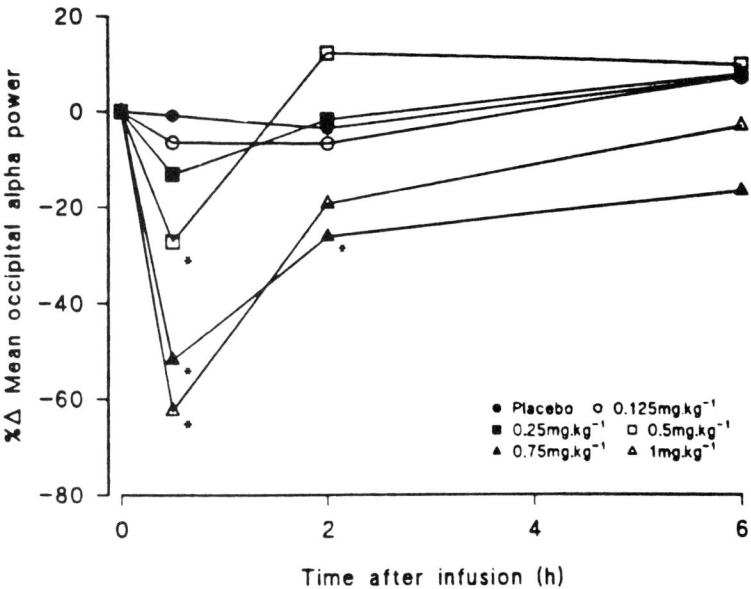

**FIGURE 1.** The dose-related effects of 619C89 on EEG alpha power. $*p<0.05$.

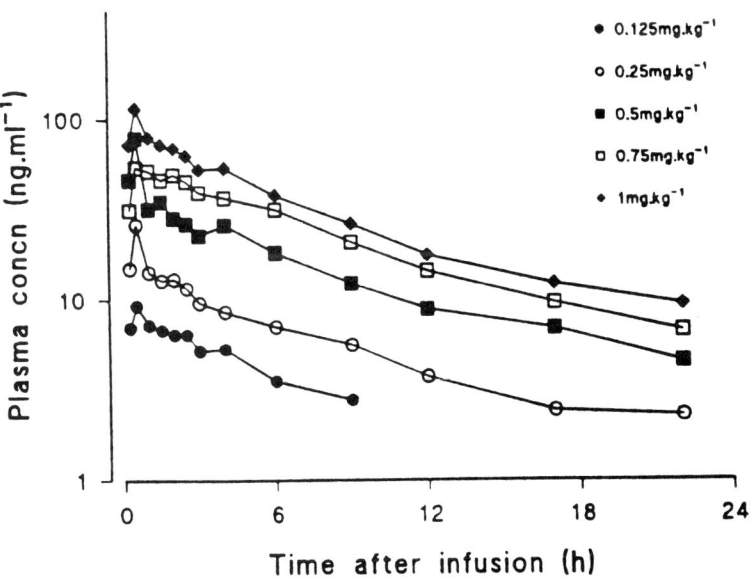

**FIGURE 2.** Mean 619C89 plasma concentrations.

of 885 (163.3) ng/h/mL$^{-1}$, CL of 1.2 (0.21) L/h$^{-1}$/kg$^{-1}$, $t_{1/2z}$ of 16.2 (5.9) h and $V_z$ of 28.1 (9.2) L/kg$^{-1}$ at a dose of 1.0 mg/kg$^{-1}$.

In order to be effective in the treatment of stroke it is important that a candidate compound penetrate quickly into the brain in pharmacologically active levels. The evidence provided by the dose-related reports of subjective AEs, by the dose-related effects on EEG power and by the time course of these events suggests that 619C89 penetrates rapidly into the brain of healthy volunteers at pharmacologically active concentrations.

### REFERENCE

1. LEACH, M. J. & J. SWAN. 1993, Stroke **24:** 1063–1067.

# *N*-Methyl-D-Aspartate Receptor Participation in Parkinson's Disease, a Neurodegenerative Disorder

ANITA VERMA[a] AND S. K. KULKARNI

*Department of Pharmaceutical Sciences*
*Panjab University*
*Chandigarh 160014, India*

Parkinson's disease is a neurodegenerative disorder associated with the loss of dopamine (DA) in nigrostriatal pathway. The antiparkinsonian efficacy of MK-801, a noncompetitive *N*-methyl-D-aspartate (NMDA) antagonist, was evaluated in a model of experimental catalepsy and stereotypy in rats and mice, respectively.

Mixed D-1/D-2 DA receptor antagonists, perphenazine and haloperidol induced catalepsy in rats. SCH 23390, a D-1 DA receptor antagonist, also produced catalepsy. Various doses of MK-801 reduced the cataleptogenic effects of perphenazine, haloperidol as well as SCH 23390. MK-801 and ketamine also produced dose-dependent increase in stereotypic behavior in naive mice. MK-801 and ketamine potentiated the stereotypic effect of apomorphine, a mixed D-1/D-2 agonist, in reserpinized but not in naive mice. B-HT 920, a D-2 agonist, reduced the stereotypic but not the anticataleptic effect of MK-801. On the other hand, SKF 38393, a D-1 agonist, enhanced the stereotypic effect of MK-801 and also its anticataleptic action against SCH 23390. The anticataleptic effect of MK-801 was also enhanced by scopolamine but not by bromocriptine or clonidine in perphenazine-treated rats.

The present data suggest that the blockade of NMDA transmission could possibly provide an efficient means for potentiating the antiparkinsonian effects of DA agonists via D-1 DA receptors, a strategy for therapeutic exploration.

# A Randomized, Double-Blind, Placebo-Controlled Ascending Dose Tolerance Study of 619C89 in Acute Stroke

KEITH W. MUIR, KENNEDY R. LEES, STEVEN J. C.
HAMILTON,[a] CHARLES F. GEORGE,[b] STEPHEN F.
HOBBIGER,[c] AND MARTIN W. LUNNON[c]

*Acute Stroke Unit*
*University Department of Medicine and Therapeutics*
*Gardiner Institute*
*Western Infirmary*
*Glasgow G11 6NT, Scotland*
[a]*Department of Medicine for the Elderly*
*Woodend Hospital*
*Aberdeen, Scotland*
[b]*Clinical Pharmacology Group*
*Southampton General Hospital*
*Southampton, United Kingdom*
[d]*Wellcome Foundation*
*Beckenham, Kent, United Kingdom*

## INTRODUCTION

Excessive glutamate release after focal central nervous system ischemia contributes to neuronal necrosis by activation of postsynaptic receptors. Compounds which block $N$-methyl-D-aspartate (NMDA) receptors consistently reduce the volume of experimental focal cerebral infarction by 50% or more, but there are concerns about the toxicity of many of these compounds, and non-NMDA glutamate receptors also contribute to ischemic injury. 619C89 blocks ischemia-induced presynaptic glutamate release. It reduces focal cerebral infarction after permanent middle cerebral artery occlusion in rats by 60–70%. Optimal neuroprotection in rats was obtained with 10 mg/kg and above. Neurological signs (tremor and ataxia) were transiently seen at 20 mg/kg and higher. Pharmacokinetic predictions from primates suggest that lower doses will be required in man. 619C89 has been well tolerated after administration to healthy young and elderly volunteers in single intravenous (iv) doses of up to 1 mg/kg.

## METHODS

Forty-eight patients with acute stroke in any arterial territory were recruited at 3 centers over 8 months. Exclusions were child-bearing potential, unconsciousness, or major coexisting illness. Treatment commenced within 12 hours of stroke onset. Subjects were randomized to a 30-minute iv infusion of 619C89 or placebo 8 hourly for 3 days in an active:placebo ratio of 3:1. A loading dose of twice the maintenance dose was given. Dose groups ascended in increments of 0.25 mg/kg from maintenance of 0.25 mg/kg/8 h. Outcome was assessed by Barthel score at 3 months.

## RESULTS

Recruitment is closed but data remain blinded until final 3 month follow-up (May 1994). Venous irritation seen in both drug and placebo groups (18/48) from low doses was partially alleviated by flushing cannulae after dosing. Vomiting occurred in 3 of 8 subjects at 0.75 mg/kg/8 h, 3 of 17 at 1.0 mg/kg/8 h and 3 of 7 at 1.25 mg/kg/8 h. Visual hallucinations were seen in 2 of 17 at 1.0 mg/kg/8 h and 3 of 7 at 1.25 mg/kg/8 h. Hallucinations occurred during and shortly after infusion early in the treatment period, and were not always seen after the first dose. No consistent abnormal laboratory indices were encountered. There were 8 deaths, 5 due directly to stroke, 2 secondary to sepsis, and 1 late death due to gastrointestinal hemorrhage complicated by inferior myocardial infarction in a patient with known peptic ulcer disease.

## DISCUSSION

Doses of 619C89 of up to 2 mg/kg loading and 1 mg/kg/8 h maintenance are tolerable after acute stroke. Further Phase II studies with this regimen and with constant infusion of 619C89 are in progress.

# Disposition and Pharmacokinetics of Remacemide Hydrochloride in Male Sprague-Dawley Rats

STEPHEN CURRY, DENNIS J. McCARTHY, KEN R. CASE,
MARK S. EISMAN, MATTHEW R. MARLER, AND
NIK A. MAHMOOD

*Fisons Pharmaceuticals*
*P.O. Box 1710*
*Rochester, New York 14603*

Remacemide hydrochloride [(±)-2-amino-$N$-(1-methyl-1,2-diphenylethyl)-acetamide monohydrochloride] is undergoing human clinical trials for treatment of epilepsy, Huntingston's disease, and neurological deficits associated with stroke and cardiopulmonary bypass. The major route of metabolic transformation of remacemide in rats yields the pharmacologically more potent desglycinate metabolite. Compared to remacemide, the metabolite has higher affinity at the NMDA receptor, is more potent as a $Na^+$ channel blocker, and is twice as potent in rodent anticonvulsant tests. It is rapidly formed *in vivo* and can be detected in the plasma as early as 2 minutes after iv dosing with remacemide hydrochloride.

The disposition and pharmacokinetics of remacemide and its desglycinated metabolite were studied in male Sprague-Dawley rats (200–250 g). Pharmacokinetic parameters were estimated using PCNONLIN V4.2 (SCI Software, Statistical Consultants, Lexington, KY). Following separate iv bolus administrations, both remacemide and its desglycinated metabolite showed a biphasic decay. Remacemide and the desglycinate were cleared at 7.1 and 8.7 $L \cdot h^{-1} \cdot kg^{-1}$, respectively. Remacemide had a shorter elimination half-life (*i.e.*, 0.5 hr) compared to the desglycinate (*i.e.*, 1.4 hr). A larger proportion of the desglycinate was distributed in the tissues than remacemide, with volumes of distribution at steady state ($Vd_{ss}$) of 15.0 and 3.9 $L \cdot kg^{-1}$, respectively. The renal clearance of both the parent drug and the desglycinate was less than 1% of the total clearance, suggesting extensive hepatic metabolism. The desglycinate has a shorter terminal half-life when administered iv compared to when it is formed from remacemide *in vivo* suggesting formation-controlled kinetics. These data were used to construct a pharmacokinetic model for the disposition of remacemide and its desglycinated metabolite in the rat (FIG. 1).

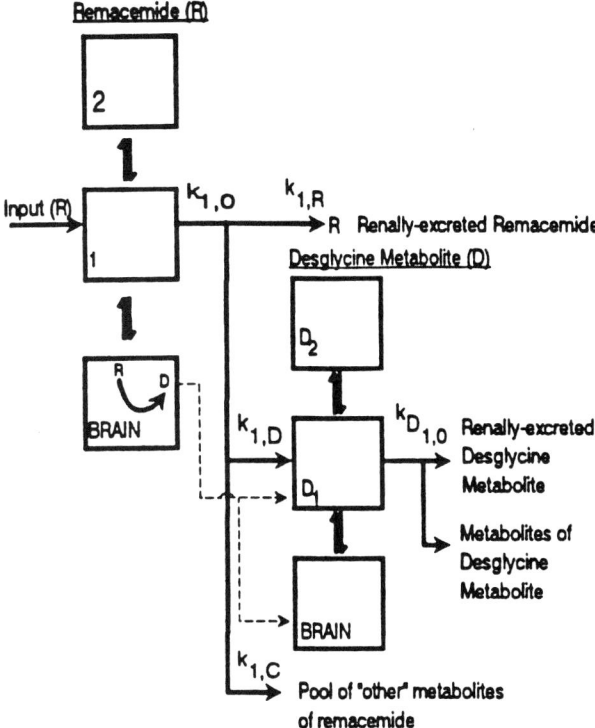

**FIGURE 1.** Pharmacokinetic model for the disposition of remacemide and its desglycinated metabolite in the rat.

# The Cerebral Hemodynamic and Metabolic Effects of the Noncompetitive NMDA Antagonist CNS 1102 in Humans with Severe Head Injury

A. WAGSTAFF, G. M. TEASDALE, G. CLIFTON,[a]
AND L. STEWART

*Department of Neuroanaesthesia*
*University Department of Neurosurgery*
*Institute of Neurological Sciences*
*Southern General Hospital*
*1345 Govan Road*
*Glasgow, G51 4TF Scotland*
[a]*University of Texas Medical School*
*University of Texas, Houston*
*6431 Fanni, Suite 7.148*
*Houston, Texas 77030*

## AIM

The aim of this study was to perform a dose escalation and safety tolerability study of the drug CNS 1102 on severely head-injured patients.

The majority of head-injured patients who subsequently die have evidence of ischemia at postmortem; this is most frequently focal ischemia associated with hematomas and contusions. The glutamate antagonists have proved very effective neuroprotective agents in animal models of focal ischemia.

CNS 1102 has a high affinity and selectivity for a binding site within the transmembrane ion channel associated with the $N$-methyl-D-aspartate (NMDA) receptors. Agents that bind to this site interfere with the function of the NMDA receptors by occluding the open channel, thereby preventing $Na^+$ and $Ca^{2+}$ ions from entering the cell.

CNS 1102 has been shown to protect cultured brain cells against toxic concentrations of glutamate *in vitro*. In animal models of acute ischemia (permanent and reversible middle cerebral artery occlusion) intravenous administration of CNS 1102 substantially reduced (by 40–70%) the amount of damage.

The cardiovascular and cardiorespiratory effects of CNS 1102 were evaluated in several species over a wide dose range, and minimal effects were demonstrated. Neurobehavioral effects observed were an increase in motor activity, incoordination, lacrimation and hypothermia. These effects lasted for about four hours.

## PATIENTS AND METHODS

Fifteen patients who had sustained a severe head injury (GCS 4-10) within the preceding 72 hours whose condition was stable and who were undergoing ventilation and intensive monitoring were given a single bolus of CNS 1102 followed by an infusion of the drug for four hours. The physiological parameters monitored were mean arterial blood pressure, intracranial pressure (ICP), cerebral perfusion pressure, jugular bulb oxygen saturation, electrocardiogram (ECG) temperature and 21 channel electroencephalogram (EEG). Assessment of outcome was made at six months using the Glasgow Outcome Score and Galveston Orientation and Amnesia Test.

## RESULTS

CNS 1102 was well tolerated by these patients. There were no adverse effects. Mean ICP and temperature fell during administration of the drug and returned to the baseline within 12 hours; no other parameters changed significantly.

## CONCLUSION

CNS 1102 is a safe drug to use in humans, up to the doses expected to provide cerebral protection.

# Effects of Nimodipine and Verapamil on Cerebral Blood Flow and Cerebrovascular Reactivity in Conscious Rabbits

GUSTAV B. WEINSTEIN

*I. M. Sechenov Institute of Evolutionary Physiology and Biochemistry*
*Russian Academy of Sciences*
*St. Petersburg 194223, Russia*

The effects of $Ca^{++}$ channel blockers (CCB) on the cerebral circulation system are known; however, there are few reports about the responses of different brain regions to these agents. We investigated the action of verapamil (Ver) and nimodipine (Nim) on local cerebral blood flow (lCBF) and cerebrovascular reactivity (CVR) in sensomotor cortex (Crt), thalamus (Th) and hypothalamus (HTh).

## METHODS

In 16 adult male rabbits Pt 100 mcm wire electrodes with 1.0–1.5-mcm bare tips were chronically implanted into these brain structures. During the following 10 recovery days the catheter was placed into a. femoralis. CCB were infused iv in the following doses: Ver, 0.6 and 1.0 mg/kg; Nim, 0.01 and 0.06 mg/kg. lCBF was measured by the hydrogen clearance method, and CVR was evaluated as %lCBF changes after 7% $CO_2$ inhalation ($PaCO_2$ raised by 12–13 mmHg).

## RESULTS

The data are shown as mean ($\pm$SD) [n]. Control lCBF (ml/100 g/min) in Crt, Th and HTh were found to be 66.3 (4.6) [51], 38.2 (2.7) [51] and 56.4 (3.1) [50]; and CVR (%) were +52 (6) [50], +59 (7) [49] and +49 (5) [49], respectively. Ver and Nim infusion changed control arterial pressure by not more than 5–10% in the first 10 min. Other changes are recorded in the TABLE 1.

## CONCLUSIONS

The actions of CCB on vessels in different brain structures are rather "mosaic." This can be related to the morphological and functional heterogeneity of these vessels, including the heterogeneity of $Ca^{++}$ channels and of their cells' membranes. Besides, the specific action of CCB on different neurons' metabolism can modulate their effect on lCBF and CVR.

TABLE 1. Changes (in %) from Preinfusion Levels

| CCB Doses (mg/kg) n = 12 | | After 15 Min | | After 60 Min | |
|---|---|---|---|---|---|
| | | lCBF | CVR | lCBF | CVR |
| Crt | | | | | |
| Ver | 0.6 | +27.7(8.0)* | +5.3(3.4) | +12.1(11.2) | +15.4(6.6)* |
| | 1.0 | +24.2(7.0)* | −19.2(6.1)* | −15.7(5.1)* | −15.6(6.2)* |
| Nim | 0.01 | −11.7(9.0) | +6.5(8.2) | −14.1(9.1) | −20.6(6.6)* |
| | 0.06 | +55.1(10.2)* | −15.4(5.3)* | +2.8(8.7) | +6.6(10.5) |
| Th | | | | | |
| Ver | 0.6 | +29.2(10.6)* | −20.9(6.7)* | −4.3(5.3) | −11.6(4.0)* |
| | 1.0 | +1.9(6.0) | −14.9(12.3) | −8.6(5.4) | −4.5(6.0) |
| Nim | 0.01 | +25.0(11.2)* | −18.8(3.8)* | +10.4(9.4) | −4.9(6.6) |
| | 0.06 | +37.8(10.7)* | −14.4(2.5)* | +7.9(8.7) | −3.8(5.6) |
| HTh | | | | | |
| Ver | 0.6 | +9.7(5.7) | +13.3(9.0) | +1.5(4.7) | −2.8(4.3) |
| | 1.0 | −15.6(3.7)* | −3.3(6.4) | −37.3(5.4)* | +7.0(9.3) |
| Nim | 0.01 | +5.2(8.4) | −4.1(9.0) | +2.2(8.5) | −5.0(7.4) |
| | 0.06 | +56.4(11.7)* | −29.4(7.8)* | +35.0(4.9)* | −13.9(5.4)* |

* $p < 0.05$.

# Clinical Pharmacology of CNS 1102 in Man

KEITH W. MUIR, DONALD G. GROSSET, AND
KENNEDY R. LEES

*Acute Stroke Unit*
*University Department of Medicine and Therapeutics*
*Gardiner Institute*
*Western Infirmary*
*Glasgow G11 6NT, Scotland*

## INTRODUCTION

Blockade of the *N*-methyl-D-aspartate (NMDA) receptor reduces the extent of experimental cerebral infarction by limiting glutamate-mediated excitotoxic neuronal death. CNS 1102 (Cambridge NeuroScience Inc, Cambridge, MA) binds to the dizocilpine site within the NMDA receptor ion channel to produce a noncompetitive use-dependent block. CNS 1102 has reduced the volume of cerebral infarction after permanent middle cerebral artery (MCA) occlusion in rats by up to 66%. We describe the results of three Phase I studies of CNS 1102 in normal humans.

## METHODS

### Study 1

Study 1 (the first administration to man) was a randomized, double-blind, ascending dose tolerance study. Twenty-seven healthy male volunteers received CNS 1102 (n = 20) or placebo (n = 7) as a single 15-minute intravenous infusion (IVI) in groups of 4 (3 active and 1 placebo). Doses of 3, 10, 30, 100, 45 and 60 µg/kg were given. Four volunteers received 45 µg/kg over 30 minutes.

### Study 2

In Study 2, 20 further volunteers received CNS 1102 or placebo as 15-minute loading and 4-hour maintenance IVI in a double-blind trial. Groups of 4 received total doses of 15, 32, 50 and 73 µg/kg as 30 µg + 5 µg/kg/h, 45 µg + 7 µg/kg/h, 20 µg + 3 µg/kg/h, and 10 µg + 1.25 µg/kg/h. Cardiovascular monitoring was undertaken throughout.

### Study 3

Study 3 was a single-blind, crossover study of 8 further subjects who received a fixed 2-mg dose of CNS 1102 as 10-ml IV bolus, 30-ml IVI over 15 minutes, and placebo in random order. Cerebral hemodynamic responses were studied by Doppler ultrasound.

## RESULTS

Total doses of 30–32 µg/kg, independent of infusion rate, were well tolerated with only minor symptoms (peripheral paraesthesia, light-headedness and flushing). Dose-dependent CNS depression, nystagmus and disinhibition, with evidence of peripheral vasoconstriction and ultimately a catatonic state comprising limb plasticity and nonresponsiveness to commands, were observed at doses of 60 µg/kg and greater. All were transient and resolved without therapy. Dose-dependent increases in both heart rate and mean arterial pressure (MAP) were seen. The peak effect was observed at 45–120 minutes following drug administration. There was no change in global cerebral blood flow, but pulsatility decreased significantly and velocity increased in the MCAs, indicating arteriolar vasoconstriction. Pharmacokinetics were consistent with a lipid-soluble agent with large volume of distribution and variable clearance (coefficient of variation 21%). Adjustment of dose by weight did not affect this variation.

## CONCLUSIONS

Total doses of up to 100 µg/kg have been administered to normal male volunteers in three separate studies. The rate of administration did not alter the incidence of symptoms, and CNS 1102 may be administered as a fixed dose bolus. Vasoconstriction of small vessels occurs in association with a significant elevation of MAP, but with no detrimental effects on cerebral blood flow. In other studies, total doses of 268 µg/kg and 90 µg/kg administered over 4 hours 15 mins have been given to severe traumatic brain-injured and stroke patients, respectively, without significant adverse effects.

# Low Environmental Temperatures or Pharmacologic Agents That Produce Hypothermia Decrease Methamphetamine Neurotoxicity in Mice

S. F. ALI, G. D. NEWPORT, R. R. HOLSON, W. SLIKKER, JR.,
AND J. F. BOWYER

*Neurochemistry Laboratory*
*Division of Neurotoxicology*
*National Center for Toxicological Research/FDA*
*Jefferson, Arkansas 72079*

Methamphetamine (METH) is one of the major drugs of abuse shown to cause neurotoxicity in rodents and nonhuman primates. Recently, we reported that METH neurotoxicity in rats depends on the environmental temperature. Here, we evaluate whether a cold environment (4°C) or drugs which affect chloride and glutamate channel function block METH neurotoxicity in mice.

Adult male CD mice received METH ip (4 × 10 mg/kg METH at 23°C and either 4 × 10 or 4 × 20 mg/kg METH at 4°C) along with 2.5 mg/kg (+)MK-801, 40 mg/kg phenobarbital or 2.5 mg/kg diazepam. Three days post 4 × 10 mg/kg METH at 23°C an 80% decrease in striatal dopamine (DA) occurred, while the same dose at 4°C produced a 20% DA decrease, and 4 × 20 mg/kg METH at 4°C produced a 54% DA decrease. At 23°C (+)MK-801 completely blocked while phenobarbital (40% decrease) and diazepam (65% decrease) partially blocked decreases in striatal DA produced by 4 × 10 mg/kg METH. Compared to the decreases in DA after METH and antagonists a similar pattern in the decreases of dihydroxyphenylacetic acid (DOPAC) and homovanillic acid (HVA) were observed. Drugs which block METH toxicity, such as haloperidol ($D_2$ receptors), pentobarbital and phenobarbital (chloride channels) and MK-801 (N-methyl-D-aspartate (NMDA)/glutamate receptors), do not necessarily have the same mechanism of action but may either induce hypothermia or block induction of hyperthermia. Therefore, it is not clear how much of their protection against METH neurotoxicity is due to the blockade of the hyperthermia produced by METH.

# Biologically Based Dose-Response Model for Neurotoxicity Risk Assessment

WILLIAM SLIKKER, JR. AND DAVID W. GAYLOR

*Divisions of Neurotoxicology and of Biometry and Risk Assessment*
*National Center for Toxicological Research/FDA*
*Jefferson, Arkansas 72079-9502*

The regulation of neurotoxicants has usually been based upon setting reference doses by dividing a no observed adverse effect level by uncertainty factors that theoretically account for interspecies and intraspecies extrapolation of experimental results in animals to humans. Recently, we proposed a four-step alternative procedure, which provides quantitative estimates of risk as a function of dose.

The first step is to establish a mathematical relationship between a biological effect or biomarker and the dose of chemical administered. To enhance the certainty of this procedure we considered the pharmacokinetics, the uptake kinetics into the target cell(s) and/or membrane interactions, and the presumed receptor site(s) interaction of the chemical or metabolite. Because these theoretical factors each contain a saturable step due to definitive amounts of required enzyme, reuptake or receptor site(s), a nonlinear, saturable dose-response curve would be predicted.

When data generated from rats administered methylenedioxymethamphetamine (MDMA) were plotted as biological effect (decreases in hippocampal serotonin concentrations) versus dose, a saturation curve best described the observed relationship.

The use of dose-response data may enhance the certainty of quantitative risk assessment.

# Role of Reactive Oxygen Species (ROS) in Neuronal Degeneration

## Modulation by Protooncogene Expression

M. ANTHONY VERITY, D. E. BREDESEN, AND T. SARAFIAN

*Departments of Neuropathology and Neurology*
*and*
*Brain Research Institute*
*University of California, Los Angeles*
*Los Angeles, California 90024*

Reactive oxygen species (ROS) may be generated by toxins, ischemia/anoxia, ionizing radiation and other forms of xenobiotic-induced cell injury. Changes in the state of oxidative stress play a role in both cell proliferation and differentiation as well as initiating irreversible cell injury. In this review, selected examples of ROS-induced neural injury will be presented with observations coupling the modification of injury by activation of early response specific genes.

Hypoglycemic neuronal injury in culture is blocked by superoxide dysmutase but only in the presence of $K^+$-induced depolarization of intracellular uptake of the enzyme, thereby identifying the genesis of $O_2^-$ as an early proximate event in the toxicity. While glutamate toxicity is considered mediated via N-methyl-D-aspartate (NMDA) receptor activation, both neuronal cell lines and immature cortical neurons demonstrate glutamate toxicity associated with inhibition of cystine uptake from the extracellular compartment. The associated decrease of intraneuronal glutathione reflects inhibition of the glutathione synthetic pathway by rate-limiting cystine leading to increased cellular oxidative stress, which may be reversed by antioxidants. Glutamate toxicity is inversely proportional to NAD(P)H: quinone reductase, an enzyme with DT-diaphorase activity. Inhibition of the reductase potentiates glutamate toxicity suggesting that reduction of intracellular glutathione may not lead to neurodegeneration if alternate pathways of oxidant metabolism are present.

The damaging effect of ionizing radiation on the developing cortex or cerebellum is associated with apoptotic cell death mediated by oxidative injury due to direct attack of ROS on DNA or via secondary activation of endonuclease cleaving the DNA backbone. In this respect, oxidative stress causes an increase in intracellular $[Ca^{2+}]$ activating a $Ca^{2+}$-dependent endonuclease. Early response gene activation is common to many forms of cell injury and closely linked to the initiation of a $Ca^{2+}$-transient.

The protooncogenes c-myc and c-fos among others are commonly expressed early during irreversible cell injury. However, the protooncogene bcl-2 is known to prevent apoptotic death in PC12 cells and neuronal cell lines. Neural cell lines transfected with a construct for the bcl-2 gene reveal considerable protection towards the prooxidants, *t*-butylhydroperoxide, and methyl mercury associated in some part with elevation of cellular GSH.

# Phospholipase A₂ Regulation in Neural Function and Injury

M. ANTHONY VERITY

*Department of Neuropathology*
*and*
*Brain Research Institute*
*Center for Health Sciences*
*University of California, Los Angeles*
*Los Angeles, California 90024*

Phospholipases A$_2$ (PLA$_2$s) catalyze the hydrolysis of glycerophospholipids at the sn-2 position with arachidonic acid and a lysoglycerophospholipid as end products. A variety of PLA$_2$s have been identified, some dependent upon mM Ca$^{2+}$. Recently, a high molecular weight cytosolic PLA$_2$ was identified containing a Ca$^{2+}$-dependent translocation domain with homology to protein kinase C.

These cytosolic PLA$_2$s are probably involved in signal transduction. Numerous pathways exist for receptor-induced arachidonate formation other than via PLA$_2$ activation including formation of phosphatidic acid via phospholipase D activation or associated with sequential phospholipase C activation, diacylglycerol formation and lipase activity. The contribution of these pathways varies between cells but a variety of agonists are known to mediate the parallel and independent activation of phospholipase C and phospholipase A$_2$.

PLA$_2$ activity is modulated by membrane phospholipid state-structure, Ca$^{2+}$ homeostasis, membrane lipid peroxidation and directly via G-protein interaction. Ca$^{2+}$ ionophores promote PLA$_2$ activation synergistically with increased oxidative stress. Moreover, intracellular Ca$^{2+}$-deranged modulation, *e.g.*, induced by low [Na$^+$]$_e$ leads to accelerated neurotoxicity in cerebellar granule cell culture. Neural cell lines have revealed PLA$_2$ activation following ischemia, anoxia, *N*-methyl-D-aspartate (NMDA) receptor activation, cyanide, α-tissue necrosis factor, etc. G-protein activation in neurons via fluoroaluminate induces dose-dependent PLA$_2$ activation associated with cytolysis. Such accelerated arachidonate formation by G-protein activation was not altered by inhibitors of protein kinase C or neomycin, known to selectively inhibit phospholipase C. Cytokines, tumor necrosis factor α (TNF-α), and lipopolysaccharide (LPS) induce PLA$_2$ expression and secretion in primary glial culture.

It is likely that controlled modulation of PLA$_2$ activation in neural systems is critical for selective neuronal function, *e.g.*, long-term potentiation, but such modulation needs strict control between abusive or physiological activation.

# Subject Index

1S, 3R-ACPD, 230
619C89
  cerebral focal ischemia and, 39
  increasing intravenous doses of, 324, 328

**A**cute ischemic stroke
  619C89 and, 324, 328
  lifarizine in, 317
  remacemide HCl and, 322
  Ro-01-6794/706 and, 249
Acute neurodegenerative processes, evaluating protection against, 50
Acute neuroprotection, adenosine and, 169
Adenosine, brain and, 163
Adenosine $A_2$ receptor, dopamine $D_2$ receptor and, 168
Adenosine receptor types, 164
Adhesion molecules, brain injury and, 65
Age dependence, dexamethasone and, 189
1-Aminocyclopropanecarboxylic acid (ACPC), 320
Animal model
  human model and, 60
  safety parameters in, 199
Antioxidant enzymes, free radicals and, 183
Antioxidants, 116
Aptiganel hydrochloride (CNS 1102), 279
Assessment approaches, 59

**B**ehavior, hypoxic rats and, 34
Biologically based dose-response model, 339
Biomarkers of neurotoxicity, 205
Blood pressure, CNS 1102 and, 287
Brain injury, TNF$\alpha$ and, 62

**C**alcitonin gene-related peptide, subarachnoid hemorrhage and, 299
Calcium, glucocorticoid receptors and, 134
Calcium antagonists, 119, 185
Calcium channel antagonists, depolarization and, 160
Calcium channels
  presynaptic, 214
  short-term regulation of, 119
  use-dependent blockers of, 210
Caloric reduction, oxidative brain damage and, 308
Cannabinoid, HU-211 as, 314
Cardiopulmonary bypass, neurophysiological test scores in, 23
Carotid endarterectomy, 23
Catalase, 184

Catecholamines, glutamine-enhanced release of, 75
Cell culture
  1,4-dihydropyridine binding assay in, 122
  disadvantage of, 111
Central nervous system, TNF$\alpha$ and, 63
Cerebral blood flow
  adenosine and, 163
  CNS 1102 and, 280
  dexamethasone and, 182
Cerebral circulation, 334
Cerebral focal ischemia, 619C89 and, 39
Cerebral hypoxic injury, 31
Cerebrovascular effects, CNS 1102, 280
Channel classification and regulation, 120
Chronic administration, adenosine-based therapies and, 170
Clinical pharmacology, CNS 1102, 279
Clinical potential for neuroprotective agents, 1
Clinical syndromes, 26
CNS 1102
  cerebral hemodynamic and metabolic effects of, 332
  clinical pharmacology of, 279, 336
CNS 1237, use-dependent channel block and, 219
Cocaine dependence, nimodipine and, 150
"Code Stroke" alert system, 2
Corticosterone, adrenal cortical hormone receptors and, 134
Corticosterone levels, variability of, 139
Corticosterone receptors types I and II, 135

**D**endritic atrophy, nimodipine and, 312
2-Deoxyglucose, dexamethasone and, 189
Depolarization, 125
Dexamethasone, neonatal hypoxic-ischemic brain damage and, 179
Dextrorphan HCl, safety of, 249
Diffuse axonal injury, 263
1,4-Dihydropyridines, binding of, 120
Dopamine $D_2$ receptor, adenosine $A_2$ receptor and, 168
Doppler ultrasound, 280
Dorsal root ganglion, radical scavengers and, 111
Dose-response models, 203

**E**lectroencephalogram (EG), recording procedures of, 145
Electrophysiology, use-dependent channel block and, 216

Energy disrupters, 116
Energy metabolism, 32
Energy repletion, neuroprotective effects of, 104
Epilepsy
  NMDA antagonists in, 12
  remacemide and, 277
Event-related potential, substance abusers and, 152
Excitatory amino acid
  severe head trauma and, 290
  excessive release of, 262
Excitotoxic effects, glutamate and, 290
Excitotoxic mechanisms, acute subdural hematoma and, 265
Excitotoxic neuronal death, CNS 1102 and, 336
Excitotoxicity, 98
  neurodegenerative diseases and, 100

**F**asting, dexamethasone and, 187
Fluid percussion injury, 264
Flunarizine, dexamethasone and, 185
Focal cerebral ischemia
  models of, 242
  prophylactic neuroprotection in, 4, 21
  remacemide HCl and, 322
  small animal model of, 301
Free fatty acids, 33
Free radical scavengers
  neuroprotective effects of, 102
  side effects and safety of, 117
Free radicals
  adenosine and, 171
  antioxidant enzymes and, 183

**G** proteins, adenosine and, 172
Gamma-aminobutyric acid (GABA), visual spatial learning in rats and, 4
Ganglioside $GM_1$
  methamphetamine-induced neurotoxicity and, 311
  perinatal brain injury and, 304
$GH_4C_1$ cells, 120
Glia, effects of glutamine on, 78
Global cerebral ischemia
  remacemide HCl and, 322
  models of, 238
Glucocorticoid, 180
  P3B and, 161
Glucose utilization, dexamethasone effects on, 188
Glutamate
  CNS and, 279
  glial cells and, 79
  hypocapnia and, 86
  putative excitotoxic effects of, 290
  use-dependent blockers controlling, 210
Glutamate antagonists, strategies for neuroprotection with, 272
Glutamate release, 619C89 and, 328
Glutamate uptake, endogenous adenosine and, 166
Glutamine-enhanced glutamate release, 72
Glycine
  hypocapnia and, 86
  NMDA receptor and, 320

**H**allucinations, 619C89 and, 329
Head injury
  CNS 1102 and, 332
  EAA release and, 290
  glutamate antagonist in treatment of, 262
Hippocampal slices, glutamate from, 75
Hippocampus
  adrenal cortical hormone receptors of, 134
  hypocapnia and, 86
  quantitative histological evaluation of neurotoxic damage in, 303
  trimethyltin and, 54
HU-211, neuroprotective activity of, 314
Huntington's disease, 14
  remacemide HCl and, 245
Hyperglycemia, dexamethasone and, 186
Hyperthermia, MK-801 and, 7
Hyperventilation, brain lactate and, 86
Hypocapnia, extracellular glutamate and glycine and, 86
Hypotension, dextrorphan and, 254
Hypothermia
  hypoxic-ischemic damage and, 182
  ischemia/reperfusion injury and, 98
  methamphetamine neurotoxicity and, 338
Hypoxia, intact dorsal root ganglion, 111
Hypoxia-ischemia, dexamethasone and, 179
Hypoxic depolarization, adenosine and, 166
Hypoxic-ischemic brain injury, role of growth factors after, 306

**I**mmunohistochemistry of neurotoxicity biomarkers, 50
Infarct volume, 619C89 and, 43
Infarction, hypoxia-ischemia and, 181
Inflammation, TNFα and, 62
Insulin-like growth factor 1, hypoxic-ischemic brain injury and, 306
Intracranial pressure, EAA release and, 294
Ion conductances, adenosine and, 167

# SUBJECT INDEX

Ischemia, glutamate release blockers and, 212
Ischemic damage, hippocampal, 263
Ischemic stroke, multicenter clinical trials and, 2

**K**ainate, glutamate levels and, 78
Kynurenate, glutamate levels and, 78

**L**-AP4, 230
L-CCG1, 230
L-channels, 120
L-SOP, 230
Lactate, brain, 86
Lifarizine, acute ischemic stroke and, 317
Limbic seizures, metabotropic glutamate receptor agonist-mediated, 230

**M**agnesium, 196
Magnesium sulfate, acute stroke and, 315
Mechanism, 98
Memory retention, nimodipine and, 312
Metabotropic glutamate receptors, 230
Methamphetamine, glutamate levels and, 78
Methamphetamine neurotoxicity, hypothermia and, 338
Methemoglobinemia, 136
Microdialysis, 291
Middle cerebral artery occlusion (MCAO), use-dependent channel block and, 218
Middle cerebral artery occlusion model of focal ischemia, 619C89 and, 39
MK-801, S-PBN and, 104
Morphometric studies, experimental design of, 47
Muscarinic receptors, 125

**N**-channels, 120
Neonatal brain damage, dexamethasone and, 179
Nerve growth factors, dexamethasone and, 196
Neurodegeneration
 adenosine $A_2$ receptors and, 167
 excitotoxic hypothesis and, 268
Neurodegenerative disease
 animal models of, 101
 EAA toxicity and, 12
Neurological deficit, 619C89 and, 45
Neuroprotection
 619C89 and, 42
 radical scavengers and, 111
Neuroprotection regimen, prophylactic pharmacologic, 22

Neurotoxicity
 assessing human, 198
 NMDA antagonists and, 268
Neurotoxicity endpoints, 200
Neurotransmitter release, adenosine analogues and, 165
Neurotrauma, CGS 19755 and, 272
Nimodipine
 auditory rare event monitoring task and, 153
 cerebral blood flow and, 334
 EEG of substance abusers and, 143, 152
 neocortical dendritic atrophy and, 312
Nitric oxide, NMDA receptors and, 310
NMDA (*N*-methyl-D-aspartate)
 depolarization in rat hippocampal slices and, 237
 ischemia and, 3
NMDA antagonist
 head trauma and, 298
 head-injured patients and, 262
 magnesium as, 315
 remacemide and, 248, 322
 safety and, 249
NMDA channel blocker, CNS 1102 as, 273
NMDA receptor
 adenosine and, 164
 amphetamine's interactions with, 309
 CNS 1102 and, 279, 336
 magnesium and, 315
 Parkinson's disease and, 327
 sensitization and desensitization of, 320
Noncompetitive antagonist, CNS 1102 as, 287
Neuroprotective agents, clinical potential for use of, 1

**O**xidative brain damage, caloric reduction and, 308
Oxidative stress, hyperthermia and, 98
Oxygen radicals, dorsal root ganglion hypoxia model and, 111

**P**-channels, 120
P3, substance abusers and, 152
Parkinson's disease
 models of, 244
 NMDA antagonists in, 14
 NMDA receptor participation in, 327
Pathophysiology and therapeutic intervention, 304
Periischemic period, hypocapnia and, 86
Perinatal brain injury, 304
Pharmacokinetics, dextrorphan, 255
Phospholipase $A_2$, 341
Placebo effects, 138
Placental insufficiency, 28

Polymorphonuclear leukocytes, brain injury and, 64
Principal components analysis, ERP and, 154
Prophylactic pharmacologic neuroprotection, focal cerebral ischemia and, 21
Protein kinase C, 125
Protooncogene expression, reactive oxygen species and, 340

Quantitative histological evaluation, neuroprotective compounds and, 47

Rapid superfusion system, $^3$H-glutamate release and, 221
Reactive oxygen species, protooncogene expression and, 340
Reflex sympathetic dystrophy, C fiber activity in, 15
Remacemide hydrochloride
 acute ischemic stroke and, 322
 mechanism of action of, 236
 Sprague-Dawley rats and, 330
Risk assessment
 biologically based dose-response model for, 339
 biomarkers and, 209
 strategies of, 198
Ro-01-6794/706, safety of, 249

S-PBN, free radical generation and, 102
Safety and tolerability, dextrorphan and, 251
Safety evaluation programs, novel therapeutics and, 319
Safety-factor approach, 201
Silver impregnation of degenerative processes, 50
Small animal model, focal cerebral ischemia, 301
Sodium channels
 neuronal voltage-activated, 213
 use-dependent blockers of, 210
Spinal cord injury, methylprednisolone in, 9
Spontaneously hypertensive rats, 619C89 and, 40
Staurosporine, 125
Steriology, 49

Stress, methemoglobin production and, 136
Striatal slices, glutamate from, 75
Stroke
 CGS 19755 and, 272
 CNS 1102 and, 287
 magnesium and, 315
Stroke rate, annual, 22
Subarachnoid hemorrhage
 calcitonin gene-related peptide and, 299
 models of, 243
 vasospasm in, 6
Substance abuse
 EEG activity in, 14
 nimodipine and, 143, 152
Superoxide, 184
Surgical retraction injury, 11
Systolic blood pressure, dextrorphan and, 258

T-channels, 120
Taurine, release of, from cultured glia, 78
Tetrodotoxin, use-dependent channel block and, 219
Therapeutics, novel, safety evaluation programs for, 319
Transcranial Doppler (TCD) ultrasound, 280
Transforming growth factor $\beta_1$ (TGF$\beta_1$), hypoxic-ischemic brain injury and, 306
Traumatic brain injury, EAA antagonist therapy in, 6
Trimethyltin, axon terminal degeneration and, 54
Tumor necrosis factor alpha (TNF$\alpha$), brain injury and inflammation and, 62

U-74689F, dexamethasone and, 185
Use-dependent blockers, 210

Verapamil, cerebral blood flow and, 334
Veratridine, 126
Vitamin E, methamphetamine-induced neurotoxicity and, 311
Voltage sensitive sodium channels, 39
Volunteers, healthy
 619C89 and, 324
 CNS 1102 in, 287, 337

"Weibel's Bible," 47

# Index of Contributors

**A**lbers, G. W., 249–261
Ali, S. F., 311, 338
Arvin, B., 62–71
Atkinson, R., 249–261

**B**amford, J., 317–318
Bär, P. R., 111–115
Barone, F. C., 62–71
Beal, M. F., 100–110
Beenhakker, M., 163–178
Beilharz, E., 306–307
Bell, B. A., 299–300, 301–302
Berlove, D., 210–229
Biegon, A., 314
Binienda, Z., 28–38
Borrelli, A. R., 236–247
Bowyer, J. F., 72–85, 309–310, 338
Bredesen, D. E., 340
Bullock, R., 262–271, 272–278, 290–297
Burton, D., 312–313

**C**arter, M. F., 163–178
Case, K. R., 330–331
Cavagnaro, J. A., 319
Chen, J., 210–229
Choi, K. T., 86–97
Chung, J. K., 86–97
Clifton, G., 332–333
Cregan, E. F., 236–247
Curry, S., 330–331

**D**aly, D., 210–229
Davies, D. L., 72–85
Durant, G. J., 210–229
Dvorak, R., 312–313

**E**isman, M. S., 330–331

**F**euerstein, G. Z., 62–71
Fischer, J. B., 210–229
Forster, M. J., 308
Fossom, L. H., 320–321

**G**aylor, D. W., 198–208, 339
George, C. F., 328–329
Gluckman, P., 304–305, 306–307
Goldin, S. M., 210–229
Graham, S. H., 210–229
Griffey, K. I., 230–235
Grosset, D. G., 279–289, 336–337
Guan, J., 306–307
Gunn, A., 304–305
Guo, X., 143–151, 152–159

**H**amilton, S. J. C., 328–329
Herning, R. I., 143–151, 152–159

Hobbiger, S., 324–326, 328–329
Holland, J. P., 301–302
Holson, R. R., 338
Holt, W. F., 210–229
Hoover, L., 312–313
Hu, L-Y., 210–229
Hussein, Z., 324–326

**I**saacson, R. L., 134–142

**J**acobson, K. A., 163–178
Johnston, B., 304–305
Jonas, S., 21–25

**K**atz, P., 249–261
Kelley, R. E., 249–261
Kertesz, A., 317–318
Kim, H. K., 86–97
Knapp, A. G., 210–229
Kulkarni, S. K., 327
Kuntz, N., 312–313
Kwak, C. S., 86–97

**L**al, H., 308
Lamb, R. J., 324–326
Lange, W. R., 143–151, 152–159
Leach, M. J., 39–46
Lees, K. R., 279–289, 315–316, 317–318, 322–323, 328–329, 336–337
Lehr, L., 249–261
Lesko, L. M., 249–261
Lin, R. C-S., 163–178
Lipe, G. W., 72–85
Liu, J., 119–133
Liu, S., 319
Lunnon, M. W., 328–329

**M**agar, S., 210–229
Magni, G., 249–261
Mahmood, N. A., 330–331
Mallard, C., 304–305
Margolin, L. D., 210–229
Marks, K., 304–305
Marler, M. R., 330–331
Marmarou, A., 290–297
Matthews, J. C., 72–85
McCarthy, D. J., 330–331
McNeill, H., 306–307
Mercer, A. J., 324–326
Mervis, R. F., 312–313
Miller, O., 306–307
Modi, M., 249–261
Muir, K. W., 279–289, 315–316, 322–323, 328–329, 336–337
Myseros, J. S., 262–271, 290–297

**N**eville, L. F., 62–71
Newport, G. D., 338

**P**almer, G. C., 236–247
Paul, K., 249–261
Perlman, M. E., 210–229
Pitman, V., 249–261
Posner, J., 324–326
Pryse-Phillips, W., 317–318

**R**ae, J., 249–261
Reddy, N. L., 210–229
Rosenbaum, D. M., 249–261
Rutledge, A., 119–133

**S**arafian, T., 340
Scallet, A. C., 47–58, 72–85, 303
Schoepp, D. D., 230–235
Schulz, J. B., 100–110
Sharma, R., 210–229
Sirimanne, E., 306–307
Skolnick, P., 320–321
Slikker, W., Jr., xi, 198–208, 338, 339
Sohal, R. S., 308
Solomon, P. R., 312–313
Squire, I. B., 317–318
Stewart, L., 332–333

Subbarao, K., 210–229
Swan, J. H., 39–46

**T**an, W., 304–305
Tandon, R., 312–313
Teasdale, G. M., 332–333
Tizzano, J. P., 230–235
Trembly, B., xi, 1–20
Triggle, D. J., 119–133
Tuor, U. I., 179–195

**V**arner, J. A., 134–142
Verity, M. A., 340, 341
Verma, A., 327
von Lubitz, D. K. J. E., 163–178

**W**agstaff, A., 332–333
Weinstein, G. B., 334–335
Willett, F., 236–247
Williams, C., 304–305, 306–307
Wood, M. S., 312–313
Woodward, J. J., 290–297

**Y**oo, K., 249–261
Young, H. F., 290–297

**Z**auner, A., 290–297

**OHIO UNIVERSITY LIBRARY**
Please return this book as so u have
finished with it. In